MASSAGE

— *a career* —
at your fingertips

FOURTH EDITION

The Complete Guide To Becoming A Bodywork Professional

MARTIN ASHLEY

ENTERPRISE PUBLISHING

Copyright © 2003 by Martin Ashley

Published by Enterprise Publishing
P.O. Box 179 / 208 Nichols St.
Carmel, NY 10512
(845) 228-0312

courtesy of Bancroft School of Massage Therapy, Worcester, MA
All other illustrations by Lorrie Klosterman
Cover design by Adventure House, New York, NY
Typesetting by PDS Associates, Allenhurst, NJ

Publisher's Cataloging-in-Publication Data

Ashley, Martin
  Massage: a career at your fingertips : Martin Ashley. — 4th
ed.
  p. cm.
  Includes index.
  ISBN 0-9644662-4-4

  1. Massage—Vocational guidance. 2. Massage—Practice. I.
Title.

RA780.5.A75   2003   615.8'22'023

10 9 8 7 6 5 4 3 2 1

Printed and bound in the United States of America

Contents

III: Sex, Gender and Touch

IV: Business, Practical and Legal Information for the Practitioner

VI: Bodywork Organizations and Trainings

VII: State-by-State Directory

This book is dedicated to my parents,
Sam and Sarah Ashley,
who gave me the luxury of a good education and plenty of slack;
to my wife Deborah who puts up with me every day
whether she likes it or not
and to my son Joshua,
a remarkable boy with a whole life ahead of him.

Acknowledgments

I want to thank Doug Brodeff, who gave me the idea to write this book. I am also grateful to Pete Whitridge, who took the time to read the original manuscript and give me many helpful criticisms and suggestions. A major debt is also due Emily Sprague, who undertook primary responsibility for assembling the state-by-state directory for this fourth edition. Another major debt is due my typesetter, Dave Saunders. This book's reference section is a typesetter's nightmare, yet Dave worked tirelessly on it and never once grumbled about the task.

In addition, the following massage and bodywork practitioners all contributed to the writing of this book by allowing me to interview them, or by furnishing useful information or reference material. Thank you all.

Paul D. Arneson
Lauren S. Bain
Kathleen Batko
Ann W. Bertland
Wes Boyce
Gordon E. Bradford
Alberto Breccia
Iris Brown
William T. Bunting
Sharon Callahan
Robert Calvert
Norman Cohen
Karen E. Craig
Paul Davenport
Jo Anne Davies
Patrick Dempsey
Doug Deyers
Bob Fasic
Adeha Feustel
Andre Fountain
A. Ann Gill
J. Joy Gottus
Roy Gottus
Ruth R. Haefer
Susanne Setuh Hesse
Pamela Hodgson
Stuart Holland
Sita Hood
Shirley Hooker
Jeff Hopkins
Jeffrey Kates
Deborah A. Kimmet
Bob King

Apara Kohls
Shivam Kohls
Scott Lamp
Mae Leone
Glenn Lloyd
Jerrine F. Manders
Danila Mansfield
Charles Mardel
Massage Magazine
Maureen A. Miller
Artie Mosgofian
Ginann Olmstead
Grieg A. Osmundson
David Palmer
Cindy Patterson
Laura Perna
Anna Pekar
Chad Porter
Cate I. Rainey
Deeta Rasmussen
Kay E. Richey
Dennis Simpson
Timothy Starbright
Christiana Stefanoff
Bruce Stephens
Kathy Tanny
Debbie Thomas
Jack Thomas
John "Shane" Watson
Dana S. Whitfield
Sherri Williamson
Carl S. Yamasaki
Etelka M. Zsiros

Introduction
Who This Book Is Written For

When I was embarking on a massage career in 1982, there was no source to turn to for information about the field, educational programs, or equipment. There has been an incredible amount of change in the field since then.

My idea in creating this book was to provide you with everything you need to know to consider, plan and execute a career in massage or bodywork. This book will not only help you decide whether to get into the field, but will guide you to the best massage or bodywork school for you, and help you make the plans and choices that bring you a rewarding career. No other source contains the information you can find in this volume.

For the novice:

For someone contemplating a massage or bodywork career, this is truly one-stop-shopping for all the essential information you will need. First you will find an overview of a career in massage or bodywork Next you will be guided through choosing a career path, acquiring a clientele, and opening an office. Business skills, bookkeeping, record-keeping, filing income taxes, receiving insurance reimbursement, massage laws nationwide, and even saving for retirement are all covered. Finally, there is a reference section that includes over one hundred equipment manufacturers and distributors, 62 forms of bodywork, and 875 massage schools arranged in a state-by-state format.

For the massage student:

If you are already enrolled in a massage school, this book will expand on your school's courses in business, ethics, marketing and legal issues, or you may be using it as the textbook for your Business and Professionalism course.

The practical information about career strategies, bodywork modalities, marketing your services, opening a massage office, ethics and boundaries, billing insurance companies, legal issues, taxes, professional associations, professional politics, and sample forms, will be useful to you for years to come.

For the practitioner:

If you are already a trained and practicing massage therapist or bodyworker, you will still find much of value in this book to help you expand your practice and be more successful. The chapters on marketing, ethics, opening a private office, working with abuse survivors, insurance reimbursement, scientific evidence for massage and income tax may give you information you do not have. You may also be interested in bodywork modalities, schools teaching different modalities, and requirements for practice in states you might move to.

You may also want to have this book in your library for the time when an aspiring massage therapist asks you how to get started in the field. It could save you a lot of time!

Browse the table of contents and see if you aren't interested in learning more. And whether you are investigating a new career, already in massage school, or already in practice, I hope you find much in this book that you value and enjoy.

Introduction to the Fourth Edition

In 1992, when the original edition of this book was published, massage was still seen as being on the fringe of society, definitely not part of the mainstream. The second, third and fourth editions of this book have documented remarkable growth in the industry and in the public's acceptance of massage.

For example, consider the number of massage schools in the U.S. The original edition listed 190. The second edition listed 316. The third edition listed 572. This fourth edition lists 875. All in just eleven years! In addition, there are these recent advances in the profession:

- Forty-one schools now offer an associate's degree in massage. (p. 240)

- The amount of scientific research documenting the health benefits of massage has grown exponentially in the last few years, largely due to the efforts of the Touch Research Institute. (Chapter 20)

- Thirty states and the District of Columbia now regulate the practice of massage, and more have legislative activity in the works. (p. 154)

- Chair massage has grown into a tremendously popular modality that has gone into the workplace, storefronts, street fairs, airports, health expos, and many other locations. (p. 30)

- The spa industry is experiencing a great surge in popularity.

- A specialized medical massage credential is being offered for the first time. (p. 134)

Massage has come out of the shadows and onto Main Street. In large and small cities, in neighborhoods, in small towns, and even on rural roads, signs advertising massage businesses are in abundance. Few places in America lack access to an establishment publicly offering professional massage.

With all of the growth that has already taken place, most Americans have yet to experience their first professional massage. Massage is still an expanding field with room for a great variety of practitioners. This book will help you understand the field, choose your place in it, and create a successful career. I wish you a wonderful journey . . .

I

An Overview
of the Profession
&
What It Takes
to Succeed in It

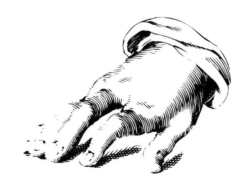

1 Is a Career in Massage for You?

Massage can be a delightful career. Your clients regard you as the person who gives them relaxation, helps relieve their pain, and assists them in improving their health. You have freedom to set your own schedule, and can earn a good living with a clear conscience.

Massage can also be a frustrating career. You have great skills and desire to help, but clients are not calling, bills are piling up, and a client has asked you for sex at the end of a massage. You may wonder whether the whole thing is worth the effort.

If you are considering pursuing a career in massage or bodywork, it is worth your while to spend a little time now examining what lies ahead and whether it is what you want. You will find information throughout this book that will help you get a fuller picture of what it is like to be a massage professional. However, certain pros and cons should be set out at the start.

First item: Money.

Many people are lured to the idea of a massage career by some simple arithmetic. The local massage therapist is charging $60.00 per hour. Eight hours a day times $60.00 per hour comes to $480.00 per day, or $2,400.00 per week. Eureka! How can I get into this!?

It is true that there are *a few* massage therapists whose economic picture is like the one in the last paragraph, but they are the exception and not the rule. The vast majority of massage professionals have a very different story to tell.

A recent AMTA member survey revealed that 57% of full-time practitioners earned less than $30,000.00 per year. A similar survey by ABMP found that the overall average for practitioners was $23,194.00 and the average first-year income was $7,700.00.

Although some massage therapists do quite well financially, it has been my experience that those who enter the field *for the purpose* of making a lot of money are not happy in the field. They either do not succeed in massage, or become so absorbed by their desire to succeed financially that they are basically unfulfilled human beings even though they earn large amounts of money.

The people in the field who are financially successful *and happy* are those who got into the field out of a sincere desire to help other people, who have good skills and who have the determination necessary to achieve success.

Those who keep at it and succeed in establishing massage careers report an extremely high rate of career satisfaction regardless of their income – the same AMTA member survey quoted above found that more than 50% of respondents were "extremely satisfied" with their careers.

Second item: Drive and motivation.

What massage has in common with other professions—such as law, medicine and accounting—is that the professional has to attract a following, a clientele, in order to earn a living.

True, there are jobs available in which you can work for an hourly wage or on commission, but these situations are usually regarded as "entry-level" positions, or situations in which you can gain experience before you are truly established in the field. Jobs where some person or institution brings you a clientele are seldom well-paid jobs; your employer might take up to 70% of the amount paid for your services.

Therefore, to succeed in the long run, you will need to establish yourself as an independent professional with a substantial client base. Every client is an individual who could choose any massage practitioner, but chooses you because of what you have to offer. To be worth choosing and to be well-known and respected take time, dedication, and organization. Know before you begin that this is the path you are choosing for the long run when you choose a career as a massage therapist.

Third item: Commitment.

From reading this far, you are getting the idea that massage is not a field you just drift into and easily start making money. Getting started will be easier if you have substantial experience in a related hands-on therapy field or a solid reputation in your community. Otherwise, you can expect that during your first year or two after massage school you will have a limited income from massage, and will be spending a fair amount of time promoting yourself in an attempt to become established.

Therefore, make a commitment to your massage career. If you approach the field in a mature way, it will be a rewarding choice for you. However, if you approach it with a half-hearted commitment, you are likely to abandon your attempt to create a practice before you reap the rewards of the marketing and promotion you do.

Making a commitment to your career means making some commitment to a place. That is not to say you must settle down in the first place you practice massage, but ultimately you should make a pledge to yourself to spend at least three years in a location as a massage therapist. If you don't take that step, you don't do justice to your chances to have a successful career in the field.

Still interested?

If none of this scares you off, you probably have a good chance of making it as a massage therapist. Other chapters will provide you with strategies and techniques that will enable you to minimize your frustration and maximize your success as a professional. If you are making the decision to undertake a career as a massage professional, may I extend a warm welcome to you, and a wish that you enjoy all the ups and downs and in-betweens that await you...

2 The Massage and Bodywork Field
Its Time Has Come

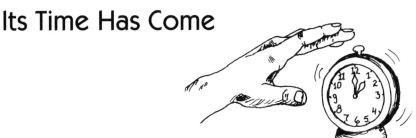

Massage is an ancient art that has been having a renaissance during the last 50 years in the United States. Many types of massage have been developed, and many types of closely and not-so-closely related therapies have evolved in recent times. In an attempt to clarify this sometimes confusing picture, I offer the following discussion of massage and definitions of various terms.

What is massage, anyway?

In one sense, the term "massage" deserves to be many words, because one word cannot be stretched enough to include the various therapeutic techniques practiced by people who call themselves massage therapists. Consider these categories:

- **Wellness massage,** for preventative general health;
- **Relaxation massage,** to remove the results of stresses of daily life, including "on-site" or chair massage;
- **Pampering (or beautification) massage,** to provide a sensuous, pleasurable indulgence or as an adjunct to beauty services.
- **Sports massage,** for training, preparation and recovery from exertion during sporting events;
- **Pain relief,** to relieve muscle soreness, minor injury pain, headaches, or the like;
- **Rehabilitative massage,** for recovery after physical injury such as broken bones;
- **Medical massage,** as an adjunct to medical treatment for illness;
- **Chiropractic adjunct,** to enhance the effectiveness of chiropractic adjustments;
- **Personal transformation massage,** to explore emotional or psychological issues or to produce shifts in consciousness;

"Bodywork" and massage

Confusing the matter still further, many people also include "bodywork" in the term massage. Such hands-on therapies as shiatsu, Trager, Rolfing, polarity, and at least 60 other forms of bodywork now available are sometimes referred to under the umbrella term "massage," especially in the Western United States.

In order to make the information in this book easier to organize and use, I have drawn a distinction between "traditional" massage, and other newly-formed kinds of hands-on therapies. With apologies to those who prefer a definition of "massage" that includes a broad spectrum of bodywork styles, I have settled on the other, perhaps more conservative definition.

In this book, the term "massage" is used to mean traditional "Swedish" massage, or systems very much like it. Swedish massage is characterized by the five strokes effleurage, petrissage, friction, vibration and tapotement. Other systems that work with the body are called "bodywork." The following definitions are offered for clarification.

Definitions

Please note: There are no "official" or widely accepted definitions of the terms "massage" and "bodywork." These definitions are offered to clarify the meanings of these terms as used in this book.

Massage. The application of touch by one person to another, using manual techniques of rubbing, stroking, kneading or compression (effleurage, petrissage, vibration, friction or tapotement), when done to produce relaxation, pain relief, injury rehabilitation, athletic preparedness or recovery, health improvement, increased awareness, or pleasure.

Bodywork. The application of touch by one person to another, to produce relaxation, pain relief, injury rehabilitation, health improvement, increased awareness, neuromuscular re-education, or pleasure, using any techniques other than those used in massage (see definition of massage, above). Bodywork does not include chiropractic, osteopathy, or any other system which has an organized licensing structure and grants the title "doctor" to its practitioners. (See the Bodywork Organizations and Trainings Directory starting on page 217.)

Massage Practitioner. Any person who publicly offers massage in return for money.

Massage Therapist. A massage practitioner who has received training in the theory and practice of massage, and is competent to use massage as a means of promoting pain relief, injury rehabilitation or health improvement.

Bodyworker. Any person who publicly offers bodywork in return for money.

The following definitions clarify the meaning of several words used in the above definitions:

"Compression" does not include static pressure applied to one spot (as in shiatsu and trigger point therapy), but does include pressure that increases and decreases or moves along the body, such as tapotement and friction.

"Health improvement" includes mental, psychological, emotional and spiritual health, as well as the health of the body's immune system, or any other system of the body.

"Pleasure" means the enjoyment of the sensations in the body, but does not include sexual arousal or stimulation of sexual organs.

Recent growth of massage—factors involved

In 1960, the average American had one of two associations for the word "massage." It was thought of either as a prelude to sex or a health club rub-down, heavy on the "karate chops." These images still remain for some people, especially older people whose personal experience of massage has been one or the other of these types. However, the last fifty years have seen phenomenal growth of legitimate, therapeutic and scientific massage. Today, for the first time in American society, massage is considered a conventional treatment for stress reduction, pain relief, treatment of medical conditions and emotional and physical well-being.

Several societal trends have facilitated the rediscovery of the ancient art of massage. The hippie movement in the 1960s, and related consciousness-raising activities, opened doors for massage as a tool for self-exploration and personal transformation. The explosion in fitness activities during the 1970s and 1980s brought acceptance for massage as both a wellness modality and a sports training aid.

In the 1990s, the widespread promotion of chair massage, (also called on-site or seated massage) introduced massage to huge numbers of people who would not have been comfortable undressing to experience massage. Chair massage went into workplaces, shopping malls, storefronts, airports, street fairs, health fairs, and many more locations. It played, and continues to play, a major role in making the general public aware of the benefits of massage, and making it more attractive to a mass market.

The medical community's view of massage has begun to shift as well. Early on, massage was considered an "alternative" treatment – something a patient might choose *instead* of medical treatment. More recently it has been referred to primarily as a "complementary" therapy – meaning one that adds to or supports other medical practices. The trend now is toward "integrative" medical clinics, which include massage and other modalities with conventional medicine under one roof. Many universities now have such integrative clinics, and hundreds of private integrative clinics have opened across the United States.

As a result of all this growth, massage schools have proliferated (one person described it as an "algae bloom"), the membership of massage organizations has skyrocketed, and massage has evolved from a service for the wealthy to a service accessible to and used by the general public.

The change has been taking place at a different pace in different places. In some parts of the West coast, massage has been popular for so long that there exists a surplus of massage therapists. In contrast, many remote or rural locations still have very little activity in the massage field. However, in most of North America, large numbers of people either have recently become aware of massage, or are ready to be shown for the first time how wonderful and therapeutic massage can be. Most areas are continuing to experience a steady, even dramatic rise in the popularity and availability of massage.

What does the future hold?

People have been doing massage for many thousands of years. Massage was something people were doing before surgery was ever performed, before medicines were prescribed, before science was even conceived, before almost any other human activity you can name. It has lasted these thousands of years because it is good. Much like gold has been the investment of choice throughout much of history because of its inherent value, massage is a part of human culture that has stood the test of time because it has real value for people.

Because massage is a service with inherent value for people, it does not need to have a market created for it in order to be in demand. Instead, massage is naturally in demand as soon as people release the artificial barriers they have against using massage services.

People's barriers to massage

These barriers are 1) anxiety about nudity and about one's own body, 2) fear of making contact with another person or oneself, 3) a belief that spending money on oneself is indulgent or wasteful, and 4) fear of the unknown.

These are significant barriers, but they are the sort of things people tend to outgrow. The more sophisticated our society becomes, the more irrelevant these barriers will seem to the general population. The general societal and scientific acceptance of massage will help these barriers continue to come down in the years to come.

Another issue is affordability. The 1980s saw an increase in income for many, and facilitated the growth of massage in part by creating a larger group of people who could afford it. Price is a factor for many people. The economy experienced a downturn immediately after the World Trade Center tragedy, but most massage therapists felt little or no effect on their practices. Even so, the economy will necessarily play a role in how much massage continues to grow in popularity, and the profession can aid the growth of massage by not pricing itself out of reach of most people.

Finally, the payment for massage services by insurance companies, if widely available, would open a whole new market for massage services. A certain number of potential massage clients will receive massage only if it is covered by their medical insurance policy. Currently, insurance reimbursement plays a minor role in the overall picture of massage therapy, but that factor might be poised to increase sharply. Whether that will change in the near future is one of the topics touched on in the next chapter.

3 Current Professional and Political Issues

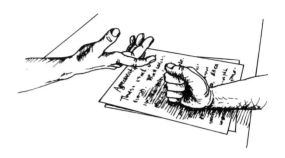

This is a very lively time in the life of the massage and bodywork profession. If you liken the massage field in the U.S. to a growing person, it has passed through its youth, survived its adolescence, and in poised to face the world as a young adult.

The 1960s saw the birth, (or re-birth) of massage as a sophisticated profession worthy of widespread acceptance in society. The '70s, '80s, '90s were a time of phenomenal growth, and a time when the profession as a whole went in many different directions looking for a sense of identity, or for its personality. Massage expanded into many different contexts, and related forms of bodywork grew up by the dozens.

Now the profession has taken root in many venues; massage therapists are commonplace in chiropractic offices, health clubs, spas, corporations, and stand-alone private offices. State regulation of massage exists in 30 states, and in many towns, cities, and counties. The National Certification Exam has been in existence for over a decade, and most of the states that regulate massage require or accept it as their written licensing exam, facilitating therapists moving from state to state.

Mainstream America has realized that massage is not sex, and that it is a scientifically-proven health modality. Related forms of bodywork have evolved and blossomed into a rich tapestry of touch therapies that present almost unlimited choices for the practitioner and for consumers. The profession is firmly entrenched on the American scene.

The purpose of this chapter is to set out the main political and professional issues currently confronting the industry. Understanding this information may not be essential to your career as a massage or bodywork practitioner, but you might find it helpful to have a broad understanding of the political issues in your chosen field. Some of this information may help you decide which school or schools to attend, and which association or associations to join. An awareness of the political process in your chosen profession may also help you avoid unpleasant surprises in the future.

What is at Stake in Political Issues?

The following scenarios are drawn from real-life experiences. While you may not experience the problems indicated by these examples, they are meant to alert you to some of the real-life situations that provide motivation for governmental regulation of massage and bodywork:

- You have a successful private massage practice. One day, your mail carrier delivers a certified letter from the State Board of Physical Therapy, ordering you to cease and desist practicing massage unless you can prove that you have a license to practice physical therapy or chiropractic.

- You want to move to a new state, but on investigation, you learn that your educational training is considered inadequate under that state's licensing law, and you must attend school at a massage school in the new state from start to finish, and then take that state's licensing exam.

- You are working with a car-crash victim who could benefit from massage therapy. She asks you "are your services covered by my medical insurance?"

- You are attempting to establish a referral relationship with a physician and when you say you do "medical massage" she says she has never heard of that and asks what credential you have that allows you to practice.

This chapter will give you an overview of the current political situation and some of the conflicting views that are being advanced, and will suggest some directions for progress in the future.

Governmental Regulation of Massage

Massage is the newest member of the group of regulated professions. Dentists, doctors, psychologists, nurses, lawyers, physical therapists, and chiropractors, among many others, have all gone through the process of establishing procedures to regulate who can and can't practice the profession. That regulation process has begun in the massage and bodywork field, but is not complete.

At present, 30 states and the District of Columbia have laws regulating massage. The requirements differ from state to state. Texas, for example, requires 300 hours of educational training. Oregon requires 330 hours. Many states require 500 hours. Ohio requires 600, New Mexico 650, New Hampshire 750 and New York and Nebraska 1,000. Most use the National Certification Exam as their written test, a few do not.

The 20 states without regulatory laws require *zero* hours, and do not restrict the practice of massage. Although some municipalities and counties in those states regulate massage, most practitioners in those 20 states do not have to answer to anyone.

Why regulate the practice of massage and bodywork?

Why not just let people do what they want, and let the free marketplace take care of who succeeds and who fails? Many in the profession believe that's the best approach and for that reason oppose governmental regulation of massage in those states where it has not yet been enacted.

Proponents of governmental regulation put forth several arguments in favor of governmental regulation of massage:

First, the public deserves protection. When a state agency regulates the practice of massage, they maintain a hearings board or grievance board to consider complaints by members of the public about how they were treated by a practitioner. In this way, the profession gives the public a quick and easy remedy against a practitioner who is incompetent or unethical. This inspires trust and confidence on the part of the public and enhances the respect of the entire profession. If there is no agency regulating massage in a state, it is much harder for an injured party to get satisfaction from the practitioner who injured her. The only remedy available is to hire a lawyer and pursue a lawsuit, which is usually a very lengthy, traumatic and expensive undertaking.

Second, state licensing protects the massage profession from other professions that claim *they* are the only ones with the right to do massage. Physical therapists in Maryland battled for many years to for the right to control the practice of massage in that state. They instituted legal proceedings against massage therapists, charging them with practicing physical therapy without a license. These conflicts finally ended with the enactment of a massage licensing law in Maryland. Similar challenges have taken place in Oregon and the District of Columbia. State regulation of massage prevents this kind of headache—the state, by regulating the field, ensures the right of massage practitioners to practice.

Third, governmental regulation of massage helps in getting rid of those who offer sexual gratification as part of a massage. Where massage is regulated by the government, there is a quick and easy process for suspending the license or registration of one who is unethical. However, where massage is not governmentally regulated, the only remedy against unethical practitioners is the criminal justice system, which is notoriously slow and inefficient. Therefore, in areas where massage is not regulated by the government, it is harder to stop those who offer sexual massage.

Finally, some believe that state regulation of massage encourages mainstream society and the medical profession to take massage practitioners seriously. The desire for acceptance as a mainstream health care provider has been an undercurrent in the licensing and certification debate for a number of years.

Why Some Oppose Attempts to Create State Regulation

Some people are against governmental regulation on principle—they are suspicious of government and don't want any outside authority taking control over their lives.

Others oppose regulation because the situation in their location does not need improvement. Perhaps the profession is well-established, unlicensed practitioners are able to receive insurance reimbursement, and there is no lack of respect and acceptance for massage and massage practitioners. Governmental regulation adds expense, burdens and restrictions. If there is no problem to be solved by regulation, then regulation is unnecessary.

For the last six years, I have subscribed to an internet discussion group for massage and bodywork practitioners. Governmental regulation of massage has been the most frequently debated topic on the list, and has evoked the most heated debate. Most of the members of the internet discussion group who express an opinion on the subject favor not regulating massage. The main issues seem to be 1) freedom to choose the amount and kind of education one wants, and 2) the desire for freedom from the tests, rules, restrictions and expenses that inevitably come with governmental regulation.

Another area of controversy in the debate, however, concerns not whether licensing is a good idea in principle, but *the way* in which the attempts to enact licensing laws are sometimes made.

Specifically, some groups within the massage profession attempt to create new licensing laws by keeping their legislative proposals secret, submitting legislation to state governments without consulting the majority of practitioners in the state where the law will be in force, and proposing legislation that favors the members of the group sponsoring the legislation, as opposed to considering the interests of all practitioners in the state.

Many groups are interested in the outcome of legislative efforts. However, two national professional organizations have some of the strongest interests concerning these issues. These organizations, the AMTA and the ABMP, sometimes have different ideas about how the licensing process should proceed. From published articles and magazine editorials about licensing issues, the following seems true of the current situation regarding attempts to create governmental regulation for massage:

The AMTA (American Massage Therapy Association) initiates attempts to create new state licensing, but does not necessarily advocate licensure for every state.

The ABMP (Associated Bodywork and Massage Professionals) is not against licensing, nor is it against the AMTA, but it opposes unilateral attempts to impose massage licensing without input from the majority of practitioners who will be affected by the law.

Currently, the ABMP is maintaining a network to alert practitioners about attempts to enact laws regulating massage. The ABMP's goal is to be included in the process of formulating the law, so the law will be responsive to all groups within the profession. In some states, AMTA representatives have invited the members of other groups to join in a coalition to formulate legislative proposals acceptable to all.

AMTA has recently instituted an official policy urging chapters to build coalitions with bodyworkers and non-AMTA members. Before the national organization will provide funding to assist in legislative efforts, state chapters must show proof of coalition-building and must conduct a survey of both members and non-members to gauge support for the proposed legislation.

In the past, AMTA supporters have sometimes promoted laws that require practitioners to get their massage education at a school accredited by COMTA (Commission on Massage Therapy Accreditation), which is an arm of AMTA (see page 129) West Virginia's licensing law originally required attendance at a COMTA school, but that provision was subsequently removed by the legislature.

Creation of laws requiring education at a COMTA-approved school has been one of the sources of discord between competing groups in the industry. In light of the current policy of AMTA to require coalition-building and non-member surveys, perhaps no future legislative proposals will include a COMTA-based educational requirement.

Licensing, Certification and Registration

These terms can be confusing. Massage practitioners sometimes are certified, sometimes are licensed, and sometimes are registered. The three terms do not mean the same thing. In order to properly understand the political issues in the massage and bodywork field, you should understand the differences between these three terms. Once you read the following, their meanings will come clear to you.

First, ask yourself this question: When you speak about licensing, certification, or registration, are you talking about what a *government* is doing or what a *private group* is doing?

Governments can create *any* of the three kinds of regulations mentioned—licensing, certification or registration. Private groups or individuals can give only *certification*.

When a government requires a *license* to practice massage, then practicing without a license is a criminal act. The licensing law sets out the requirements for obtaining a license and establishes a procedure by which qualified individuals can apply for a license.

When a government *certifies* practitioners, that is usually a voluntary procedure that carries some benefit. For example, in Maine, certified practitioners may use the title "Massage Therapist" and non-certified practitioner may not. In Delaware, certified practitioners are exempt from the "Adult Entertainment Law" but non-certified practitioners fall under its authority.

When a government *registers* practitioners, they generally do not restrict the practice, but keep track of practitioners by requiring them to submit certain information to the government. (However, Texas requires registration as a mandatory condition to practice massage, so registration operates much the same as a license in that state.)

Private groups can give only *certification*. They cannot give a license or registration. Private groups that give certification are giving an individual their private approval. They are certifying that the person has completed a specific course of study or passed a specific test.

Certification is never a legal requirement to practice massage, but it can be a legal requirement to practice forms of bodywork that are protected by trade-name or service-mark protection, such as Rolfing, Trager, Feldenkrais, etc. As to those forms of bodywork, certification from the owner of the name is required to use that name in connection with your work.

Now that you understand the differences between registration, certification, and licensing, I have to add that the National Certification Exam complicates the picture by being part "certification" and part "license".

The National Certification Exam (NCE) is a standardized written test that is created by a private group (not by a government). However, it has been chosen as the written exam by governments in most of the states that regulate massage (see page 154). These states have other requirements, such as educational requirements, licensing fees, and sometimes character references, but they use the National Certification Exam as their written exam for massage.

The National Certification Exam (NCE) therefore operates both as a *private certification* and as a *governmentally-required exam*. A brief history of the creation of the NCE is the subject of the next section.

A Brief History of the National Certification Exam

During the late 1980s, the AMTA announced its plan to create a voluntary, nationwide certification exam for massage. It was initially to be an AMTA project, and was to be a Swedish massage certification exam. Although the exam was to be voluntary, many therapists became concerned that it would nonetheless become a practical requirement, since the goal of the exam was to standardize the qualifications of professional massage therapists throughout the United States.

Some non-AMTA massage therapists became resentful that a standard was being created without their input, which could impair their ability to earn a living. Some were angered that this action was being taken without consultation with any industry leaders outside the AMTA.

In the wake of this initial controversy, some organized attempts at reconciliation took place, without much success. As time went on, AMTA decided to make the certification project separate from the AMTA. When it was launched as an independent organization, the certification project was funded by a loan from the AMTA, and seven of the nine members of the steering committee were AMTA members. These connections to the AMTA caused some non-AMTA members to believe that the project was still an arm of the AMTA.

After the exam had been created, the steering committee was dissolved and replaced by the National Certification Board, which now administers the test. The National Certification Board is incorporated in the state of Virginia, and Board members are elected by mail ballot from all nationally certified practitioners. The Board has a stated commitment to cooperate with the AMTA toward mutual goals, but it is administratively separate from AMTA.

The National Certification Exam certifies basic competence in massage, and does not test for competence in any specific area of practice, such as sports massage, medical massage, shiatsu or the like. There is no practical portion of the test, i.e., no test of manual skills is involved.

The exam is given on a continuous basis at locations with interactive computer terminals. It was first administered in June 1992. As of 2002, more than 40,000 practitioners had passed the exam, and over 900 practitioners were taking the exam every month.

To be eligible for the exam, a practitioner must have completed 500 hours of education in massage or bodywork. Professional experience can substitute for a portion of the educational requirement. The exam covers anatomy and physiology, clinical pathology, massage assessment and technique, business practices and ethics. Continuing education is required to maintain certified status, but not to maintain state licensure in states that use the test as their written exam. For further information about the NCE, you can contact National Certification Board for Therapeutic Massage and Bodywork at (703) 610-9015 or Infoline (800) 296-0664 or on the Internet at **www.ncbtmb.com**.

Suggestions for the future

In Chapter Two, I noted that the term "massage" is used to cover many different approaches to this kind of work. Boiled down to the most fundamental issue, the massage community is divided between viewing massage as a "personal service" and viewing massage as a "health care service". In other words, some identify with the idea that massage is mostly about wellness and relaxation, or "personal service". Others identify with the idea that massage is a medical or quasi-medical therapy, i.e., "a health care service".

A recent AMTA survey of public attitudes about massage found that roughly half of the general public thinks of massage as a health service and roughly half thinks of massage as a non-medical stress-reducing service. This same duality exists within the profession.

Therefore, I have for many years advocated for *specialized credentials* for massage therapists and bodyworkers, just like there are specialized doctors (surgeons, psychiatrists, dermatologists, etc.) and specialized dentists (orthodontists, periodontists, etc.). Specialists must achieve a separate certification to practice their specialty.

The licensing, regulation and certification of professional competence for "relaxation" massage should be viewed very differently from the licensing, regulation and certification of specialties, such as medical massage.

State licensing of massage aims at basic, or entry-level credentialing. Licensing is designed to assure basic professional competence so the public is protected from untrained practitioners. 500 hours of training (or the 300 hours required in Texas) is enough to provide this entry-level competency in massage, including basic anatomy, massage techniques, contraindications, proper hygiene, and basic business skill. However, 500 hours is not enough to provide training both as a massage practitioner and also as a specialist in a particular branch of massage or bodywork.

Forms of bodywork that are protected by trade-name or service-mark protection enforce advanced educational standards by limiting use of the trade name (such as "Rolfer" or "Trager Practitioner") to those who have met the governing organization's educational requirements. The possibility also exists for creating standard credentials for non-trade-marked modalities, such as medical massage, reflexology, sports massage, polarity, and others.

The newly-created American Manual Medicine Association, or AMMA (see page 134) is attempting to establish a standardized credential for medical massage. In fact, AMMA is promoting two medical massage credentials; an entry level medical massage certification and an advanced medical massage certification.

If the medical massage credentials being created by AMMA become widely accepted, it will become easier to convince physicians, hospitals and insurance carriers to use credentialed therapists to offer this healing modality to medical patients.

If the massage profession evolves so that state governments license the practice of massage to assure basic professional competence, and the massage profession itself certifies specialists in the major modalities that are practiced, massage will have truly grown into its potential as a profession, and will have achieved a real maturity.

II

Career Options, Strategies and Tactics

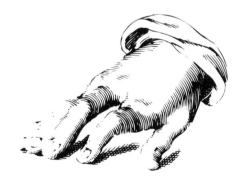

4 Your Career in Massage or Bodywork
Let's Get Organized

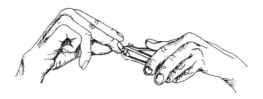

A surprising fact is that most massage school graduates never create a massage practice that supports them financially. They either never make an organized effort to practice massage professionally, or they give it a try but abandon their efforts before they achieve a successful practice.

The purposes of the four chapters in this section are:

1. To help you gain clarity about what it is you want from your professional life in massage or bodywork.

2. To help you make a sensible plan for achieving your goals.

3. To help you follow through on that plan with a minimum of wasted effort and a maximum of success.

Common misconceptions

Many would-be massage therapists have certain wrong assumptions about the paths their careers will take. One very common expectation about a massage career goes like this:

> I will attend massage school, where I will learn everything I need to know to be a successful massage therapist. When I finish school, I will set up a practice. Clients will come to me and I will be busy and happy.

Several misconceptions are evident in this scenario. First, massage school will not teach you everything you need to know, either about giving a good massage or about operating in the business world. In fact, you should look at your first 1,000 professional massages as completion of your education as a massage therapist. Your skill level and confidence level will grow for years to come.

Second, you probably will not be in a position to set up a practice right out of school. Unless you have a very good reputation in the community, it will take time and effort to build your reputation sufficiently to establish a clientele.

Third, clients will not come to you just because you make yourself available. If you get yourself an office and say "Here I am, world!" the world will respond with a deafening silence. In order to be a busy massage therapist or bodyworker, you will need to take organized, affirmative steps to let people know you are there and make them want to take advantage of your services.

Finally, being busy and being happy are not necessarily the same thing. You want to attract those clients that most suit you. Even when you do not have enough work, there are still clients out there whom you do not want to have. Your clients will be a significant part of your life when your practice is going, so take the time to attract a clientele you will enjoy serving.

Typical career paths

In imagining what your career will be like, and taking logical steps to reach your goals, it will help you to have the benefit of the experiences of those who have walked the path before you. Numerous interviews with successful massage therapists and bodyworkers have disclosed many common elements in their career paths.

Below are capsule versions of the careers of some actual massage therapists and bodyworkers. Some are more successful than others. All are earning their sole livelihood at massage or bodywork.

"A" started his career in massage when he had a wife and a baby and was very poor. His wife was very supportive. During the early years, he did very little else to earn money, except some painting work for Christmas money. He chose this approach so that he would be fully immersed in the profession and would be forced to overcome any obstacles. It took two years to achieve a steady client load. After four years, he was so busy he was turning away clients, and now travels with world-class athletes to international sporting events.

"B" went to massage school, then went traveling in Asia for 15 months. On his return to California, he found he was seriously depressed. After three months of depression, he pulled himself out of it and began working at a health spa and promoting himself locally, working out of his home and doing house calls. Newspaper coverage of him and his Asian trip helped his practice grow, and within eight months, he was doing upwards of 20 massages per week. His business is growing, yet he plans to spend only one or two more years in the area before moving on to some other location.

"C" had a marketing background, and when she graduated from massage school, used newspaper ads, coupons and flyers to gather a practice quickly. She worked out of her home in San Diego, and had 10 to 15 clients per week within a month of starting her marketing program. After two years, she got out of massage completely, finding she was "fed up" with dealing with men who were asking her for sexual favors. She currently works as a receptionist in a wholistic health center.

"D" opened a store-front massage office in Chicago right out of massage school. She did a great deal of personal promotion in the neighborhood. Almost all of her clients in the early days were men, many of whom presented her with requests for sex. Her husband supported her financially for the first few years, and despite aggressive promotion, it took about three years for her practice to reach a profitable level, especially in light of the very high rent she had to pay for a corner store-front business location. After four years in practice, she is seeing 20 to 30 clients per week.

"E" did massage for about five years as a hobby, accepting donations, before ever attending massage school. He has been out of massage school eight years, and does 6 to 15 massages per week. The slow growth of his practice and his current pace of activity are exactly to his liking.

"F" spent quite a few years not succeeding in the massage field. He worked as a physical therapy assistant for three years, and also tried to establish a massage practice in a hair salon. Then he "took some time off" from the profession. He returned to the profession and became involved in his state massage associations. He became active in the AMTA and went into practice with a prominent sports massage teacher and practitioner. His massage practice reached full capacity within three months of starting in this office, and he has since taken on a significant leadership role in the AMTA.

"G" had 10 years experience as a swimming trainer and worked as a case manager in a chiropractor's office while she attended massage school. She did some massage in the chiropractor's office for a few months after graduation. A cardiologist who had heard of her invited her to rent an office in his tasteful, downtown practice building at a very reasonable rent. She accepted, and once there, she was able to work on some very influential community members who spread the word about her skills. Within three months of moving to the cardiologist's office, she had a thriving practice.

"H" started out in the field as a new mother, and very poor. She was always moving from one home to another in search of cheaper rent. Her main priority was to be very good at her work, and it took her several years to begin to earn a living at massage. She has now been in practice 10 years, specializes in pregnancy massage, and works at a birthing center. She sees 15 to 20 clients per week, most of whom are regulars. She would welcome having more clients.

"I" made a point of having non-massage work that supported her when she began her massage career. She was concerned that if she were financially needy, clients would sense that neediness and be put off. Instead, having her financial needs met, she could approach her clients with warmth and openness. Within one and a half years, she was seeing 20 clients per week, and only then did she quit her other job. She has kept her practice at that level ever since.

"J" did house cleaning at the beginning of her massage career to meet expenses. The first year brought only enough massage income to pay expenses such as office rent and supplies. After fifteen months, she was earning enough from massage to stop doing cleaning work. After 18 months, her client load was 10 to 15 per week.

"K" was a public school teacher. She started gathering a practice during after-school hours, and as the practice grew, she switched to substitute teaching, and eventually was able to let go of substitute teaching, and be a full-time massage therapist. The entire process took four years, which was longer than she thought it would take. She currently sees 15 to 20 clients per week.

"L" has a practice as a polarity therapist, which she took six years to build. For the first year, she kept her job as a university teacher, and saw one to three clients per week to decide if she wanted to pursue polarity more seriously. For the next three years, she held a consulting job two days per week, and built her polarity practice up to about six clients per week. She currently sees 12 to 15 polarity clients per week, teaches four yoga classes per week, and markets her own yoga instructional tapes.

"M" opened a practice in the town she grew up in immediately after finishing massage school. During the next two and a half years, she worked in at least six different locations in and around the area, gaining experience and slowly gaining a client base. She then opened an office in a charming, wealthy seaside resort town a few miles away. She coordinated this new office with a direct mail promotion and a public speaking engagement. Within weeks of moving, her practice doubled, and within two months she was seeing 30 or more clients per week.

"N" worked for four years as a physical therapy assistant and sports therapist before going to massage school. She has been supporting herself with massage work during the first year after massage school, doing house calls and working in a chiropractor's office doing massage for $14 per hour. Her goal is to be a physical therapist.

"O" worked full-time for AT&T, and practiced massage in her off-hours, doing house calls in an affluent community. After about one and a half years, she left her job and went into massage full-time. She went to work in a hotel health spa to supplement her practice, and has a busy practice.

"P" went to massage school after several years in practice as a lawyer. After graduating from massage school, he took a job teaching law, and did one to three massages per week on the side. He did this for three years, and then set out to establish a massage practice in a new location where he knew very few people. It took two years for the practice to produce enough income to meet his living expenses. He used some of his spare time to work on a book about the massage profession. After three and a half years of practice, he is seeing between 12 and 20 clients per week.

Elements these career paths have in common

The experiences summarized above display several elements that are repeated in more than one story. Consider the following:

- Those who had substantial experience in a hands-on field before going to massage school became established massage therapists much more quickly than those who had no such experience.

- For those without such prior experience, the average time needed to establish an income-producing practice varied quite a bit, but two years was about average. Some made it in a year, some took three or four years. Those taking longer than four years probably were not making an organized attempt to become established.

- Attempts at rapid growth through advertising tend to bring sexually-oriented male clients.

- It appears to take longer for most men to become established massage therapists than it does for women.

Main causes of career failures

What factors explain the failure of most massage school graduates to create a successful professional practice? The two main ways in which would-be massage therapists sabotage their careers are moving too often, and being reluctant to promote themselves.

As you can understand from reading the career capsules above, success as a massage therapist comes only after a period of building a reputation in the community. The two essential elements in this process are 1) doing things to become known and 2) giving the process some time.

Recent massage school graduates are often very unsettled. Perhaps you are "in transition", having moved away from home to attend massage school, and not knowing where you want to settle to start a new life. Perhaps you are living in your home town, and you are apprehensive about becoming established, for fear that if you acquire a successful practice, you will never leave your home town and see the world. Perhaps you do not have confidence in your ability to give a professional massage.

If you are in such a situation, or in a similar situation that makes you unsure or reluctant about becoming established, you have at least three logical approaches you can take:

1. **The side-step.** Do some other kind of work to earn a living, and do massage on the side. This will give you the opportunity to see if you really enjoy massage work, and will give your skills a chance to slowly improve. It also will give you time to become better known in the community. If and when you decide to move to full-time massage work, you will have a stronger local reputation.

2. **The trial balloon.** Take any job you can get doing massage, such as working in a health club, resort, spa or chiropractor's office. These jobs will give you substantial experience doing massage, will give your skills a chance to grow, and may yield some contacts that can lead to a different job opportunity. While the pay usually will not be high, you retain the opportunity to leave town without sacrificing any time and energy spent in reputation-building.

3. **The leap of faith.** Act as if you have decided to stay in town for awhile. Commit yourself to staying for two or three years and take some steps to build a clientele.

If you don't know where you'd rather live, and you can't figure your life out, there is a good chance that three years from now you will either be right where you are now, or will move to a new place and still not be sure what you want to do. If you decide to take a stand wherever you are now, you may find that any major issues in your life are just as easy to wrangle with while you build a massage career as they would if you moved somewhere else or did something different.

The golden keys to career success

Having discussed what holds some people back from succeeding in the field, what is it that generates success for those who succeed? There are four keys to success in this field, and all four are indispensable. Imagine them like the four legs of a table. If any of the legs is short or missing, the table is not of much use.

The four golden keys to success in this field are:

Location   Personality   Skills   Desire

Location. You might be the greatest massage therapist on earth, but if you are in a town filled with people who cannot afford your services, or who have overwhelming resistance to trying massage, you will not do well.

Location refers also to the part of town your office is in. Neighborhoods have characters, as do streets, as do individual buildings. The character of the surroundings seeps into people's attitudes about you and your office.

Personality. Your clients are not simply coming to you for a physical treatment. They are coming to you for your presence as well as your skills. They may come in for work on the body, but it is the whole person who decides whether to come back for another massage.

Not only should your clients feel completely comfortable in your presence, they should look forward to coming to see you as a chance to be with you for an hour. Successful massage therapists develop personal, often warm relationships with their clients.

Skills. You need to have the ability to do a good treatment. The client must feel better leaving than coming in. The client must also feel there is some good reason for choosing your therapy over the competition.

In short, whatever type of massage or bodywork you practice, you need to know what you are doing and do it well. This can mean not just education, but experience. Your skills as a massage therapist will improve throughout the first few years of your massage career.

Desire. Consider whether you whole-heartedly want to succeed in your practice. If not, what is it that is holding you back? Your deepest and most honest desires deserve expression. If you honestly want to be a professional massage therapist, you will focus your efforts efficiently and effectively.

Do your best to look inside and discover what you really want from your massage career. If you have reluctance to really put yourself in the public eye and build a clientele, ask yourself why, or talk it over with a trusted friend. Understanding yourself is a valuable asset in making choices that will bring you a career you can really enjoy.

How do you rate yourself on the Four Golden Keys?

Re-read the four golden keys to success. This is the most important information in this book. If you embark on a massage career with a significant weakness in any of these four areas, you should understand that you need to work on this area in order to become successful. Before you put yourself through any needless hardship, consider very carefully your assessment of yourself and your career.

Make a commitment to strengthen your weaknesses

If any of these four keys is missing or deficient in your assessment of yourself, make a commitment to yourself that you will work on this area. Here are some suggestions for how to improve.

Location. Do some research about the town, neighborhood and building you are planning to be in. Find out about the residents' income and standard of living. Find out how well any massage therapists in that area are doing.

Generally speaking, it is more difficult to be the only massage therapist in town, because that indicates there is no established massage clientele in that area. On the other hand, if you are the first and only practitioner in an area, you will have a secure professional foundation once you do become established.

Imagine the best neighborhood, street and block for your massage office. What other businesses are on the street? What is the look of the neighborhood? Imagine yourself as a client coming to this office. Is it difficult to get to? Is it on the way to other places you may want to go? As you come onto the block and into the building, what thoughts do you have? How do you feel?

Coming to your office is what every client will do at the start of your sessions. Evaluate the experience of coming to your office, and make sure you choose a location that makes coming to see you a pleasant and comfortable experience.

Personality. If you have an abrasive personality, make a commitment to yourself to soften it. If you are shy, make a commitment to yourself to be a little more outgoing so you can put your clients at ease.

You yourself enjoy being around people who are caring, accepting, warm and easy-going. These traits are important for the massage therapist. If you are too talkative, judgmental, sarcastic, crude or angry, these traits will tend to discourage your clientele and make it difficult for you to become established.

Of course, you cannot become someone you are not. However, you can choose to suppress the aspects of your character that would interfere with your career. Remember that the tongue often acts as a sword, so when in doubt, say less rather than more.

Skills. Understand that your skills will continue to grow for years to come. Take continuing education workshops and professional trainings. Get massage often, not only to feel good but to learn from the skill of others. Continue to grow psychologically as well, as growth and maturity will lend their own added value to your manual skills.

Look for opportunities that match your skill level, and understand that your fees will rise with your skills and reputation.

Desire. Take steps that are consonant with your true desires for success—don't reach for the stars if you heart is not in it. You may not be ready for success today. If you are not ready, don't struggle—do something else for awhile and do massage on the side. When you have the desire that fosters organization and commitment, it will be much easier for you to get started in this profession. Be honest with yourself about what you want.

Weaknesses can be worked into strengths if you have the commitment to do so. These are the keys to success in your career. Use them well.

5 Career Options in Massage

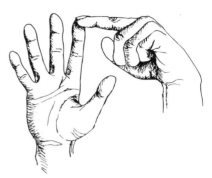

This chapter's purpose is to expose you to the broad range of options for the kinds of massage work you can do, the types of clients you can work with, opportunities for self-employment, and what you can expect in various employment situations.

Kinds of massage, types of clients

The six categories described below pretty much cover the field of massage at the present moment. Each of these types of massage attracts its own type of client, and requires its own set of skills on the part of the practitioner. You might practice several of these types of massage, but in most cases you will not practice more than one or two types in any one location.

1. Relaxation/stress reduction. The most common kind of massage, relaxation or stress reduction massage includes the types of treatments common in resorts, spas, private offices and clients' homes. This category would also include wellness massage, or preventative health massage.

2. Sports massage. This rapidly growing field encompasses athletic training massage and massage designed to help an athlete prepare for competition and recover from competing.

3. Medical massage. Working by prescription, or in a hospital, or in a physical therapist's office, the medical massage therapist works with pathologies, pain or recovery from injury. Medical massage can also be adapted to a non-medical clientele, and practiced in a home or office setting.

4. Chiropractic adjunct. Working in chiropractors' offices is becoming more and more common, especially on the West coast. Some practitioners operate relatively independently from the chiropractor, with a cross-referral agreement. Others work by prescription of the chiropractor, working on specific parts of the body that the chiropractor designates.

5. Psychotherapeutic massage. Some massage therapists focus on shifts in awareness and psychological insight that can be brought about with massage. These therapists often work by referral from psychotherapists, and usually work out of a private massage office. They often combine another form of bodywork with massage.

6. Pampering. Probably a branch of relaxation massage, pampering refers to the type of treatment that might be found in some spas and hair salons. This treatment is usually thought of as more of a beautification treatment than a health treatment, and might include salt glows, loofa rubs, and light Swedish massage.

7. Chair massage. Massage or shiatsu done with clothing on, client seated, in any location. This can be done as an introduction to massage for clients who may not come in for an office massage, or can be a continuing form of stress-reduction therapy when done on a regular basis, as in the office setting.

Settings for the practice of massage

The following are locations where massage is currently practiced. Some of these locations are traditional locations for massage, and the arrangements establishments make with massage therapists are fairly uniform. Others are not so well established, and the arrangements may vary from place to place.

In general, the more the owner of the location provides in terms of linens, booking service and client base, the less she or he will expect to pay the massage therapist. If the location has a built-in clientele, such as a resort, the owner will usually take at least half of the fee, and sometimes quite a bit more than half.

At the other end of the spectrum, if the massage therapist brings additional business to the location, or adds a sense of uniqueness to what the location has to offer, the owner may make a very favorable deal with the massage therapist, on occasion even allowing the therapist to retain 100% of the fee.

Health clubs. Home of the "rub down" in the old days, health clubs are increasingly being staffed by well-trained massage therapists, who may practice relaxation massage or sports massage.

Some clubs will hire a therapist for an hourly wage, usually between $8 and $15 per hour. Some give an hourly wage plus a small percentage of the price of the massage, and some pay the therapist anywhere from 45% to 100% of the price of the massage.

Generally, clubs where the massage therapist has to cultivate the clientele will offer the therapist a larger percentage of the proceeds. Clubs where massage is an established part of the routine, especially where there are two or more treatment rooms, will usually pay less to the therapist, since they are supplying the clients.

Common disadvantages of health clubs are relatively low pay, noisy environments, and clients who may not have a sophisticated understanding of the value of massage.

A major advantage of health clubs, especially for newly trained massage therapists, is the chance to get lots of experience in a short period of time. If your health club will allow you to bring outside clients in, it can also serve as an office location for you while you develop a private practice, and this can be a substantial advantage.

Spas and resorts. Many of the same comments that apply to health clubs apply to spas and resort facilities. When compensation is based solely on an hourly rate, spas may pay anywhere from $10.00 to $38.00 per client hour. When compensation is based solely on percentage, spas may pay anywhere from 15% to 50% of the client fee, although one therapist in Texas reports that resort hotels in his area pay between 50% and 70% of the fee charged to clients. Some spas may pay a combination of a small hourly wage plus a percentage.

The therapist in a spa or resort usually does not need to supply anything. The massage room will be equipped, and the spa or resort will do the bookings. The clients are supplied for you, but since they are vacationers, they seldom will become repeat clients for you in your local practice.

Spas usually have clean, comfortable and quiet massage rooms, and the clients are there for vacation or healthful relaxation, so their mood is usually conducive to enjoying a pleasant massage experience. Tips are usually good, and the costlier the resort, the better the tips are likely to be.

Hair salons. There are no reliable generalizations to make about the practice of massage in hair salons. Sometimes the service offered is a pampering-style light Swedish massage, and sometimes it is expert massage therapy.

Some salon owners expect a large percentage of the proceeds or a fixed monthly rental from the massage therapist, and some offer more reasonable arrangements to the therapist. It may depend in part on whether the salon owner sees the massage therapist as bringing new business or prestige to the salon, or as simply relying on the salon's established clientele.

The salon owner will often offer a "day of beauty" or "day spa" experience which includes a massage, usually a half-hour full-body massage. The price of the package will be discounted, and the salon owner will usually expect the massage therapist to offer her services at a discount for the day of beauty clients.

Common disadvantages of practicing in hair salons are noise, noxious odors, and an approach to massage as a "pampering" or beautification service. Advantages include a strong clientele for referrals (in an appropriate salon) and an atmosphere in which massage stands out as a unique service.

If you practice in a salon, some practical suggestions are: give demonstration massages to the stylists, who can be good sources of referral; give hand massage to salon clients during slow times; do chair massage in a location visible to salon clients; and confirm all appointments by phone, as no-shows and cancellations can be a particular problem at salons.

Cruise ships. The main advantages of working on a cruise ship are the excitement and exploration available to one traveling the seas of the world, and the opportunity to get a great deal of experience in the massage field in a short period of time.

Working conditions are usually cramped, a ten to twelve hour work-day is the norm, and pay is usually low. Many therapists on cruise ships concentrate on selling skin care products and their work may be classified as "beauty" treatments. Because of the long hours, low pay, and transient lifestyle, working on a cruise ship is usually considered a temporary job, although some individuals do choose this work as a long-term career option.

Hiring is usually done through a separate company. By far the largest of these is Steiner TransOcean (**www.steinerleisure.com**), which hires for the major cruise lines. Steiner employees work 12 hour days with 1½ days off per week. Assignments last four to eight months. Weekly base pay is low—perhaps $50.00 per week—and most of the therapist's compensation comes from tips and sales of a proprietary line of oils and beauty products.

It is possible to apply on-line for cruise ship work. Visit **www.cruiselinejob.com** and check under "Beauty Salon." Their listing for massage therapist has the following job description: "Extensive experience required. Must be qualified in Swedish Massage. Any additional qualifications like Aromatherapy, Shiatsu, Reflexology, Reiki Healing or Sports Therapy is a definite plus. Good English Language skills required. Salary range: $2,600–3,600 U.S. per month, depending on gratuities and cruise line."

Chair massage or on-site massage. Chair massage, also called on-site or seated massage, has grown rapidly into a substantial part of the massage industry. On October 17, 1989, the Wall Street Journal ran a front-page story about chair massage, and its growth has accelerated ever since. On August 15, 1990, the Associated Press carried a photograph of an on-site massage session being given to a customer waiting in line at the new McDonald's in Moscow. Since then, the locations for practicing chair massage have become practically unlimited.

Large and small corporations recognize the value of on-site massage. It can improve employee satisfaction, reduce absenteeism, reduce repetitive stress injuries, and improve employee retention rates. These can all directly contribute to the profitability of the company. Major corporations such as Reebok, Rockwell International, and Boeing offer on-site massage to employees, and thousands of medium-sized and smaller companies are doing likewise.

A recent study found that about six percent of workplaces offer on-site massage, but where it is provided, 60 percent of employees take advantage of the service.

When practiced in the workplace, the practitioner usually offers a ten to fifteen minute session to employees. Sometimes the company hires the practitioner and provides the service as a fringe benefit, and sometimes the employees pay individually for their massages.

Other locations for chair massage that are gaining in popularity are shopping centers, airports, fitness fairs, craft shows, and store-fronts. A company called "Massage Bar" (**www.massagebar.com**) has two locations at the Sea-Tac airport, one at the Nashville airport, and a concession at the Seattle Convention center, and hopes to expand substantially. For the first week of 2001, riders of the Paris subway received complementary 6-minute chair massages, along with green tea and crackers.

A chair massage treatment is usually a shiatsu-like treatment, using a specially designed chair that supports the client's chest and face, exposing the back and shoulders. Massage chairs were once a side-line for massage table companies, but have increased in popularity and sales of chairs now rival sales of massage tables.

There are two ways to approach on-site — as a practitioner or as an entrepreneur. As with other forms of massage practice, the hardest part of the job is acquiring a clientele. In this case, that means convincing a corporate executive that your services would be beneficial to his or her workers. The strongest incentive for a corporation is financial, so emphasize how on-site massage can reduce absenteeism, assist with repetitive stress injury, improve workplace satisfaction and increase productivity.

Once you have a contact to perform services in a workplace or other location, you can perform them yourself, or hire others to do so. If you establish a large number of clients, you can keep yourself and others busy, often making a percentage profit on the work done by those you hire.

Many massage schools include courses on practicing and marketing chair massage. Additional educational resources are listed on page 222.

Chiropractic offices. Especially in California, business relationships between chiropractors and massage therapists have become quite common. Chiropractors typically employ massage therapists to work in the chiropractor's office. The chiropractor most often prescribes massage for his or her patients, handles the insurance billing procedure, and pays the therapist either a commission or an hourly wage.

Some chiropractors pay the therapist 50% of the amount charged for massage. Some pay 50% but require the massage therapist to pay a monthly rental out of the therapist's 50%. Those who employ therapists at an hourly rate often pay in the neighborhood of $15 to $20 per hour.

Chiropractors have traditionally had great reluctance about prescribing massage for their patients. Some clients enjoy massage much more than chiropractic, or believe they benefit more from massage, and choose to stop going to the chiropractor and go to the massage therapist instead.

Chiropractors combat this by having the massage therapist in their office, and prescribing massage so that insurance reimbursement will cover the cost. The client receives massage as a no-cost added benefit of chiropractic care, and therefore has an added incentive to keep coming to the chiropractor.

The chiropractor not only gains a unique service to offer, but makes a large profit, since chiropractors can bill massage services to insurance companies at far more than they pay the massage therapist (often $80 per hour or more). The massage therapist, usually a recent massage school graduate, has a way to make a living wage and to gain a great deal of professional experience quickly.

The massage/chiropractic relationship varies greatly from state to state. In some states, like California, New York and Virginia, no restrictions exist on practice relationships massage therapists and chiropractors may enter into. In other states, some barriers do exist. Maryland and New Jersey chiropractors have all received a letter from their state boards advising them that only chiropractors can perform massage services in a chiropractic office, disrupting established relationships between chiropractors and massage therapists.

Hospitals. Hospital-based massage is experiencing a long-overdue phase of growth. Massage programs based in hospitals have existed for about twenty years, but until recently they were few in number. One writer estimated in 1993 that 50 U.S. hospitals had one or more massage therapists working in some capacity with patients. (*Massage* Magazine, March/April 1993) Three years later, in 1996, the newsletter of the Hospital-Based Massage Network estimated there were 100 to 150 hospitals using massage. That number has been swiftly rising since then.

Several different kinds of hospital-based massage programs exist. Some involve working only on staff members, giving chair massage for stress reduction. Some involve working on the general public, usually in a wellness center, in association with the hospital. Some involve working on hospital patients by physician referral as a part of the hospital's health care team. These are sometimes paid positions, sometimes volunteer. The paid positions may be employee positions or independent contractor positions. The departments most likely to employ massage therapists are pre-surgery and post-surgery, obstetrics & gynecology, ante-partum and post-partum, neonatal intensive care, oncology, physical therapy, occupational therapy, orthopedics, cardio-pulmonary, rehabilitation, out-patient pain management, speech therapy, HIV/AIDS, and fitness or wellness centers.

The acceptance of massage in hospitals is usually the result of a good working relationship between doctors or administrators at the hospital and educators or practitioners in the massage community. The exchange of information and ideas in personal and professional relationships brings about the possibility of establishing a hospital-based massage program.

Those who wish to work in hospital settings or who want additional information about this area of practice can contact:

> Hospital-Based Massage Network
> 5 Old Town Square, Suite 205
> Fort Collins, CO 80524
> (970) 407-9232, **www.hbmn.com**

The Network produces a quarterly publication (sample issue $6.00). The network lists the following individuals who may be hired as consultants on creating or joining a hospital-based massage program:

> Xerlan Geiser, Oklahoma: (918) 622-6644
> Karen Gibson, Colorado: (970) 945-3060
> Susan Hughes, California: (415) 383-7731
> Martha Brown Menard, Virginia: (804) 984-5046
> Susan Ogg-Cormier, Louisiana: (318) 989-2148
> Marianne Segal, Florida: (813) 521-5079
> Arlene Reinking-Hanf, New York: (914) 667-6980

The following massage schools are listed by HBMN as offering externships in hospital-based massage:

> Arizona: Desert Institute of the healing Arts
> California: California Pacific Medical Center

> Colorado: Boulder College of Massage Therapy
> Nevada: Ralston School of Massage
> Oregon: Oregon School of Massage
> Washington: Brenneke School of Massage

House Calls. If you talk to massage therapists about house calls, you will find that most therapists either love them or hate them. The majority seem to hate them. I personally love them.

All of the massage therapists I have talked to who hate house calls charge only a few dollars more than they charge for studio massage. Those who love house calls generally charge 40% to 50% more for a house call than for a studio massage.

Clients expect house calls to cost more. If your price is $60.00 for a studio massage, consider charging $85.00 or $90.00 for a house call. Another method of pricing is to start with your basic fee for massage; add $5.00 for carrying and setting up your table, and add 50 cents per mile for your commuting fee.

House calls have several advantages. First, there is no office rental to pay. Second, the higher fee includes compensation for your time driving to and from the client's home. It's nice to be paid for driving time, especially if your body is feeling the effects of a busy massage schedule. Third, the client usually finds it easier to fit a house call into their schedule, and may have an easier time relaxing at home than she or he would in an office environment. Finally, you get to visit lots of people's homes, many of which are quite interesting.

Certain disadvantages exist as well. First, you have little control over the environment. The phone might ring, the kids might cry, the dog might bark, the room might be cramped and it might be too hot or too cold.

Second, people dawdle more at home than they would if they came to your office. They will take a phone call, or someone will come to the door, or they will be late getting home. It is not uncommon for a one-hour massage to extend to an hour and twenty minutes. Add commuting time, and you might spend well over two hours doing a one-hour massage.

Third, carrying the massage table in and out of the car, in and out of the house, and up and down stairs can be tiring. It helps tremendously to purchase a light table and a carrying case with side handle and shoulder strap.

The real beauty of house calls comes when you can establish yourself in a community, so that you have enough business to go from one house call to another, thereby reducing your commuting time. Another advantageous situation is the couple, each of whom wants a massage at home. Some therapists do house calls exclusively, and when they become established can make a very good living.

Suggestion: Keep your oil bottle in a zip-lock plastic bag when traveling to avoid messy leaks and spills.

Office in your home. Home massage office practice has major advantages and major disadvantages. The advantages are fairly obvious—no commute and complete control over your massage environment. One disadvantage is the increased vulnerability of your home because of contact with the public. Another is that some zoning boards prohibit massage as a home occupation, fearing either that you will conduct a prostitution service in you home or that your business traffic will disturb the neighborhood.

A practitioner operating in a home office must have all the permits and licenses that would be necessary for any massage office. However, some communities will not issue a permit for a home massage practice, even though they would issue a permit to a dentist or psychotherapist in the same location.

In communities that refuse to permit massage practices in the home, some practitioners simply keep a low profile and hope they do not get caught violating the law. It is a shame that professionals are required to do this, but it results from local government officials who believe that massage equals prostitution. Consider organizing the home practitioner massage therapists in your town and trying to work through the governmental process to get the zoning restrictions changed. If you choose this option, consult your professional association for guidance and support.

Another potential obstacle to a home office is liability insurance, also called "slip and fall" insurance. Most homeowners' policies do not cover a home business. It may be possible to purchase a rider for your home business at a small additional cost, or you may have to purchase business liability insurance. See Chapter 17 for more information.

The challenge in a home office is to create a professional massage environment. This means no dogs barking, no music or television sounds wafting into the room. It also means keeping your massage environment separate from your living environment, and if possible, having a separate entrance so that clients do not have to walk through your living space to get to the massage room. If there is no separate entrance, the massage room should be the first or second room one comes to on entering the house.

If you are going to base your business in your home office, treat it as professionally as you would any other office space. Charge the going rate, have a separate phone line, and create the ideal massage room. Your efforts to create a professional atmosphere are just as important in a home office as in any other office you practice in.

Group Practice. Joining in practice with other massage therapists or other health practitioners can be a great way to share expenses, generate cross-referrals, and create a sense of community in which each member draws support from belonging to the group.

One difficulty with a group practice is that everyone shares the responsibility for making decisions that affect the group, so there is a need for regularly scheduled meetings in which everyone must participate. This can be time-consuming, and can take lots of energy, especially when it comes in the middle of a busy week.

Some group practices hire a receptionist, and others use the group members to answer the phone on a rotating basis. A receptionist is a substantial expense that has to be split among the practice members, so sharing phone duties substantially lowers the overhead. However, for a well-established practice, having a receptionist can be a luxury for the practitioners who would rather not deal with telephones and scheduling. The presence of a receptionist also designates the office off as a successful and professional operation.

Entrepreneur with associates. Similar to a group practice, several massage therapists or other kinds of therapists practice in a single location. Instead of being a group venture, however, it is the business venture of one or two who lease or own the establishment. The other practitioners either rent space or pay a percentage of the fees they charge. Payment of rent is much more common than fee-splitting.

The entrepreneur can often arrange things so that the rents paid by the other therapists cover the entire expense of the building, giving the entrepreneur a rent-free office. Generally, the entrepreneur is someone with a strong reputation in the community and good business skills.

Individual massage office. In an individual office, you have complete control over your environment and your schedule. You also have complete responsibility for getting done everything that needs to be done, including paying the rent and all other expenses. You have the most freedom and the most responsibility; the most potential for debt and the most potential for large income.

Legal relationships

Any two people who have a business relationship also have a legal relationship. These relationships can apply to people in all of the categories discussed above.

Sole proprietor. When you are the only one in charge of your business, you are the sole proprietor. In the eyes of the law, you and the business are one. Business income and personal income are pooled together for income tax purposes, as are business deductions and personal deductions.

If you work in another person's office, you will need to understand whether you are working as an employee or as an independent contractor.

Independent contractor/employee. This refers to the two different legal relationships you can have when you make an agreement to work in another person or organization's location.

The main difference to you lies in how your income taxes are handled. If you are an *employee*, your employer is responsible for paying social security tax on your earnings, and must withhold money from your pay for this purpose.

However, if you are an *independent contractor*, you are responsible for paying your own contribution to the social security system, called a self-employment tax, and nothing is withheld from your pay. This can make a significant difference to you and to the person who may have to pay social security tax on your wages.

Another difference between employees and independent contractors relates to insurance. The person you are working for will normally have business insurance that covers employees but *not* independent contractors. For this reason, some massage employers will hire only employees, so that they will be covered under the business insurance policy.

The key fact that distinguishes between your status as an independent contractor or employee is who has *control* over the way in which you perform your services. If you are in charge of setting your hours and your fees, and choosing the specifics of the treatments you give, then you are an independent contractor. If the person or organization you work for controls your hours, your prices, and your therapeutic services, then you are an employee. You are more likely to be considered and *employee* if this is the only company you work for, or if you do not use your own equipment or supplies, or if massage is the main business of the person you work for.

If your situation has elements of both employment and independent contracting, then you have to examine it to see which definition it more closely fits. If you are truly an employee but your employer treats you as an independent contractor, the IRS can charge substantial penalties to your employer for failing to withhold the appropriate taxes.

6 Career Strategies

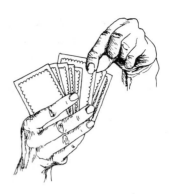

The purpose of this chapter is to help you acquire a "big picture" of your possibilities for a massage career. This chapter will examine the ways you can organize your career, from the investigation phase through the building of a practice.

The following four steps form a framework for your massage career:

1. Investigate the field — explore the field to see if you are interested in pursuing a career.

2. Go to massage school — make a choice based on geography, educational standards, or specialization.

3. Choose one of three approaches for professional growth: cautious exploration, planned transition or total immersion.

4. Create a business plan and follow it through.

1. Investigate the field

This book contains some of the flavor of a career in massage, but your own experience is the most reliable guide you can consult. Supplement the resources and ideas in this book by finding people who can complete your picture of the field. Get a professional massage. Talk to professionals about their careers. Listen to what people say about massage.

Imagine yourself in the profession. Can you? Is it easy, enjoyable and exciting, or awkward and unnatural? Ask yourself why you want to go into the field. Are your motives based in service and a desire to connect with other people, or are you thinking more about what you can get from the profession?

This is the time to be as honest with yourself as you can. Choosing massage as a career can be very rewarding for the person who wants to grow and serve. It can be frustrating for the person who does not have the determination to make a commitment and follow it through.

2. Going to massage school

Some massage schools offer evening programs so that you can go to school without changing your life. Others require full-time attendance.

If you are unsure about pursuing massage as a career, you might consider taking some adult education massage classes, or classes for the general public offered by the massage school in your area. This can be an excellent way to "get your feet wet" without risking your whole lifestyle. It may also have the advantage of making the rest of your professional education tax-deductible (See Chapter 19).

Your choice of a massage school will set the tone for your career. The items to look at in selecting a school are:

A) Consider the licensing requirements of the states you are interested in living in.

If your chosen state has a licensing requirement, you will probably find it easiest to attend a massage school in that state. The school will be aware of the licensing requirement in its home state, and will tailor its curriculum to those requirements.

If you go to an out-of-state school, be sure their training is acceptable to the authorities in your home state. The specific requirements for licensing in each state are unique. Even states with the same number of required hours of education may require study of different subjects.

B) Give yourself a strong educational foundation to support your career in the years ahead.

You might choose a 100-hour massage program, learn all you need to establish a career, and enjoy tremendous success in the field for years to come.

You might choose a 100-hour massage program, and on graduating find out that the state or locality you want to practice in has adopted a 500-hour educational requirement.

The trend among states licensing the practice of massage seems to be toward 500 or more hours as a "normal" amount of professional training. All things being equal, it would be prudent to obtain at least 500 hours.

Of course, all things are not equal, and more training costs more time and money. You will have to gather all the information you can, and use your own judgment and intuition to make the best choice for yourself.

C) Choose a school that offers the approach to massage and the specializations that most interest you.

Some schools listed in the State-by-State directory did not respond to a request for program information. However, as to those that did, their listings contain enough information to understand the emphasis, or general orientation of the school. Almost all schools will send a brochure or catalogue upon request, which will give a more complete picture. You may find it useful to compare several schools' catalogues before making your decision.

Some schools require a personal interview, and even for those that do not, it is a good idea to visit the school before making a commitment to attend. Get the flavor of the place. See how you feel there. See if you would expect to fit in comfortably with the students currently there, and with the overall atmosphere. Get the details of the financial arrangements, including the school's refund policy for those who leave early.

Massage school is very often a "different" sort of school than the ones you are used to. Since students practice on each other, a large part of your curriculum will consist of giving and receiving practice massages. Receiving massage can bring about emotional responses and unexpected changes. Receiving massage several times a week during your massage school program can accelerate the process of change.

Many massage schools recognize this and integrate this aspect of learning into the program. In fact, many schools consider a student's personal growth an essential component of the curriculum. These schools will recognize the psychologically transforming effect massage can have for clients.

Other schools emphasize "medical massage" or the "medical model." Schools with this emphasis present Swedish massage with an emphasis on medical applications. These schools tend to minimize the focus on consciousness and personal growth.

Still other schools present a focused approach to career growth, emphasizing a strong work ethic. These schools will place a greater value on building technical skills, business skills and practical experience. Their programs will be more directed toward the goal of achieving professional competence and career placement in the most efficient way.

The trend in recent years has been for degree-granting institutions, most often community colleges, to create programs to train massage therapists. These programs tend to be much less costly than private schools, but may also lack an element of personal attention, and may be narrower in focus than some private school programs.

Think about these issues, but also let your intuition guide you to the best school for your needs. Going to massage school can be a very special and life-changing experience. Choose with your mind and your heart, and have a great time.

3. Choose your approach:
permanent part-time, cautious exploration, planned transition or total immersion

Your massage career will take some time to grow. Your skills as a therapist will mature for years after you finish massage school. Your reputation in the community will likewise take time to build. It is best to have a plan that will allow you to integrate that period of career growth into the context of your life.

Plan A: Permanent Part-Time

Massage is a career that lends itself well to part-time practice, and a great many massage therapists—possibly more than half—choose to keep their career permanently part-time.

In 1999, ABMP conducted a survey of its members and found that about half of those surveyed had a second, non-massage job. In 2000, AMTA did a survey of its members and found that more than half of the respondents practiced massage part-time. A 1999 job analysis conducted by the National Certification Board found that 65% of massage practitioners earned $20,000.00 per year or less.

Full-time massage work can be physically demanding. Repetitive strain injuries can be a problem, and giving out your energy all day can be depleting. While some practitioners can give six or seven massages per day with no ill effects, others know that they must stop after three or four massages per day in order to stay healthy.

If you can acquire either a house-call practice or an office practice with low overhead costs, a part-time massage practice can support you, and can give you the freedom to pursue your other interests as well. For parents of small children, those with other part-time jobs, aspiring writers, dancers, actors, and people in a variety of other work situations, a part-time massage career can make a lot of sense.

Plan B: Cautious Exploration

This is a low-risk alternative. The idea is to make no significant changes in your current lifestyle, but integrate massage education and exploration of massage practice into your life.

You can do this by going to a massage school that has evening or weekend classes, and using your after-hours time to experiment with doing massage profession-ally. You can charge for your services or not, as you see fit. (In states that require a license, you can charge only after licensure) The idea is to gain experience, and to learn whether massage is a field you want to put some real energy into.

After exploring the field in this way, you will be in a position to know whether it is something you enjoy and can commit to pursuing for a living. At this point, you can move to Plan C or Plan D, or make an informed choice to remain a part-time massage practitioner.

Plan C: Planned Transition

This is for those who are committed to pursuing a career in massage, yet want to do it in a way that creates a minimum of disruption in their lives. It is a plan that is particularly well suited to teachers, part-time and flex-time workers, and others with substantial free time to pursue a massage career.

A teacher might build her massage practice after working hours. When it reaches a good level, she can switch to substitute teaching. When the practice will sup-port her fully, she can quit teaching and rely fully on massage. Similarly, a waiter or waitress can cut back on hours as the massage practice grows, eventually giving up waiting tables completely.

In order to make this option work, you will need to be committed. Making a living at your "day job" can take a lot out of you, yet you need to have the energy and drive to become established in your new field during your after-hours time. In the next chapter, you will read about the many marketing techniques available to you. Make sure you will have the energy to keep your current job and also apply yourself to building a massage practice. The transition may take several years, so be sure you are prepared.

Plan D: Total Immersion

This is a sink-or-swim approach in which you quit your job, rely on whatever financial support you have, and focus 100 percent on establishing yourself as a professional massage therapist. This option requires some means of financial inde-pendence—either a bankroll, a generous spouse or benefactor, or a talent at living without much money.

Most marketing techniques require you to have an office setting for the practice of massage. To pursue Total Immersion, you should have an office. This will of course add a significant expense for which you must be prepared. Give some thought to the economics of the situation, and decide whether you could essentially go without any income for a year. There is a good chance that your first year will be a very lean one, and that your second may not be a great deal better.

Some prefer this approach because it forces the person to do everything possible to make a success of their massage career. To pursue this option requires a clear sense of commitment, and also an understanding of the balance between self-promotion and patience. You should also be prepared for some long, lonely days.

This option will be easier for the individual who has lots of contacts and a strong local reputation. Such a person will have the best chance of establishing a practice relatively quickly. It is not advisable for someone who is new in the community.

4. Create a Business Plan and Follow it Through

A business plan is like a blueprint. You can build without one, but having one is likely to make your task easier and your result better.

The specifics for creating a business plan, and a form you can use to create your own, are provided in the next chapter.

7 Marketing Yourself as a Massage Therapist

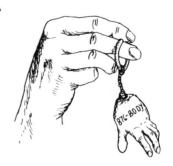

This topic mystifies more massage therapists and bodyworkers than any other. Books, marketing kits, seminars, instructional videos, and other items are on the market to teach you how to acquire a following in your chosen profession.

This guide will give you the benefit of my experiences, as well as those of many other therapists I have interviewed, as to principles and techniques you can use to market your professional services. Before examining the specific techniques you can use, however, there are a few questions you should ask yourself.

1. Preliminary questions

Are You Ready?

Do you feel your massage is worth $60.00 per hour (or whatever is the going rate in your area)?

How would you feel about having a strong clientele in the town you are now living in? Are you prepared to call this place home?

Imagine introducing yourself to a variety of people in your town. You tell them you are a massage therapist. How does that feel to you?

The above questions touch on the chief reasons that massage practitioners, even after they have gone to massage school, are reluctant to make a commitment to building a massage practice. If you are not ready to present yourself to the public as a professional deserving their time and money, take the time to grow before making a sincere effort at professional marketing.

That growth may mean gaining new professional skills. It may mean confronting issues of self-image or self-esteem. It may mean learning to be comfortable relating to a broad variety of people. Your growth on all these levels will continue for a long time, well into your professional career. You do not need to be perfect to succeed as a massage therapist — just ready.

How Long Do You Expect This To Take?

How much of a hurry are you in? Are you expecting to throw yourself into a marketing campaign for six months and then have a thriving practice? Are you willing to spend two years or longer creating a practice for yourself? If you are looking for the six-month version, you will probably be disappointed in the results. These things take time.

Consider advertising, for example. One study has shown that the average consumer will notice your ad only one out of three times you run it, and that the same consumer has to *see* your ad nine times before she is ready to purchase the advertised goods or services. Therefore, you may need to run an ad 27 times to have your client actually come in for a massage.

Word of mouth can be similarly time-consuming. A client coming to me for the first time told me that a friend had been urging him to try my massage for *two years.* Two years is an exceptionally long delay in accepting a referral, but I include this example to give you the idea that some aspects of marketing simply cannot be rushed. Successful marketing involves a blend of *commitment* and *patience.*

What's your plan?

Make a plan for your career—what your practice will be like in six months, one year, two years, three years, five years. Use the form below or create your own planning form.

All sources of professional business guidance will tell you, as a business person, that a business plan is an essential part of your growth process. Advantages of a business plan are:

- It helps you know where you want your career to go;

- It helps you keep track of your progress toward your goals;

- It helps you organize your efforts toward meeting your goals;

- It gives you the clarity to express your goals to others so that they will help you find opportunities.

At the same time, it is important to stay flexible and be quite willing to depart from the plan. In fact, every few months or so, you may want to completely rewrite your plan to reflect what you have learned or how your goals have changed.

For example, let's say you make a business plan that emphasizes house calls in an affluent suburb. It includes working at a health spa in that area part-time and using advertising in a community newspaper to try to break into the house call market. Midway through this project, you meet a cardiologist who offers you an office in his group practice. This is a terrific opportunity that you had not even realized was possible.

Do you pass up the cardiologist because you are in the middle of a different plan? Of course not. You change your business plan. At the same time, it was important to have the business plan even though you changed it; you might never have met the cardiologist.

When you make your plans for six months, one year, two years, three years and five years from now, be as detailed and specific as you can. Include your best predictions about all of the following:

- Location for doing massage

- Target clients

- Type of work you want to be doing

- How clients will learn about you

- Number of clients you want or expect to have

- Workshops, professional trainings and meetings to attend

- Advertising and other promotional plans

- Expenses you are likely to incur

Mark on the top of each plan the date you write it, and the target date for the goals you create. Take your group of plans out every few months and see how things are going. Revise your business plan at least once a year.

Sample Business Plan

On page 45 is a sample business plan for Mary Jones. Mary has been out of massage school one year, and is seeing 8 to 12 clients per week. Some of these are house calls, and some are in a resort 15 miles from her home. She has a part-time job doing cleaning work to supplement her income.

Create Your Business Plan

Use the form on page 46 as a sample to create your business plan. If you feel the form does not suit your particular needs, by all means modify it to take into account the planning you need to do.

You will be creating more business plans as time goes by, so you may want to create a form that suits you and make a few copies of it. Keep your business plans in a folder and keep the folder with your other business materials, such as business receipts, client records, and professional books.

2. Nuts and Bolts of Marketing for Massage and Bodywork

You have examined your readiness for success, your expectations about your career path, and your plans for making your goals take shape. You now have an understanding of the larger picture that your marketing efforts will fit into.

Before discussing the specific marketing techniques you might use, there is one broad principle to consider:

Person-to-person contact is the most effective.

Because massage is a personal service, and because it is relatively expensive, people want to have a good idea that they are going to like both the person and the person's treatment before they come in for a massage. It is much harder to convey this level of confidence with impersonal contact, such as advertising, than it is with person-to-person contact.

To overcome people's natural shyness and resistance to the idea of nudity and being touched, you need to let people know enough about you to trust you, and enough about your work to have confidence in it.

Keep this in mind as you consider the following techniques you can use to promote your professional services.

MARY JONES' BUSINESS PLAN   May 7, 2004

Goals:

> To increase clientele to 25 per week
> To keep commuting distances to a minimum
> To emphasize sports massage in my practice

Target clientele:

> Amateur and professional athletes
> Local residents
> Professionals and their spouses

Possible new locations to work in:

> Hospital wellness center
> Sports injury clinic
> Country club

Means of reaching new clients:

> Ads or feature story in country club newsletter
> Person-to-person contact with physicians and attorneys in the area
> Contacts with personal fitness trainers and athletic trainers in the area
> Ads or feature story in local circulation newspaper

Six month goals:

Acquire a local office at a low cost where I can see clients; meet at least four personal fitness trainers or athletic trainers and give them complimentary demonstration massages; meet at least four doctors or lawyers in the area and introduce them to myself and my work.

One year goals:

Take advanced trainings in neuromuscular therapy and sports massage techniques; expand contacts with personal fitness trainers and athletic trainers; expand athletic clientele to at least 12 per week; obtain a quality office environment where I can create the ideal setting for sports and rehabilitative massage as well as doing relaxation massage.

Two year goals:

Have firmly established sports/rehabilitative massage office, seeing 20 clients per week. Supplement practice with occasional house calls for professional clientele. Work with world-class athletes in preparation for competitive events.

Three year goals:

Travel with athletes to sporting events, hire other sports massage therapists to work in my clinic when I am away.

Five year goals:

Offer sports massage trainings; employ at least one full-time massage therapist in my clinic; work exclusively with competitive athletes.

SAMPLE BUSINESS PLAN   date _____

Items to consider:
      Location for doing massage
      Target clients
      Type of work I want to be doing
      How clients will learn about me
      Number of clients I will have
      Current fee structure
      Workshops, professional trainings and meetings
      Advertising and other promotional plans
      Expenses I am likely to incur

Goals:

Target clientele:

Possible locations to work in:

Means of reaching target clientele:

Six month goals:

One year goals:

Two year goals:

Three year goals:

Five year goals:

A. Person-to-person Marketing Techniques

All professions depend chiefly on referrals, or word-of-mouth, and massage is no exception. A certain amount of word-of-mouth marketing happens naturally. If you give one client a great massage, she naturally wants to tell her friends, and some of them may be curious enough to try you out sooner or later.

The art of marketing yourself, however, lies in accelerating this process as much as possible. The main task to accomplish in that regard is to become widely known and accepted within as many groups as possible in your community.

The following are some proven methods for making people familiar with you and comfortable with you, and interested in trying your therapy:

1. Demonstration/lecture at health clubs, professional groups and social groups

These can be a very effective way to become known and accepted, and to increase your clientele. The idea is to present a short speech on the nature of massage, the benefits it can have, and what is to be expected during a session. This is followed up by a brief demonstration on a volunteer.

If you are doing it in a place where a massage room is available, such as a health club, you might consider following it up with an offer to do a ten-minute foot massage on anyone who is curious.

A presentation of this sort accomplishes many marketing goals all at once. As you establish rapport with the group, you become known, familiar and accepted. They learn the theory of massage and how it can help them, and they gain an understanding of the process and what to expect. Then, after your demonstration, they see and hear from your client how wonderful a person feels after one of your treatments.

For someone who is curious about massage but fearful about nudity or about being touched by a stranger, the lecture/demonstration is perhaps the only marketing tool that will give that person the confidence to try a massage. By creating confidence in yourself, taking the mystery out of the massage process, and giving the person a clear idea of what she has to gain by having a massage, you can effectively break down some strong barriers to using your services.

One therapist gave several lecture/demonstrations at her health club, a women-only club. She made such an impression that practically each time she went into the club for a workout after that, one or more members came up to her asking to schedule a massage appointment.

Other locations for this type of presentation are civic, professional and social groups. Ask your friends and clients about any groups they are members of, such as the Rotary, local women's club, yoga group, exercise class, or toastmasters. These groups are often glad to have outside speakers, and the fact that one of their members recommends you will be an advantage.

Many people have a great fear of public speaking, and will feel it is impossible to do a lecture/demonstration in front of a group. If you can't, you can't. However, if you can't you are missing out on one of the most effective and successful marketing opportunities you can use. Remember that the group you speak to will be there because they are interested in you and in massage. They are on your side and they want to like you. Prepare in advance what you are going to say and do, and just be yourself.

A group that can help you overcome your fear of public speaking is Toastmasters International. They have regional meetings everywhere, usually early in the morning, and each participant gives short talks and receives constructive criticism. You can find your local groups at **www.toastmasters.org**, by calling Toastmasters at (949) 858-8255 or writing to P.O. Box 9052, Mission Viejo, CA 92690.

2. Free introductory massages for selected individuals

Anyone who is likely to be the source of repeated referrals should be cultivated as a contact. Such people are psychotherapists, medical doctors, chiropractors, acupuncturists, wholistic practitioners of all sorts, team coaches and sports trainers, dancing teachers, real estate agents, other massage therapists and bodyworkers, and people who are well-known and well-respected members of the community.

Any of these people, who are in a position of trust with their friends, neighbors, clients, and patients, will generally be listened to by those they know. Therefore, once they believe in you and your work, they can be a good source of referrals.

You may wish to seek out these people and try to introduce yourself, or you may wait until you meet someone in the natural course of events. Either way, offering a complimentary massage can be an excellent way of introducing that person to you and your work. Once they know you and your work from their own experience, they will be more willing to refer clients to you.

3. Gift Certificates as a mass marketing tool

Consider using gift certificates creatively as a promotional tool. Some ways to do so are:

- give out gift certificates with your business card

- give gift certificates to charities and fund raisers to use as prizes

- give gift certificates to a local radio station to be given away to callers

Even though you may give out a large number of gift certificates, most will probably not be redeemed. You may find that only about one in five certificates is actually used. The recipients who do use the certificates are interested in becoming massage clients, and a significant percentage of these are likely to become repeat customers.

Hopefully, at least ten percent of the people who redeem your gift certificates will become repeat clients. If so, you will have acquired a very valuable practice boost for no cost to yourself, and the publicity generated by your promotion will have boosted your reputation and good will in the community. Consider the following true story about using gift certificates as a marketing tool:

> In 1999, I did a small mailing to CPAs at tax time, empathizing with their stress and enclosing a gift certificate for massage. Of the ten CPAs I mailed to, only two responded. Only one actually made an appointment, and, after several cancellations and reschedulings in a

row, I was about ready to give up on her. However, after her massage, she made regular appointments for herself and her husband through the end of that year, then referred her neighbors, both of whom come every week for massage ... and then *they* referred some folks ... short version of the story is that one give away ended up providing about ⅔ of my income that year! Since that time I have formed a relationship with a local high end real estate agent. I have given her probably a hundred or more certificates to give to her clients as closing (or other) gifts, and she continues to send me a small but steady flow of folks who like and can afford massage.

4. Discounts to clients for referrals

One therapist gives a ten-dollar discount on the next massage to any client who refers another client. She believes this fosters referrals, as it gives clients a motivation to spread the word about massage.

In a similar vein, one therapist offers a "buy two gift certificates, get your massage free" promotion. I have not tried either approach. My hunch is that clients have a natural desire to tell their friends and neighbors when they like you and your service. However, it is possible that a financial incentive would give them more of a reason to do so. Those of you who do try it, let me know your experiences.

5. Join the local Chamber of Commerce

Consider joining the Chamber of Commerce in your community. These are local business people who are getting together to share matters of common concern. You are such a person, and there is no reason you should not be involved in such a group.

The contacts you make in a group like this will be valuable for your career, since these people know many members of the community. The more you become known and accepted as a "normal" business person, the less resistance people will have to the idea of coming to you for a massage.

6. Do on-site promotional massages

This means going where the people are and working either for free or for a small amount, doing brief treatments.

You can rent a booth at a health fair, craft fair, workshop center or convention and offer five or ten minute massages. You can arrange in advance to set up at the end of a sporting event, or at a shopping center during busy times. If your office is on a busy street, consider doing chair massage on a volunteer in front of your building to draw attention to you and your practice.

The exposure you get from such activities may bring you clients immediately, and also may have a long-term benefit in getting you known in the local community.

7. Join as many organizations as you comfortably can

The goal is to meet large numbers of people and to become known. Don't join organizations just to accomplish a marketing goal. You won't have fun, and you may seem pushy. Join organizations you are interested in, but don't be shy about telling people what you do, and never get caught without your business card handy to give out to an interested person.

B. Person-To-Paper Contact

There are some people who are your potential clients, whom you cannot reach in person or through a personal recommendation. Reaching them through the printed word may be your only means of making contact.

Advertising is a quick way to reach large numbers of people. The difficult aspects of using advertising effectively are *avoiding* the people you do *not* want to find you, and making a persuasive impression on the people you do want to find you.

Advertising has the disadvantage of being impersonal contact. It will let people know who you are and where you are and perhaps what you offer. However, it will not tell them that they will like you, that they can trust you, that you have a great touch and tremendous skills, or that they will feel much better after one of your treatments.

Therefore, advertising will most effectively reach those clients who are already familiar with massage but do not currently have a massage therapist whom they go to. This is a relatively small percentage of the general population. However, it takes only one new regular client to make any advertisement worth its cost.

The biggest disadvantage of advertising is that it opens you to sexually-oriented massage clients. A great many men have had sexual experiences that were billed as "massage." In many areas of the United States today, it is easier to find sexual massage than it is to find legitimate massage. Though great progress has been made in legitimizing the profession in recent years, confusion persists.

Doing any general advertising virtually guarantees that you will be confronted by at least some men calling to find out if they can get sexual services from you. Every massage therapist I know finds this to be draining, degrading and infuriating. However, at this point in the history of massage, it is an unavoidable side-effect of using advertising as a tool to build your practice.

Suggestion: In any person-to-paper advertising you do, consider including a photo of yourself. This will do several things. First, it will help dispel any idea that you are offering sexual massage. Second, it will convey some information about you—it is the best substitute available for personal contact. Finally, it is an eye-catcher. In a print medium, a photo tends to draw attention, and it can help clients see an ad they might otherwise miss.

1. Flyers and Business cards

Flyers and business cards are best used after you have made person-to-person contact, to further explain your work or to serve as a reminder about you and your services.

Most therapists who have tried leaving flyers for the general public and posting business cards in places like health food stores and supermarkets find that the results are poor. You may find that your business cards mainly reach the other therapists who see your card when they post theirs.

One flyer that worked was the one used by Wes Boyce in southern California. That is reproduced on the following page. Wes used this flyer as part of his plan to become established quickly from the ground up. This flyer brought him 100 clients within seven months, and at that point he canceled the promotion. His promotion had raised $1,000 for Meals On Wheels.

He did not make much money directly from these massages, although some clients tipped him, and a few became paying customers. However, he was able to get a lot of practical experience in a short time, and also generated a great deal of public awareness about himself and his work.

2. Direct mail

This refers to those packets of ads and coupons we all get in the mail from time to time. Some massage therapists have used these very effectively to build their practices.

These direct mailings generally go to 10,000 homes at a time. The cost to have your ad or coupon included will usually be a few hundred dollars. This may sound like a lot of money, but consider that one weekly client will repay the entire cost of the promotion in two to three months.

Two useful approaches to direct mail are to use it when you open a new office, and to use it at holiday times to advertise gift certificates. It can also be used as a major promotion to boost an existing practice.

To get in touch with direct mail companies, look in the mailers for their phone number and address, or get the Business-to-Business Yellow Pages if there is one for your area. (available free from your local phone company's business office) Look in the listing for "Marketing Programs and Services."

The direct mail sales person will help you design your promotion. Most such promotions include a special offer or coupon, such as an introductory massage for new clients at a reduced price.

3. Yellow Pages

All of the massage therapists I interviewed who have yellow pages listings agreed that the listing more than paid for itself with the business it generated. However, they also agreed that the quality of calls that came from the listing was poor. A large percentage of these calls are from men seeking sex, and a significant amount of time and energy is taken in screening these calls.

Some localities have two listings in the yellow pages — one for massage, and one for massage therapists. The idea behind the distinction is to tip off the sex-seekers that those listed as massage therapists are legitimate. Unfortunately, the sex clients either don't see the distinction, or figure that you're really offering sex and you put the listing under "massage therapist" to fool the police. If your listing has the word "massage" in it, you can count on sex calls.

You can help create the image you want by carefully selecting the name and information you present in the yellow pages. One practical option is to choose a

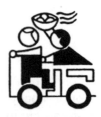

business name at the beginning of the alphabet, since you will get more calls if you are listed first.

Another practical option is to choose a name like "wholistic health center" to attract only legitimate callers. The business name you choose for your yellow pages listing need not be the same as the one on your business cards or bank account. The people who publish the yellow pages will accept most any business name you supply.

Yellow pages ads are expensive. A basic listing with no more than name and phone number will cost around $20 per month. A small block ad with some basic information can cost around $60 per month. Larger ads can cost a great deal more. This will be more economical for a group practice than for an individual.

Getting into the yellow pages requires some advance planning. In my area, the deadline for new orders is in March, and new books are distributed in July. If you are opening a new office, or changing locations, you may want to coordinate your move with the schedule of the yellow pages publisher to minimize the disruption in your practice.

4. Newspaper coverage of you and your practice

One way to become better known is to have a local newspaper reporter write an article about you, about massage, and about any particular aspect of you or your work that is unique or interesting.

Make contact with a reporter for your local newspaper, and give her or him a massage. Discuss anything about yourself or your work or training that may be of interest, and let the reporter decide what angle might serve as the basis for a story.

After the story appears in the paper, frame it and put it on your office wall. Your clients will be gently reminded that you are a special person worthy of respect.

5. Placing ads in newspapers

Many successful massage therapists never advertised in newspapers and never will. Others have found newspaper advertising to be a way to shorten the time needed to build a practice to a self-supporting level. Others have advertised and been so frustrated by the clients who responded that they have burned out on massage as a profession. The following information about newspaper advertising should help you make the most of newspaper advertising.

Two types of newspaper ads — classifieds, display ads

Two types of massage ads are available in newspapers — display ads and business classified ads. Display ads (also called block ads) appear in the body of the paper, with the news and features articles, and therefore are seen by more readers than business classifieds. Display ads are larger and substantially more expensive than business classifieds. Display ads make sense in small-circulation newspapers, when you are trying to break into a new market. In larger newspapers, massage ads almost always run in the business classifieds.

Business classifieds

Business classifieds is a separate section of the classifieds, devoted to business services such as painting, carpentry, cleaning and hauling. While these ads are much cheaper than display ads, they cost a great deal more than a normal classified ad.

The response to advertising in the business classifieds tends to be immediate. If the response to your classified ad is going to be good, you will know within the first few days. Start with a short run for your ad, so that if the response is not good, you have the opportunity to try a different newspaper.

Generally speaking, business classified advertising is cost-effective for massage therapists. In other words, you will generally make more money as a result of placing the ad than you spend on the ad. The other question, however, is how much grief you will have to put up with in the process.

Display advertising

Display advertising is quite different from business classified advertising. Someone looking up massage in a business classified is ready for a massage — today, if possible. Someone just reading the news or features, who sees your display ad in the newspaper, was not thinking about massage until she saw your ad. She may not be ready for massage for quite a while.

In fact, it may take many exposures to your ad before this person feels you are sufficiently "familiar" to give you a try. After seeing your ad a few times, she will begin to get the idea that you are not just a passing fad, but a true fixture in the community.

The more times a person sees your ad, the more familiar and accepted your name will be to that person. After five to ten exposures to your ad, the person may be sufficiently comfortable with your print image that she would consider trying a massage. The more nervous the person is about massage, the longer it may take for her to begin to feel comfortable about you by repeatedly seeing you ad.

Therefore, display advertising is generally best used in small circulation newspapers, where you have a particular desire to break into a new market that you feel has a good potential for your practice. Choose your newspaper and plan to place your ad many times. Keep your ad the same each time you run it, so that the "familiarity" factor works best. Use a picture of yourself in the ad — this will be an eye-catcher, will help the person feel she knows you and will give more of a sense that you can be trusted.

Types of Newspapers

Many types of newspapers exist, and you can use each differently in aid of your marketing goals. The different types of newspapers are general circulation dailies, special interest newspapers (usually weekly or monthly), and local or regional papers (usually weekly).

General circulation newspapers

These are the daily newspapers read by the general population. The general circulation newspaper I advertised in is the Asbury Park Press, which serves a region within about a 25-mile radius of Asbury Park, New Jersey. Their business classified directory includes a listing for massage, and at the top of the massage listing each day is the following notice:

> ATTENTION ADVERTISERS: The only copy permitted in a massage ad is: name, address, phone number, rates & hours. The only exception is a licensed spa listing their facilities (sauna, steam room, etc.)
>
> The terminology 'Professional or Licensed' can be used if customer sends copy of certificate from a school of massage prior to ad running.
>
> Ads must be paid in advance.

This notice appeared for the first time shortly after the same newspaper ran a story about a prostitution ring that had operated through the massage classifieds. The management placed the notice at the top of the massage listing in an attempt to prevent the use of its massage ads for prostitution.

I advertised in this listing immediately before and immediately after the story about the prostitution ring operating through the massage classifieds. Despite the notice at the top of the listing, and despite the story in the same newspaper about prostitution arrests, roughly ninety percent of the calls I received from this ad were men looking for sexual massage. This percentage did not seem to change as a result of the prostitution story or as a result of putting the notice at the top of the massage listing.

Phone calls at 7:00 A.M. and 11:45 P.M. in response to my ad were not uncommon. I chose to answer my own phone, although some therapists who advertise leave the answering machine on and selectively return calls. I found that, in general, people calling at unusual times were looking for unusual massage services. My first name (Martin) indicated I was a man, and my ad apparently attracted a great many gay or bisexual callers. Calls for sexual massage dropped off dramatically after the first week.

Most of the clients looking for sex had the sense to stop trying when I explained in no uncertain terms that my massage was completely legitimate and did not include any sexual contact. A few, however, apparently regarded that as a challenge and made appointments anyway.

These men would wait until the end of their massage, or in some cases until their second or third massage, to verbally or non-verbally make their wishes known. This was quite a growth experience for me, as I had to learn how to deal with my own feelings of anger and resentment in such a situation.

My growth brought me to a point where I could comfortably take charge of the situation. I learned to discuss any suspect signs of arousal immediately, carefully watch the client's attitude about the subject, and terminate the massage immediately if the client was being inappropriate. Once I realized that I had control of the situation, my emotional response lessened dramatically.

The several regular clients I acquired through this advertising exposure are lovely people whom I appreciate very much as clients, and who never would have found me without the ad. The total expense for the ads I ran was about $250 over a period of several weeks. Despite the irritation factor, on the whole it was well worth doing.

Special interest newspapers

There may be newspapers for special interest groups in your area that can be good sources of massage clients. Such papers include:

- New age or holistically oriented newspapers

- Religious or community oriented newspapers

- Homeowners' association newsletters

- In-house newspapers for corporations

- In-house newspapers for institutions such as retirement communities and hospitals

- Magazines or newsletters targeted to women, mothers, families, athletes, or other groups

- Real estate mailings sent out by local agents

The cost involved is usually low, and the response level probably will also be low. However, such exposure can be useful in gaining entry into a new market. I placed small ads in two local newspapers targeted to the Jewish community in my area. These generated enough new business to at least pay for the ads, and also served to gain some name recognition.

If there is a corporate headquarters or large corporate office near your practice consider advertising in their in-house corporate newspaper. This can be a good source of clients who can afford your services and are near your office on a daily basis.

Local and regional newspapers

Many communities have small local papers, which are published once or twice a week. These are sometimes mailed to all households in the community at no charge. These papers often have a "business classified" section similar to the one in general circulation newspapers.

Before advertising in one of these, get the flavor of the other ads in the paper. If a massage ad would seem distinctly out of place in comparison to the other types of ads that are currently running, it may not be a good idea to place your ad in that paper.

As with special interest newspapers, the circulation of local papers will be small, as will be the cost to advertise. One advantage is that you can be sure that any potential clients who see this ad will be close to you and able to conveniently reach your office.

C. Broadcast Media

Radio, broadcast television, and direct access cable television are also possibilities for massage marketing. Generally speaking, the cost of commercial advertisements on radio and television is too great for an individual massage practice.

Direct access cable, however, can provide opportunities for exposure. A pair of chiropractors in my area produced a multi-part feature on wholistic health modalities that was broadcast on direct access cable. One segment was on massage, and the therapist they chose for that segment received significant exposure at no expense to her.

D. Internet Marketing Opportunities

The Internet, at least at the present, will not provide a majority of your massage referrals, but it can provide your practice a boost if done properly.

How successful is Internet marketing? There's an old saying "The more things change, the more they remain the same." With the Internet, as with pre-Internet massage marketing, there are some success stories and some flops, and many in-betweens.

One massage therapist in Southern California has a successful website at **www.MassageDirect.com**. She has actively promoted the website and has also listed her practice with several referral websites (referral websites are discussed below). She reports receiving several clients per month from the Internet. A practitioner in Denver has a website which is listed with many search engines, yet he has received only one Internet client in six months. Another practitioner has entirely given up on Internet referrals because most of the clients who found her from the Internet were seeking sexual massage, and most of the appointments made were not kept.

A husband and wife who are both bodyworkers in Rutland, Vermont have a website, and although they are listed on many search engines, their community is so sparsely populated that the Internet does not provide them with client referrals. However, their website has proven to be a good marketing tool in other ways; when a new client calls, after giving some preliminary information, they can refer the person to the website for further information and details. They believe this gives them an edge over other local practitioners who do not have a website. In addition, they have sold gift certificates to out-of-town people who want to give gift certificates to their central Vermont friends and relatives.

As far as I know, no one supports a massage practice exclusively with Internet referrals (at least not yet). How successful your site becomes will depend partly on where you live, partly on how well you produce your site, and partly on the skills and services you have to offer to the public.

There are two basic strategies for using the Internet to market your practice. One is self-promotion and the other is getting listed on sites that promote your practice for you. Following are some of the basics for each approach.

Strategy #1—Make a website and promote it. If you have ever created a website, you know it is not as intimidating as a novice might think. Free software is available on the Internet that you can use to create websites. Even Microsoft Word can be used to create a basic web page.

If you have never made a website, you may think of it as an impossible challenge. Some people just don't get along with computers. If that describes you, then find someone who is computer-savvy to make a website for you. It's not that big a job for someone who knows how to do it—you can hire someone to make your website, or you may even find someone willing to trade massage for website creation services.

Designing your website

Your website should reflect who you are and what services you offer. Design it the way you would design your massage room—think about how the visitor will feel at your site and choose words and images that reflect the best about you and your work. Your website should also "sell" you to potential clients; it should convince them that you have something valuable or unique to offer them, and it should give them a sense of personal connection with you and a basis for trusting you.

One crucial element of a successful website is a good quality photograph of yourself. The old saying "a picture is worth a thousand words" has some truth in it. Don't you get a "feeling" about a person when you see their photograph? With a service as personal as massage, it is crucial that a potential client has a reason to trust you and feel comfortable with you, and putting your photograph on the site goes a long way to starting that personal relationship.

Your site should also act like a good résumé does; it should get across your strengths and talents so the potential customer feels interested about trying your work. Put your best foot forward when you describe yourself. Be positive and self-confident without misrepresenting yourself or your work.

Finally, make sure your site is attractive and easy to use. If you are not talented in this way, invest a little money in a graphics person who can give your site an appealing overall look and a functional design. A site that is beautiful and well-organized will make the visitor feel comfortable and attracted to you and your work.

For a good sample practitioner website, visit **www.MassageVermont.com**. When I visited this site, it opened with a professional-quality photograph of the two practitioners that own the site, and their names, phone number, address, and certifications. Following that were their fee schedule displayed in a very easy-to-follow format, and a brief bio of each of them. Next came a brief description of the types of work they do and the benefits of the work, accompanied by the logos of all the professional organizations they belong to. Finally, there was a brief "Q & A" section.

Your website's "address"

Most "Internet Service Providers" offer a free website as part of their service. However, I suggest you not have your website on their server, but instead create a "domain name" that becomes your permanent Internet identity. You may think the good ones are all gone, but think again—if you invent an unusual name, it may still be available. For example, when I was writing this chapter in April, 2002, the domain name "mygreathands.com" was still available! You can also choose your own name or a variation of your name as your domain name.

A domain name that has some relation to you or your practice will be easier to remember and publicize. In addition, the name is yours forever, and you can take it with you when you move or change Internet Service Providers. This allows you to build "brand name" recognition over a period of years.

The owner of a domain name must pay an annual fee to register the name. Shop on the Internet for the best price—you can find domain name registration services for as little as $15.00 per year. Likewise, shop around for a company that will "host" your site on their server. You can purchase this service as cheaply as $10.00 per month or less.

Promoting your website

Now that you have put the time and energy (or money) into creating your website, you want people to come and visit. There are two ways of promoting your website on the Internet—through search engines, and through links. The links that will most directly help you promote your professional website are "referral" sites discussed below.

Search engines, such as google.com (my favorite), altavista.com, lycos.com, and many others, actually gather and compile as much of the Internet as they possibly can, and then search their compilation upon request by visitors.

Once you create your website, you can manually submit it to search engines, or use services (some are free, some charge a fee) that submit your site to multiple search engines. Alternatively, you can just wait for the search engines to find you, since all of them routinely "sweep" the Internet to update their compilations.

When you design your website, investigate how to choose the "meta-tags" that describe your website. These are words that are invisible to the users of your site, but are read by the computers accessing your site. Some search engines use these words to rank your site's usefulness to the users doing a search. Choose key words for your meta-tags that people would use in searching for you, such as the type of work you do or your location. If your meta-tags match the terms used in a search request, the search engine will place your site at the top of the list of results for that particular search.

You can also seek out local websites, such as city websites and local directory websites. These sites focus strictly on what is available in your local or regional area, so any visitors to these sites are there because they are interested in your location. These sites have less traffic than sites of national interest, but may provide you with better results, since all the visitors to a local area website are potential clients for your practice.

Strategy #2—Join referral websites. A number of websites provide searchable "directories" of massage practitioners. The owners of these websites may do publicity or advertising to attract potential clients to their websites. Alternatively, they may have a domain name that a potential client might "guess" at and visit on a hunch, such as "iwantamassage.com"

Someone seeking a massage practitioner visits the website and searches the site's database for a massage practitioner in a particular location. They are then provided with a list of all the practitioners in that location who have signed up with the website. It is then up to the person seeking massage to reach out and contact the practitioner.

Most of these referral websites are fairly new, so they don't have well-established track records. These are the referral websites I was able to locate by searching on the Internet. Next to each web address is the cost to a practitioner for listing with that site.

www.danke.com/Orthodoc/mtlisting.html	free
www.health-alt.com	free
www.holistic.com	free
www.iwantamassage.com	free (insurance required)
www.MassageResource.com	free
www.qwl.com/mtwc	free
www.FitnessFinderUSA.com	$29.95 to $49.95 per year
www.MassageDirect.com	$25.00 per year
www.MassageReferral.com	$25.00 per year
www.MassageNetwork.com	$20.00 per year
www.MassageOutpost.com	$75.00 per year
www.abmp.com	members only
www.amta.org	members only
www.imagroup.com	members only
www.NCBTMB.com	NCE certified only

Some of the sites listed as "free" may offer a basic listing (name, address, phone) at no charge, but then offer to sell you a "complete" listing consisting of your practice details and fees. Some of the sites will include a link to your personal website and others will not.

The Internet, like the Yellow Pages, is used by both legitimate clients and clients seeking sexual massage. In particular, I have heard that **www.iwantamassage.com** has been used by clients seeking sexual massage. As with any massage advertising, you must be prepared for the occasional errant caller who must be re-directed.

Will Internet marketing pay for itself?

As you can see, Internet marketing is not expensive. You can create your website for no cost if you know your way around computers and software, or you can have someone create a site at a modest cost. The only out-of-pocket expense I had when I created **www.CareerAtYourFingertips.com** was $40.00 for the software (called "WS-ftp") needed to communicate between my computer and the computer hosting my website.

At $15.00 per year for domain name registration and $10.00 per month for hosting services, you can have a basic web presence for $135.00 per year. You could subscribe to practically all of the referral services listed above and still have a total Internet budget of about $250.00 per year. Keep in mind that since this is a business expense, it is tax-deductible, so you will receive a tax credit worth about 30% of this amount when you do your income taxes the following April 15th (see page 157).

The Internet is still growing, and will continue to grow in importance for a number of years. At this time, it may be a "judgment call" whether an Internet presence is cost-effective for a massage or bodywork practice. However, just being able to refer potential clients to your website for "further information" is a big plus in credibility and prestige. In a few years, I suspect that practitioners without websites—even in this "high-touch" profession—may be looked on as not being serious about their careers.

Even if you are already an established practitioner, creating a website for your practice will help you continue to thrive by attracting new clients to your practice. As a relatively inexpensive way to lend prestige and credibility to your practice, I recommend establishing an Internet identity to anyone seeking to earn a living practicing massage or bodywork.

E. Ethereal Marketing Techniques

"There is more to the world" says Shakespeare, "than is dreamt of in your philosophy." Many successful practitioners believe there is more to making contact with another person than operating in the world of the physical senses.

These are some of the unorthodox marketing tips used by some successful massage practitioners:

- Visualize an open field, and see clients coming across that field to you.

- Meditate, tell the universe you are ready for people to come into your life.

- Imagine that you have a dial you can turn to control the flow of your practice. Turn it up to become busier, turn it down when you need freedom from your practice.

If this sounds like so much hocus-pocus to you, don't bother with it. You may find, at some point, that it has meaning for you. For example, several therapists have said that when they find themselves feeling frantic and wishing they had spare time instead of appointments, their clients often call in and cancel.

A skeptical person can always see something like this as coincidence. It is not scientific and cannot be proven. If it intrigues you, simply suspend disbelief. Allow the possibility that it is hogwash and allow the opposite possibility that it is a real phenomenon. Then stay with your experience, see how things go and form opinions later.

F. Joining Managed Care Networks

Reimbursement for massage by insurance companies is covered in Chapter 21. This section deals with becoming a provider in a managed care network.

Massage and Managed Care

In recent years, the medical insurance industry has developed a means of offering massage to its customers without actually reimbursing for massage. The "managed care" movement in the insurance industry has come to regard massage therapy as an added service it can offer to attract customers to its medical insurance plan. Massage, acupuncture, chiropractic, and some other "alternative" or "complementary" therapies are being added by HMOs and PPOs to make their plans more attractive to consumers.

A few of these companies cover massage as a reimbursed service, usually by offering a "rider" to their customers at an additional cost to cover alternative therapies. However, most HMOs and PPOs do not actually pay for massage services. Instead, they offer massage to their customers by creating a discounted referral network.

Massage offered by HMOs and PPOs usually works as follows: First, a network of "providers" is assembled by the insurance company. These networks usually include chiropractors, acupuncturists, massage therapists, and other kinds of practitioners. Either the insurance company assembles the network or they make a contract with an independent company to assemble a network for them.

The members of the network must agree to offer professional services to clients of the insurance company at a discounted rate. Sometimes the fees are set by the insurance company; more commonly, the provider agrees to work on the company's clients at a discount, usually approximately 20% less than the provider's regular fees.

The insurance company offers this discount network at no cost to its members, and supplies all its members with a directory of network providers whom they can contact directly to make appointments for services at discounted prices.

Clients use the directory to locate a practitioner in their area. They call the therapist directly for an appointment, and all future arrangements are between the therapist and the client. Usually no paperwork is required by the insurance company. The insurance company does not pay the therapist; its only role is to assemble the network of providers and give the directory of providers to its customers.

Advantages and disadvantages

The major advantage to the massage therapist in participating in this type of network is having a source of client referrals without any marketing effort on the therapist's part. This can be an advantage for a new massage therapist or someone who has not built their practice to the level they would like it to reach.

Some therapists receive a substantial number of referrals from these programs, while others receive only a few calls as a result of being listed. I have been listed with Oxford Health Plans, Inc. as a participating provider for several years. During the first year I received very few calls. More recently, I have been receiving about one call per month. Participating in this network has not been a major source of clients. However, I live in a non-metropolitan area, and I suspect that therapists in a more urban setting may do better with these referrals.

Another benefit to being on a referral list of this type is that you can use the listing in your marketing materials. For example, if you have a brochure that describes you and your work, you can state that you are an official provider for the "such-and-such" insurance company. Additionally, if you are on one or two insurance company lists, this may lend additional credibility when you contact physicians to seek referrals for insurance reimbursement work.

There is no limit on how many companies' lists you can be on; you could theoretically be on all the referral lists in your area, and get clients from all the companies that offer referral services in your region.

The main disadvantage is that you must give a substantial discount from your regular fee. The discount is fixed by the referring insurance company. Busy therapists may regard working at a discount as an imposition, since they have to take time away from other clients who would pay full price for their services.

Some therapists also find that the clients referred by these networks are "bargain hunters" who may be looking more for a price break than for a professional relationship with a qualified therapist. For this reason, you may find a difference in the quality of client you receive from these networks compared to other sources.

The Credentialing Process

All of these programs use some type of credentialing process to assemble the network of massage therapists providing services for their clients, to assure they are referring their clients to trustworthy professionals.

The pioneer of this trend on the East Coast was Oxford Health Plans, Inc., a large HMO/PPO that was the first to offer discounted alternative therapies to its members. Oxford has the most rigorous credentialing process I know of. They require proof of national certification, massage school diploma, malpractice insurance, liability insurance, résumé, photographs of the inside and outside of your office, examples of your record-keeping system and progress notes, and a personal visit by an Oxford representative.

Many insurance companies hire outside companies to create their network. These companies take on the job of finding massage therapists and making sure they are qualified providers. The largest of these network credentialing companies is American Specialty Health Networks (ASHN).

You may have received one or more mailings from American Specialized Heath Networks with an application to join their network. (I've gotten two) They provide credentialed networks for some branches of AETNA/US Healthcare, Blue Cross/Blue Shield, CIGNA Health Care, Health Net, Kaiser, PacifiCare, Prudential, United Health Care, and Intel. If you want to become a provider for ASHN you can contact them at 8989 Rio San Diego Dr., Suite 250, San Diego, CA 92108, 888-511-2743, fax 619-297-1717, or **www.ashn.com**.

Two of the many other credentialing companies are OptimumHealth, Inc., 980 North Michigan Ave, Suite 1400, Chicago, IL 60611, 312-214-4924, fax 312-214-3510, (**www.OptimumHealthOnline.com**) and Complementary Care Company, P.O. Box 11264, Baltimore, MD 21239, 888-862-3223, 410-254-2134, fax 410-426-5297, (**www.c3online.com**).

The Trend Is Toward More Massage

A recent study indicated that about 11% of HMOs offer massage services, usually in the form of a discount plan. Most HMO directors surveyed said that "consumer demand" was the main reason they offer these services to their members. This same survey also showed that the trend is toward greater and greater inclusion of "alternative" or "complementary" therapies in the managed care industry.

Is Managed Care For You?

If you are in need of increasing your clientele, and willing to offer a discount on your services in return for referrals, this may be something for you to pursue.

To become listed in a referral network, contact either a credentialing company or one of the health insurance companies in your area that maintains a massage referral network. The company will guide you in the process of becoming credentialed and being added to their network. This process can take several months, so start early if this may be something you want to do.

G. Fostering Repeat Business

The first goal of your marketing efforts is to get potential clients to try you out. The next goal is to have them realize they should come back and make massage a regular part of their lives.

Client retention, or fostering repeat business, is an extremely important part of success in your career as a massage practitioner. You will spend a great deal of energy getting your clients to know you, trust you, and try your services. The extra energy you devote to client retention will produce major rewards by giving you a full schedule of regular clients.

The main ways you can foster repeat business are to create an understanding of the benefits of massage, encourage re-booking, and stay in touch with your clients.

Create an understanding of the benefits of massage

After receiving a massage, the client's body will understand how healthful it is, but the person's mind may not. Many people guide themselves primarily by their mental processes, and unless these people have an understanding of the value of massage, they may not become repeat clients.

You can help them understand the process by honestly explaining how massage benefits people in general, and how they specifically could benefit from a regular program of treatment. There is no need to be a salesman, or to be pushy. If you are honest and forthright, people will respect your professionalism and appreciate the information — they want to take care of themselves once they understand how.

Your massage school education will teach you the benefits of massage (see Chapter 20 for further information), and your work in particular will take on certain unique characteristics that promote health and well-being. Part of your job as a massage practitioner is to educate your clients about the benefits your work offers them. Teach them enough to understand the value of your work, and why they should come to you on a regular basis.

Encourage re-booking

Keep client retention in the back of your mind from the moment of your first contact with a client and at all times thereafter.

Make sure you find out what each client needs each time a client comes to you and do your best to provide it. Make sure the client understands the value of your massage for her specific issues or conditions. Create a treatment plan tailored to this client. Emphasize the importance of consistency and follow-through.

Finally, ask the client to make her next appointment before leaving your office. After receiving your work, the client is in a receptive frame of mind and is relaxed. Rather than relying on phone messages in the future to communicate, this is the best time to make the client's next appointment.

Many massage practitioners are uncomfortable doing these things, feeling they require too much "salesmanship." But the fact is, you have something of value for this client, and you should do all you can to create the opportunity to provide your unique services to this person. If that includes mastering communication techniques to educate your client and encourage her to return regularly, you should embrace those techniques as part of your therapy practice.

Stay in touch with your clients

Some therapists call their clients a day or two after their first massage to ask how they are feeling. This is especially appropriate with clients who have come in for relief from a specific condition.

Other ways to stay in touch with clients are:

- Send birthday cards

- Photocopy an article of interest about massage and send it to all your clients with a short note

- Send holiday greeting cards at Christmas or Rosh Hashanah

- Send a flyer or post card reminding clients that you offer gift certificates at holiday time

- Send flyers or post cards advertising any special offers you are making on your services

- Send announcements to your clients when you begin working in a new location or take on an associate in your office

- If you have a seasonal clientele, send thank-you letters to your clients at the end of the season for their patronage.

Other ideas on client retention

- Send a "Welcome" card after a client's first session offering $5.00 off on the next session; this lets the client know you value them and encourages them to re-book.

- Give out promotional items with your name on them. One such item is a bottle of spring water with your label on it; clients can re-use it, and will have a constant reminder of your name and phone number on hand.

- Send clients a gift certificate on the yearly anniversary of their first visit.

Make sure your sincere desire to help shines through in all your promotion. People will see through a tactic that is insincere, but will respond to your communications if they sense that you are motivated by a real desire to help and to be of service.

For further information about marketing

Magazine articles and books about marketing massage appear on a regular basis. For the most part, they all have basically the same advice presented in this book, although each author filters and expresses the information through their unique perspective. An excellent new book called *Marketing Massage* by Monica Rose-berry (Milady Publishing, $31.95) provides a book-length discussion of the subject matter covered in this chapter, and it presents its own version of the "golden keys to success" (see page 24) with a different slant.

You will also see marketing kits and seminars on marketing advertised in trade journals. These tend to be expensive, and you should be cautious about them. The best marketing devices you can obtain are education and motivation—these turn *you* into your own best resource.

It is more worthwhile to invest in training yourself about marketing than it is to buy the expensive videos and packets you may see advertised. Even the best materials, ideas and suggestions will not create your career success—it is your own energy, effort, enthusiasm and talents that will ultimately bring you a full practice.

8 Opening a Massage Office

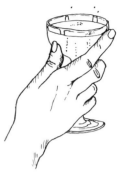

Opening an office is a big step. It is the mark of maturity of a massage career. It requires confidence in your professional skills, your business ability, and your commitment to your practice.

When the time comes in your career to open your own office, it should be a joyous venture. It will bring you the chance to make a better living and have a clear professional identity. This chapter will help you be fully prepared and ready to take this step, and will give you the basic information you will need to make the best choices in bringing your office to life.

The topics covered in this chapter are governmental requirements, practical requirements, and business decisions. Business decisions include measuring your readiness to open an office, choosing a location, and negotiating a lease. In addition, you will find a checklist for office opening, and discussions of opening a group practice and buying an existing practice.

Governmental Requirements

You are becoming a local business owner, and as such you are taking on a new identity in the eyes of your local government. One of the main functions of local government is to regulate the operations of businesses. By the same token, a substantial source of revenue for local government is license fees and taxes paid by local business owners.

So you are in a two-way relationship with your local government. On one hand, the government wants to exert its authority over you to make sure you do things to their liking. On the other hand, the government wants to see you succeed, so that you will make money and share it with the government.

Your first step is to visit your local government, whether it is a town hall, city hall, municipal complex, or village governmental center. Bring a note pad and pen. Ask for assistance about the following items:

1. Massage licensing law

Most towns and cities do not have laws regulating the practice of massage, but many do. These laws often were written more to guard against prostitution than to realistically regulate massage practice. You may find that the local law regulates massage quite heavily. Some local laws prohibit massaging members of the opposite sex. A few towns prohibit the practice of massage completely.

If your town has a restrictive law, you will have to choose 1. meeting all of the restrictions, 2. giving up the idea of practicing there, 3. fighting to have the law changed, or 4. practicing there and risking being penalized for violating the law. If you think you may choose number 4, it is probably not a good idea to march into city hall and identify yourself as a way of getting information.

2. Practitioner license, establishment license

If the town has a licensing law, it will probably have two parts to it. One will give the requirements for a massage practitioner license, and the other will give the requirements for a massage establishment license.

The practitioner license applies to your right to practice massage within the town, and the establishment license applies to the office in which you will practice massage. Each will have a separate procedure and a separate fee.

3. Zoning requirements

Almost all towns have zoning laws, which regulate the types of "uses" that may take place in different "zones." In other words, zoning laws restrict the kinds of businesses you can operate in different neighborhoods. Certain neighborhoods are set aside for residences only. Others may be zoned for industrial uses, such as factories and warehouses. Others will be for stores or professional practices. A sample zoning map is on page 69.

Before committing to a particular location for a massage office, you should be sure that the location has the proper zoning for use as a massage business.

Different communities will use different zoning classifications for massage. Some will call it a personal service. Others will call it a profession. Others will call it a health service. Still others refer to it as "adult entertainment." What they call it will have an effect on which zones you will be allowed to locate in.

The town clerk can direct you to the zoning map for the city. If the zoning board can tell you exactly which category massage is considered to be for zoning purposes, you can check the map to see which neighborhoods are open to you for an office location. If there is doubt about which category they consider massage, you may need to go before the zoning board to get a definitive ruling before choosing your office location.

If you are opening a home office, the zoning board may require a hearing before deciding whether to allow you to operate a massage practice in your home. They may consider factors such as the burden placed on neighborhood parking, the percentage of space in the home devoted to your business, and whether you will be the only one who performs massage services in your home. If you need to appear before the zoning board, consider consulting an attorney beforehand to advise you about how to proceed or to represent you before the zoning board.

4. Health, police and fire department inspections

Inquire of the health department, police department and fire department what their policies are about inspecting a massage office before it opens. Ask about any

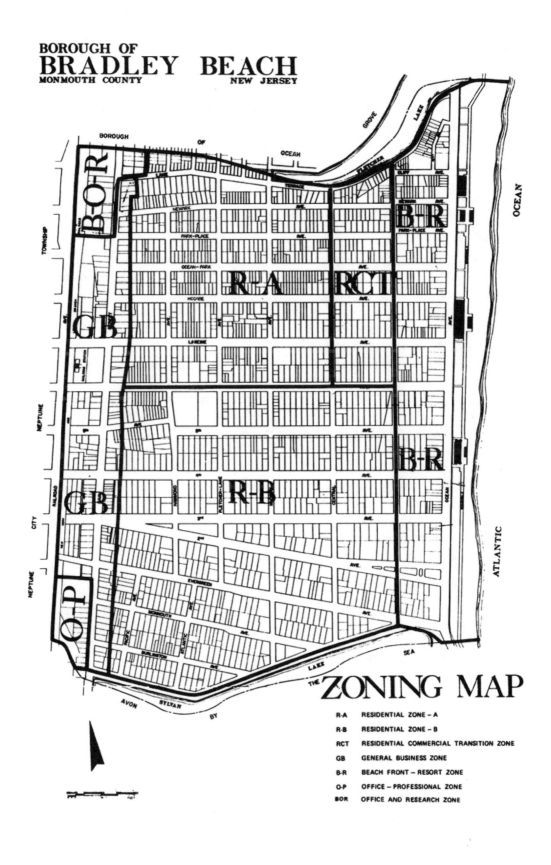

BOROUGH OF
BRADLEY BEACH
MONMOUTH COUNTY   NEW JERSEY

ZONING MAP

R-A	RESIDENTIAL ZONE – A
R-B	RESIDENTIAL ZONE – B
RCT	RESIDENTIAL COMMERCIAL TRANSITION ZONE
GB	GENERAL BUSINESS ZONE
B-R	BEACH FRONT – RESORT ZONE
O-P	OFFICE – PROFESSIONAL ZONE
BOR	OFFICE AND RESEARCH ZONE

requirements you will need to meet. Write down the answers you receive, the name of the person who gives you the information, and the date.

5. Local business taxes

Ask the clerk about any local taxes, such as sewer tax, business property tax, or other local business taxes. Make a note of this information, as you will want to know what your expenses will be in operating your business.

Practical Requirements

1. Fictitious name statement (also called "assumed name" or "doing business as")

If you will give your business a name other than your own name (such as "Wholistic Massage Center" or "Beams of Light Massage") you will need to register your fictitious name with the county government. This allows the public to know who owns a business when the owner's name is not included in the business name. This certificate does not give you exclusive rights to the name. For that you must seek trade-name or service-mark protection.

To register your fictitious name, you must go to the county seat, the town in your county that houses the county government offices. If you do not know where that is, someone in your bank or city government office can tell you. Contact the county clerk, and find out the cost for registering a fictitious or assumed name, the hours you can go and do so, and the procedure for doing so. In some places, the procedure includes advertising your fictitious name in local newspapers.

In most cases, you will be required to do your own checking through the county's records of business names to make sure that no one has already chosen that business name. This can take awhile, so give yourself enough time to take care of this. After you have checked the records, you pay your fee (bring cash and keep your receipt) and you will receive a "fictitious name certificate" (or "assumed name certificate").

2. Business bank account

Your bank will require a fictitious name certificate in order to open an account in the name of your business. It is a good idea to have a business checking account, and to pay for all business expenses with your business checks (or business credit card). Your business will appear more credible and established than it would if you pay for business purchases with your personal checks or credit cards. Having a separate account will also make your task easier when it is time to prepare your year-end income taxes.

3. Business stationery, cards, gift certificates, flyers

Choose a print shop that you can be comfortable with. You will probably be a repeat customer for your printer. You should have a printer that you have confidence in, as to quality, prompt completion of orders, and competitive price. Consider recommendations of others and your own observations when in the shop.

The bare minimum you will need to open your office is business cards. Consider whether to also invest in customized gift certificates and business stationary.

Also consider: A rubber stamp with your business name and address, a rubber stamp with your bank account number to endorse the back of checks, flyers that describe you and your business, a printed coupon for purchasers of pre-paid series of massage, and promotional items to publicize your office.

Business Decisions

1. Financial and Professional Readiness

Start-up costs

First consider that you will need some money up front in order to open an office. You will need money for office furnishings, first month's rent, security deposit, telephone and utility deposit, printing needs and advertising or other promotional costs. If you have established credit, you may be able to get a loan. Otherwise you will need to use your savings to meet these start-up costs.

As a guideline for planning purposes, the following figures are estimates of the amounts you will need to spend on start-up costs:

Massage table	$500	Desk	$175
Table or shelf	80	Hamper	35
Phone/ans. mach.	75	Music system	250
Sheets/towels	200	First month rent	400
Security deposit	400	Phone deposit	150
Utility deposit	75	Printing	100
Ads/promotion	300	Miscellaneous	100

Any of these items can be more or less than the amounts shown, depending on your particular circumstances. The start-up costs in the sample above total $2,840.

Monthly expenses vs. income

Next examine your ability to meet the continuing financial obligations of operating a professional office.

Perhaps you work in a health club, hair salon, or doctor's office. Would most of your clients stay with the new massage therapist who replaces you or would they follow you to your office?

Estimated Monthly Business Income

Take an honest look at your client list, and imagine the first month in your new office. Examine your records to see what your business income has been for the last few months, and any upward or downward trends you notice.

Consider, also, that once you have an office of your own, it may be easier for you to create new growth. First, you will have strong motivation to do so. Second, you will have a location that is conducive to the kind of work you want to do. Third, you will have an established office that will serve as the focus of your marketing efforts—promotional ideas such as direct mail, lecture/demonstration and advertising will be more open to you than they would be if your were working in an employer's space.

Make an estimate of your first month's income. If in doubt, choose a lower figure for planning purposes. For purposes of making a sample financial projection, we will assume you can start in your new office with an income of $1,200 per month. This is your "estimated monthly business income."

Other Monthly Income

Calculate your other sources of income, apart from your business. Include any sources of income you know you can count on, such as interest, alimony, pension, or the like. Total all this income, and figure how much you receive in an average month. For purposes of this example, we will use the figure $150 per month for your "Other Monthly Income."

Total Estimated Income

Add your "estimated monthly business income" to your "other monthly income." In this example, the total is $1,350.

Estimated Monthly Business Expenses

Calculate the amount you must spend each month for your office rent, telephone, and yellow pages. Also include a twelfth of your annual business expenses, such as advertising, oils and linens, business taxes, professional association dues, accountant fees, insurance costs, and the like.

The total of your monthly business expenses is likely to be between $300 and $1,200. This is the amount you need each month to support your business. We will use the figure of $600 per month as an example of "estimated monthly business expenses."

Estimated Monthly Personal Expenses

This is the amount you need to live on each month, for such essentials as home rental, food, automobile, health insurance and taxes. One way to calculate this is to look through your checkbook for last year. Add up all the money you spent on personal expenses, plus your best guess for how much cash you spent, and divide by 12. Another way is to add up your fixed expenses and then add an estimate for your spending money.

Let's say you come up with a total of $1,000 per month for your "estimated monthly personal expenses."

Estimated Total Monthly Expenses

Add the "estimated monthly business expenses" of $600 per month to "estimated monthly personal expenses" of $1,000 per month to find your "estimated total monthly expenses." This is the amount you will need to earn each month in order to support your new office and your current lifestyle. In our example, this is $1,600.

These estimated figures are summarized in the chart below.

New Office Financial Projections

INCOME		
Estimated monthly business income	$1,200	
Other monthly income	150	
Total estimated income	1,350	
EXPENSES		
Estimated monthly business expenses in new office location	600	
Estimated monthly personal expenses	1,000	
Estimated total monthly expenses	1,600	
NET DEFICIT	$250	per month

This projection shows expenses will be higher than income. Subtracting income ($1,350) from expenses ($1,600) shows an estimated deficit of $250 per month for this person's overall lifestyle after opening the new massage office.

If your financial planning estimate shows a net deficit per month, you should plan to have a reserve of at least one year's worth of deficits before you decide to open your office. It may take a year for you to see any significant increase in your business, so plan to start with the ability to sustain your practice at its current level for at least a year.

In this example, that would mean you should have a capital reserve of $3,000 to supplement your income for the first year.

Consider choosing a larger figure for your capital reserve, since it is possible your second year may also produce a net deficit.

Additional Reserves For Business and Personal Expenses

In addition to the predictable expenses, you should ideally be prepared for the unforeseen ones as well. For example, your car's transmission falls out. You need $600 to fix it. You decide it would help business to do a direct mail promotion. You need $400 for the cost of the mailing.

This kind of expense can come up without warning, so you should plan on at least another $1,000 to draw on for such emergencies.

Total Needs for Financial Readiness

Add your Start-up Costs, your first year's Net Deficit, and Additional Reserves. This is the amount you can expect to need in the first year to start your business and supplement your income. In the example above, this total would be $6,840.

If your skills, personality and location are good, and you approach your marketing with commitment and organization, you should find that after the first year you begin to see some increase in your practice. You may still have a net deficit each month in the second year. If you proceed with organization and commitment, you should have a net profit after the second year, and have a net operating profit for the rest of your massage career.

2. Location

There is an old joke in the real estate business:

> *Question:* What are the three most important factors in the value of real estate?
>
> *Answer:* Location, location and location

This expresses a basic truth about the business world. Location counts for a great deal in business. Choose a location that is central, easy to get to, enjoyable to go to, and that conveys a positive image for your practice.

WIZARD OF ID

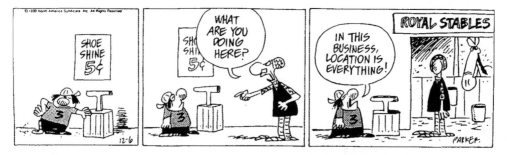

Take your time finding a location. Consider a broad range of questions.

Consider the town:

- Is the town one that can support a massage therapist?

- Are any massage therapists currently earning a living in this town?

- Will I be in direct competition with them or will we draw on different client bases?

- Is there another town in the area that would afford a better image or a more receptive client population?

Consider the neighborhood and building:

- What is the ideal location within my town for my particular practice?

- Will this location be one my clients are comfortable coming to? One they will look forward to coming to?

- Is the building attractive and well-maintained?

- Is the building visible to large numbers of people on a daily basis?

- Are the other offices in the building ones whose images fit comfortably with the image I want for my practice?

- Is the neighborhood safe and pleasant?

- Is parking convenient?

- What other businesses are nearby?

- Will this location support my plans for future growth?

- Do I feel comfortable thinking of this as "my" office?

Your choice of an office location can make your whole professional life easier or more difficult. Do yourself a favor, and make the selection of an office your highest priority. Investigate, think, feel and take some time with this decision. Your efforts will pay great dividends for years to come.

3. Negotiating a Lease

Look for items in a lease which give you flexibility and control and avoid items which give power to the landlord and obligate you excessively.

For example, your lease should include a statement that the office provided will be suitable for use as a professional massage office — as to noise level, temperature control and good repair of all fixtures. This gives you a legal right to complain if the landlord fails to provide you with a quiet and warm massage environment.

If you have any doubts about the zoning for the location, put in the lease that it becomes void if the city refuses to approve zoning for a massage business at that location. Otherwise, you could be stuck with a lease on an office in which you cannot open your business. Also consider making the lease conditional upon being granted a local massage practitioner license and a massage establishment license.

You also may want to negotiate for a lease that is renewable at your option. After all, you do not know for sure that you will succeed in your business, or that you will like the location. Give yourself the option to leave after a year. At the same time, give yourself the option to renew for a second and third year at the same rental (or a small increase) so that you know you will be able to enjoy the reward for your efforts if your practice is very successful.

Spell out in the lease any other items that you consider of special importance to you, and make sure you understand all of the provisions of the lease you sign. As a precaution, it is good practice to show the lease to a lawyer or experienced business person to get an informed opinion before signing.

One further thing to keep in mind is that, while your lease gives you legal rights, these may not amount to anything in practical terms if you wind up having a conflict with your landlord. If you need to hire a lawyer and file a lawsuit, your expenses in suing will almost certainly be more than you would recover even if you win. You can sue in small claims court if you meet the local requirements. However, even that takes preparation, time, energy and expense. While your lease should afford you legal protection, steering free of conflict is worth much more than having right on your side.

The lease on page 76 is the one I signed when I moved into a massage office in a beauty salon. It's not perfect, and the rent was too high, but it is as an example of the kinds of items you may want to include in a business lease.

LEASE CONTRACT

This contract is entered into this 15th day of January, 1988, between Martin Ashley (Martin) and Anthony Marzarella, doing business as Anthony Louis (Anthony). The parties agree as follows:

1. Anthony will furnish a massage room in Le Club salon on Route 88, Brick, New Jersey. He will also furnish a receptionist to take appointments for massage and to collect clients' payments for massage. The receptionist selected shall be a courteous individual who presents a positive image of massage and of the massage therapists employed to work at Le Club.

2. Martin will pay a monthly rental to Anthony of $400.00 per month, payable on the 1st day of each month. Martin will also pay Anthony 17% of the cost of advertising which advertises massage at Le Club.

3. This contract shall be for a period of three months, and shall be renewable at Martin's option for additional periods of three months, up to a total of one year. In addition, after the first year, the contract shall be renewable for an additional year at a monthly rent not to exceed $500 per month.

4. Anthony shall obtain a Brick massage establishment license, and Martin shall obtain a Brick massage practitioner license. All massage therapists employed by Martin at Le Club shall have Brick massage practitioner licenses. Martin shall have the right to transfer or sell his rights under this contract to any other individual who has a Brick massage practitioner license.

5. Permanent improvements to the premises made by Anthony shall be the property of Anthony, and furnishings placed in the massage room by Martin shall remain the property of Martin.

6. Collection of the amount due to be paid for massage shall be the responsibility of Anthony. The receptionist shall collect payment from massage clients.

7. Liability to clients and customers for any accidents or injuries shall be Martin's if the accident or injury occurs within the massage room, and Anthony's if the accident or injury occurs elsewhere on Le Club premises.

_____
date   Anthony Marzarella

_____
date   Martin Ashley

4. Taking Credit Cards

Consider taking Visa and MasterCard in payment for your services. The disadvantage is the cost—there are setup costs, either purchase or rental, and transaction costs for each charge. If you process a small amount of business on credit cards, the setup fees may make it too costly for you. But if you process a large amount of charges on credit cards, these costs are spread out over many transactions and will not be much of a burden.

In order to take credit cards, you first need to establish a "merchant account", and you next need either software or hardware that will allow you to process credit transactions. Hardware (the "swiper" and printer) can be purchased for several hundred dollars or leased for $15.00 to $50.00 per month. There may also be a monthly minimum processing fee, a per-transaction fee, and a percentage of each sale taken as a processing fee. Shop around, as prices vary considerably from company to company. As a target price, try to find a merchant account costing $15.00 per month plus 1 to 2 percent of credit charges.

Clients usually find it convenient to write a check or pay cash, but you may find there is some business you will do only if you take credit cards. Credit cards make it very easy for clients to buy gift certificates — they can order them much as they do flowers from a florist. It also facilitates sales of series coupons, and can make it easier for a client who finds herself without checks or sufficient cash. An office that takes credit cards also presents a very established and professional image.

To investigate taking credit cards in your business, go to the bank where you have your business checking account, and ask for assistance. Check with other banks, and check the Business-to-Business Yellow Pages under "Credit Card Equipment and Supplies." Costco offers low-cost merchant accounts to executive members (1-888-474-0500).

You should also search the Internet if you are seeking a merchant account. There are literally hundreds of websites offering merchant accounts, with terms that vary greatly. Some sites offer accounts that operate only on your website, and others offer accounts you can use in your office.

One final option to consider is to "piggy-back" on someone else's merchant account; make a deal to use someone else's merchant account for a fixed per-use fee. If you are a low-volume credit merchant, this type of arrangement will almost certainly be the cheapest alternative you can find.

5. Furnishing Your Office

The furnishings you choose for your office will reflect your personality and your preferences for a setting in which to practice your particular type of work. You might choose pastels and crystals if you lean toward the ethereal, and whites and stainless steel if you lean toward the clinical. Only you know the atmosphere you want for yourself and your clients. Certain basics, however, apply to most or all massage rooms:

- In general, you should keep your office spacious and uncluttered, as this generally promotes a more comfortable and relaxed feeling.

- Arrange for lighting that is not harsh. Avoid ceiling lights, as these will be too bright for clients when face up. Dimming switches are inexpensive and easily available. One type installs in the wall switch and another screws directly into the bulb socket. Also consider stained glass lamps designed to hold low-watt bulbs and night lights that plug into wall sockets.

- Your diplomas will add an air of professionalism to the walls. Consider also some artwork to create an appropriate atmosphere.

- Keep a desk in your office. The desk is the place for your telephone and answering machine, phone books, schedule book and client files.

- Linens can be kept on a shelf, in a cabinet, or under the massage table. Choose your linens after you decide on a color scheme for the office, or use white linens, which can go with any office colors.

- Have a mirror available to your clients.

- Give your clients ample hooks for their clothing. Create a private space for dressing and undressing or leave the room while clients are dressing and undressing. Have a table or counter where clients can put their jewelry and personal belongings.

- Have a computer, word processor or typewriter in the office so you can do paperwork between appointments if necessary.

- Have your business cards out in a spot where clients will see them and can take one.

- Consider having bottled water available for you and your clients in your office.

Checklist for office furnishings

massage table	mirror
linens	desk
hamper	table or counter space for client's use
oil	
chair	music system
clothing hooks for clients	
business card holder	telephone and answering machine
bottled water cooler or other dispenser	computer
lighting system	artwork, diplomas or other decorations for walls

6. *Telephone Reception*

One advantage of a group practice is that the group can pool resources to either hire a receptionist or rotate duties on phone reception. This assures that callers will reach a person who can answer their questions about massage and schedule an appointment.

If you are practicing alone, it is much more difficult to answer your own phone. Hopefully, you will be too busy doing massage to be serving as your own receptionist. The choices available to you are hiring an answering service or using voicemail or an answering machine.

Practically all therapists, faced with this choice, choose voicemail or an answering machine over an answering service. The service may seem to have the advantage of presenting the caller with a live human to talk to, but the person who works for the answering service is not likely to be familiar with massage. Therefore, she or he cannot answer the potential client's questions about your services. The answering service can take messages for you, but that is about all.

A new service has recently come on the market, "My Receptionist." This is a company in Eau Claire, Wisconsin that provides your personal phone line, so that their employees can answer your line with your business name, answer questions about you and your services, and schedule your appointments. Cost for the service starts at $29.95 per month, with additional charges for individual calls and for credit card transactions. Contact information is in the reference section on page 209.

Caller I.D.

Caller I.D. has become a very common feature, and is a standard feature on most cell phones. Some Caller I.D. devices store the numbers of the last twenty or so people who have called your number, which can be useful information.

When you have caller I.D., and you are making an appointment with a new client for the first time, you can say to the person "Can I call you at 555-3456 to confirm?" The fact that you know their phone number will be a strong deterrent for any sex clients who may be calling you. If the caller has chosen to block his identity from caller I.D., this may be someone you want to be especially careful with.

Checklist for office opening

The items in this checklist are arranged in chronological order — in other words, do number one first, number two second, etc. Begin this process three to six months before your target date for opening your new office.

Three to six months before opening:

1. Contact local government for information about zoning, and any regulations of health, fire and police departments

2. Contact direct mail company to learn the date of their next mailing; contact phone company to learn deadline for next yellow pages listing

3. Consider possible locations and look at offices for rent

4. Negotiate a lease for your office location, select starting date with enough lead time to make all preparations

5. Obtain all necessary governmental approvals, licenses and permits

Two to four weeks before opening:

6. Register fictitious name with county

7. Establish business checking account

8. Contact telephone company to connect new service

9. Order stationery, business cards and any promotional items you plan to use to publicize your office's opening

10. If appropriate, plan an advertising push when you open to create an increased clientele for your new venture

11. Shop for office furnishings

12. Notify all your clients of your new office opening and any introductory promotions you may be having

13. Get to know the neighbors in your new location and use any opportunities to gain clientele through your neighbors

Opening a group practice

Group practice refers to several massage therapists or related professionals sharing a suite of offices. Group practices have some significant advantages over individual practices, as well as some disadvantages.

The two main advantages of group practices are shared expenses and cross-referrals. The main disadvantage is the group decision process.

Renting an office suite and sharing the cost usually results in a lower price to each member than she would have to pay for a similar office space rented individually.

A group practice has the potential to become well-known as a center, thereby attracting a larger clientele through the reputation of the group. Once such a reputation is established for a group practice, it will generate a significant walk-in trade, and all the group members will benefit.

The disadvantage of a group practice is that decisions must be made by the group as a whole. This usually means devoting one evening per week to the process of group decision-making. After a busy week of massage, an evening of group process can seem like a burden. However, if you choose carefully which other practitioners you associate with, these group meetings can be an enjoyable opportunity for learning and socializing.

Buying an Existing Massage Practice

Occasionally, practitioners sell their practice. You may have an opportunity to purchase an existing practice. This may seem like an appealing way to have a ready-made practice. However, buying an existing practice is risky, and you should be extremely careful if you choose to do so.

Ask yourself several questions:

1. Why is this person selling her practice? She may not be giving you the real reason. Ask to see her appointment book, and take a minute to look at it. See how busy the office really is.

2. Will she take any of her clients with her? This can be a problem if the selling therapist plans to stay in massage and to stay in the area. You could find you have paid for a practice that evaporates as soon as you arrive.

3. Will her clients like you? It was the selling therapist's style of massage and personality that attracted her current clientele. If your massage and your personality are different from hers, her clients may be dissatisfied with you and may leave to try other therapists.

If I were buying an existing practice, I would want to first become an associate, and work in the office on a part-time basis. By so doing, I would get the feel of the clientele, and know whether they would accept me, and whether I would feel comfortable working with them. I would also have the opportunity to see first-hand how busy the practice is.

Ask the seller if such an arrangement is possible. You could try it for a couple of months, at which time you would decide whether to buy the practice for a pre-set amount of money.

The real value of an established practice is the client base, the group of people who are in the habit of coming to this practice for massage on a regular basis. The client base can be a valuable asset if you are new to a community and want to become established quickly. I suggest you base a purchase price on the number of clients you believe will stay with you after you take the practice over. You will need to make your best estimate of this.

If the client base will give you only enough income to meet the office rent, it is not worth much to you. On the other hand, if you will be able to step in and immediately earn enough to meet expenses and take home an income of $500 per week, that has a substantial value.

Figuring the value of an existing practice is tricky, but consider this formula. Project the income you expect to earn immediately after taking over the office. To do this, you must have some basis for knowing how many clients will stay with you after the selling therapist leaves.

Assume your projected income for the first month is $1300. Next, total the expenses you will have for rent, phone, yellow pages, insurance, taxes and supplies.

Assume this is $750 per month. Subtract the expenses from your expected income. You can project your estimated profit to be $550 for the first month.

Offer the seller three to five times the amount you expect to take home as profit for the first month. If your assessment is correct, you will be able to recover your investment within a year or so, and you will then have a successful practice with a minimum of marketing effort on your part.

The figure you offer will probably be less than the seller was hoping for. The seller may hope for a figure that represents a year's profit, or even more. In the "business world", a going business is commonly sold for three or four times the net annual income. However, it is hard to imagine a situation where that would be an appropriate formula for the value of a massage practice.

If the business is very attractive and you can afford it, you may want to agree to more than a few months' net income. However, you should only offer what the business will be worth *to you*. If you were buying a store that sold brand-name goods, the established trade would be reliable. In your case, the value of this business depends very much on how much it will change after you take it over.

III

Sex, Gender
and Touch

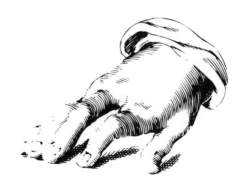

9 Sex and Massage

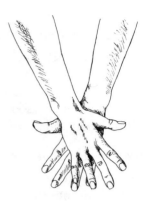

About half-way through my massage school course, I began to wonder when we would have the class about sexuality and massage, to help us understand and deal with sexual feelings that may arise for the client or the therapist during a session. I kept waiting for such a class, but it never arrived.

When I set up a practice in the "real world," I encountered sexual issues that deserved to be discussed in schools. While some schools now include a discussion of sexuality and massage in their programs, many programs still do not give students meaningful preparation for what they can expect in the "real world."

Differences in approach

The approach I suggest for a professional massage therapist or bodyworker is to set up clear boundaries for the therapeutic session. Any sexual intention by the client or the therapist is outside those boundaries. A client who presents sexual intentions should be confronted, and if the client acknowledges sexual intentions, the treatment should be ended.

Some authors and some educators differ with that approach, and regard a client's sexual desires not so much as a problem, but as an opportunity to foster the client's growth by exploring the psychological issues he has concerning sexuality. Be aware that if you choose such an approach, you are crossing the line between massage and counseling. If you have psychological training and the therapeutic skills needed to work in that way, there is nothing wrong with doing so. I don't, and most massage therapists don't. Therefore, my advice is to simply terminate a massage when a client presents the wish for sexual gratification.

Clients who want sexual massage

Occasionally, a woman massage client attempts to initiate sexual contact, either with a male or female massage therapist during a massage session. Instances in which men attempt to initiate sexual contact, either with a male or female massage therapist are, unfortunately, much more common.

It is likely that at some point in your career, you will have a client attempt to initiate sexual contact. The following suggestions and observations are offered as guidelines for what to expect and how to deal with what takes place. Since the great majority of sexually oriented clients are men, the male pronoun is used throughout this chapter.

Arousal need not be considered a problem

A few men experience a partial erection at some point during a massage. These men are not necessarily after sex, and may actually be somewhat embarrassed by their arousal. The simple fact of a male client having an erection should not be seen as a problem, as long as the man's attitude is appropriate and he presents no verbal or non-verbal sexual expressions.

Arousal plus inappropriate action is a problem

Signs to watch for if a male client has an erection are: touching the genitals; grinding the hips into the massage table; moving the hips in any way; using muscular contraction to flex the penis.

These activities should alert you that this client will probably present a request for sex. You should confront him immediately about his arousal. Unless he can explain his actions to your satisfaction, terminate the massage immediately.

Other, subtler signs to look for are very shallow breathing or sighs of appreciation or pleasure. If you have some experience with clients who want sex, you will learn to "feel" that desire coming from them. It may be a subtle change in the mood in the room, or a change in *your* breathing or thinking that you cannot explain.

If in doubt, confront

If a client has an erection and you perceive signs that lead you to believe this client wants sex, ask your client questions to find out if you are right. Mention that he seems to be aroused and ask his feeling about that.

If the client's response tells you his attitude about the arousal is one of enjoyment, terminate the massage immediately. If the client continues to make any voluntary movements of a sexual nature, such as grinding the hips or touching the genitals, terminate the massage.

Your massage room is your environment, and you are in control of what does and does not happen there. Do not allow a client to threaten that control. Do not be afraid of losing business—any client who is sexually oriented is a client you want very much to lose anyway.

If you are alone in your office, you may want to have a phone number handy for someone you know you can reach in an emergency. It may help you to feel more at ease to know someone is available to help you if necessary.

Understanding the big picture

Sex and massage have undoubtedly been linked for thousands of years. One explanation for the persistent connection between the two has been offered by David Lauterstein, co-director of the Lauterstein-Conway School of Massage in Austin, Texas:

> … we rather awkwardly encounter the one good reason massage and prostitution were ever associated. Both address people's need for love. However, prostitutes simply don't deliver—selling sex as love is robbery. That's a good reason why it's illegal. Massage therapy recognizes that underneath each person's tension, stress, even illness and injury, is an unmet need for energetic nourishment, i.e., love.

Unfortunately, many men are not aware of the distinction Mr. Lauterstein refers to. They *think* that what they need to be happy is sex, and there are plenty of "practitioners" who are willing to indulge them in their illusion.

In some parts of the world, a manually-stimulated orgasm is the normal and accepted conclusion of a professional massage. In many parts of the United States, a sexual massage is more common and easier to find than a legitimate massage. In some areas (San Diego, for example) the sexual massage ads in the yellow pages completely overwhelm the few listings for massage therapists.

In recent years, newspapers have carried stories of "acupressure" parlors fronting for prostitution in Los Angeles County, California, and massage parlors fronting for prostitution in the Oyster Bay area of Long Island, New York. The New York parlors were closed only after a march by licensed massage therapists, who announced plans to hold a press conference in front of their local senator's office unless action was taken.

Millions of men have had sexual massage experiences, and continue to have them today. As such, it is understandable that they would have some confusion about what it is you do. That is why you should be 1) non-judgmental and 2) completely clear in your communications before beginning a massage.

Screening new clients

It is a good practice to ask anyone who calls you how they heard about you. First, you want to be able to thank clients for referrals, and keep track of how successful your various promotional activities have been. Second, if the person does not come as a referral from a trusted client, you want to be able to make sure the person does not have the wrong idea.

Most sex clients will find you either through the yellow pages or through a newspaper ad. With male callers who have located me through advertising, I make a point of stating at the beginning that my massage is strictly non-sexual. I may use terms like "legitimate" or "therapeutic" to reinforce the message. I then ask them if this is the type of massage they are looking for, and pause to give them an opportunity to answer.

Massage clients understand the need for such an explanation, and are not put off. Most of the sex callers will hang up at that point, but some persist. During the conversation that follows, I have learned to watch my breathing. If my own breathing becomes shallow, and my heart starts beating fast, I have learned that this means my unconscious is getting the message that there is something dishonest about the caller.

Clients looking for sexual massage will try to find out what they can get without saying anything incriminating. Typical questions the sex caller may ask, in an attempt to find out if he can get a sexual massage, are these:

> Is this a nude massage?
>
> Is this a "complete"?
>
> What will you be wearing during the massage?
>
> Is tipping allowed?

Are there extras?

Can I get a release?

What else is included?

Does a girl give the massage?

If you hear any of these questions, politely tell him he has the wrong office, and hang up.

To minimize sex clients, get a first *and last* name for any first-time clients, and a phone number you can call to confirm the appointment.

Try to avoid same-day appointments with first-time male clients. Clients who want same-day service are less likely to become regular clients and more likely to demand same-day booking again. In addition, a significant number of same-day appointments turn out to be no-shows.

Be cautious with male internet referrals. If the client will not give his name and phone number, be suspicious. These calls may have a high no-show rate as well.

Phone to confirm the appointment the day it is to take place. If any difficulty or confusion results from your attempt to confirm the appointment, be prepared for a no-show or a client who may be using a fictitious name.

One Massage Therapist's Story

The following essay is one of four essays in a work called Massage Portraits, originally published in 1984 in CoEvolution Quarterly/Whole Earth Review, issue No. 43. It is written by Anneke Campbell and is reprinted with her permission. I include it here because it captures well many of the aspects of dealing with a client seeking sex.

CHIP

It was nine in the evening when the phone rang, and a male voice asked if he could come for a massage. "How did you find out about me?" I asked, always cautious. "Connie usually works on me when I'm in town, but she's out for the evening."

I knew Connie did good work, so I relaxed. "My old football injury is acting up," the man continued, "Could you see me tonight?" "Well ..." I didn't much feel like it, but my rent was due at the end of the week. "Alright then." "I sure do appreciate it."

The fellow who walked in my door was a massive six-foot-four, dark-haired, jowly. I was going to have to work for my money. Chip had played football at college in the sixties, and nearly gone pro. Partly due to his back problem, he had opted for business, and was doing quite well, if he did say so himself. He also told me he was divorced. He took off all his clothes with bravura, as if to let me know he had no hang-ups about his body, not him.

His back was a sheet of lumpy, tight muscle. I stood close to the massage table and leaned all my weight into my hands. I began by pushing on the bunched-up erector spinae, and to my surprise, they softened up right away. Chip was responsive. I concentrated with my fingers on the vertebrae, which were buried in fibroid connective tissue. While I worked, Chip told me about the injury which had left him with some weakness in the sacral area. He had experienced both numbness and aching in his legs for years.

"There's nothing I can do about nerve impairment, if that's what the problem is," I explained, "but your entire back is a mess, probably due to compensating for the injury. And I can do something about all these tense, bunched-up muscles." I used long, firm strokes down the erector spinae and up the latissimus dorsi. I kneaded the well-padded abdominal obliques and trapezius. I worked so hard that the muscles in my own arms started aching, and drops of sweat ticked at the small of my back.

After about forty minutes, he began to moan. I was feeling pleased with the results of my work; his back was definitely less rigid than when I started. "Doesn't it feel better?" I asked. "It does, oh yes, but you're not getting to where most of the pain is." "Which is?" "Lower down."

I chased an uncomfortable thought from my mind, and moved my hands down to his sacrum and pelvic brim. I focused on the tiny muscles that lie over the sacrum; they were mushy in texture, a mushiness I associate with damage, and I could see that these could well be the source of his "weakness." Underneath, my fingers discovered some cyst-like formations. Here I worked carefully, but thoroughly. "Lower," he said.

I ignored the request. Chip's heavy body seemed suddenly disgusting to me. "Massage my thighs, that's where the problem is, on the inside of my thighs." "I've only a few minutes left." "How about another hour?" "I don't work two hours in a row," I lied.

I did some long, firm strokes down the length of his legs, trying to ignore the slight grinding of his pelvis into the massage table. I moved up, and took his bullish neck into my hands. Muscle like rock. He needed another hour, that was clear, but he wasn't going to get it from me.

"My masseuse in Florida, she does a full-body massage." I felt a sudden stab of hatred for the masseuse in Florida. "Yep, but she's a strong lady," Chip continued, "bigger than you are. You're just a little thing, aren't you. Well, what this lady does, it doesn't take much strength really."

I remained silent, kneading away at his sterno-cleido-mastoids. "She massages me down there, you know …" "I don't do that kind of massage." "I'll give you fifty dollars." "Thank you, but no," I say, clear I would never do such a thing. "One hundred dollars then." "I don't do that kind of massage," I repeated, thinking, good Lord, one hundred dollars for a hand-job, he must be filthy rich.

"Please," he said, "One hundred and twenty?" Half a month's rent, I thought. Is it really that different, rubbing his penis or rubbing his trapezius? What's a little come on my hands? And what difference would it make to anyone but me?

"No," I said, and left the room. As I washed my hands, I noticed they were shaking. I felt a little sick to my stomach, and worried about being alone in the house with this huge man. I sat down in an easy chair in the living room. After a while, Chip appeared, fully dressed. He handed me a twenty-dollar bill. "Thanks," he said, "my back feels a hell of a lot better."

For the first time in that hour, I looked him fully in the eye. The cringing I saw there took away my fear. He was obviously embarrassed, but more to the point, terribly lonely. I knew what he needed was not sex, but warmth, contact, friendship. I nearly wished I could help him, but I had no desire to be his friend. "I'm glad your back feels better." I said, getting up. I opened the door, and extended my hand. Chip held it between his for a moment. "Good hands," he said.

Therapists who have sexual feelings toward clients

Very likely, at some point in your career, you will feel sexually attracted to a client on your table. It is your responsibility to your client and to your practice to work with your own feelings and control your thoughts and actions.

Your touch transmits your thoughts

Your touch communicates an unbelievable amount of information to the person you are touching. If you are viewing them with sexual intention, they will feel that in your touch. They may not be consciously aware of what they are feeling, but the communication will take place nonetheless.

If you have ever had the experience of receiving a massage from someone who had sex on their mind, you know what I mean. You can feel it in their touch. It is a totally different experience than being treated by a therapist.

Transmitting sexual feelings in your massage can sabotage your practice. The client whom you approach sexually will feel uncomfortable, and is not likely to become a repeat client. He or she is also likely to communicate to others a feeling of discomfort, uneasiness, or general dissatisfaction with your massage.

As you practice massage with clients where there is the potential of a sexual attraction, either by you or by the client, monitor your own thoughts and feelings. If you start to slip into sexual thoughts about a client, try to determine whether these are originating with you or the client. If you find that you are responsible for originating these feelings, simply choose to stop. Remind yourself of your therapeutic intention, and focus your thoughts on your techniques and therapeutic goals for this client.

The fact is that all massage practitioners and all clients are human beings, and human beings are sexual beings. Neither the client nor the massage therapist leaves their essential nature outside the massage room. The challenge for both people in a massage is to be who you really are, which has many, many facets – including a sexual nature – but understand that a professional massage is a context in which any expression of your sexual nature or your client's sexual nature is inappropriate.

Create a safe and non-sexual environment in your practice

Be alert to your own feelings of sexual attraction and to signs that a sexual attraction may be taking place for clients. Subtle signals and comments that pass unnoticed can create an ambiguity which invites confusion about these issues.

Make sure your dress and general appearance convey a professional, not a sexual intention. Make sure there are no items in your massage room that could invite sexual confusion, such as suggestive artwork.

It is advisable to outline in advance what the client can expect during the massage session, including draping. Communicate in advance about whether to massage the abdomen and other potentially provocative parts of the body.

Choose language that does not invite confusion. Use scientific names for body parts, and avoid personal or evaluative comments about the client's body, such as making statements about how they look.

Avoid careless contact with the client's body. Do not contact the client's body with your trunk or legs.

If you feel sexual attraction while giving a massage, do not deny to yourself that you have these feelings; do not act on the feelings; acknowledge the feelings and make a conscious choice to sacrifice this sexual attraction for the sake of your career and the client's therapeutic experience.

Never initiate sexual contact with a client

Occasionally, stories are reported about professionals, including massage therapists, who sexually accost their clients. This is damaging to the profession as a whole, and disastrous to the lives of the therapists involved.

It is one thing to decide to date a client, to become friends, and make a transition from a therapist/client relationship to whatever personal relationship you both decide to have. That presents no particular moral or ethical problem.

It is another thing to attempt to initiate sexual activity with a client *during* a professional massage. This is immoral, unethical, and illegal. The massage relationship involves trust on the part of the client, who becomes vulnerable to the therapist. In this sense, the relationship resembles that of a doctor and patient, or priest and penitent. The trust placed in you by your client gives you a greater responsibility to be honest and above board in your dealings.

If you feel a desire to initiate sexual activity with your clients, seek professional help. You may be able to learn something about yourself in the course of working with this desire. If you are unable to control this desire, your best course of action may be to stop practicing massage, or to limit your practice to men only or women only.

10 For Men Only

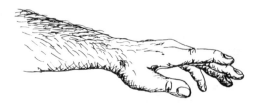

The challenge for a male massage therapist

In the massage field in general, attracting clients and becoming established is more difficult for a man than for a woman. This is not true in certain specialties, like sports massage, on-site massage, Rolfing, Trager, polarity, and other forms of bodywork that do not involve nudity and stroking. It is also not true in some other countries, such as Germany, where men tend to be accepted as massage therapists more easily than women.

However, in the field of Swedish massage in the United States, experience shows that most clients prefer having a woman give them a massage. Most women are shy about becoming undressed and being touched by a man they are not intimate with. Many also have self-image issues and are embarrassed to have a man see their bodies. Many men feel uncomfortable being touched by another man, and prefer the nurturance they receive from a woman's touch.

Some groups of clients that prefer male therapists

Some men prefer a male therapist because they want to avoid any possibility of arousal. Such groups include Catholic priests, orthodox Jewish men, and men with strong moral principles.

Many gay men prefer a male therapist, apparently because they are more comfortable in the company of men.

Many athletes and very muscular men prefer a male therapist, having the belief that most women lack the strength to give them a satisfyingly deep massage.

Some clients are gender-neutral

A certain number of clients do not care whether their massage therapist is male or female, but choose a therapist on personality and skill level. Such clients are a minority. Generally speaking, such clients are probably more common in cosmopolitan areas and on the west coast.

The task for a male massage therapist

Because the available client pool for men is smaller, men have to try harder, be better, and have more patience than women when establishing a massage practice.

Men can and do succeed in the field, and some men become tremendously successful. Do not allow the challenge to discourage you. Knowing the situation in advance will allow you to better plan your career and focus on target groups which are likely to produce clients for you.

The male as pursuer

Societal conditioning, and perhaps instinctual patterns, result in men generally pursuing women sexually and initiating sexual contact in relationships. As a result, men tend to be in the habit of seeking sexual encounters.

One very successful male therapist told me that he considers it a great advantage to him that he is married. His desire to couple is focused on his wife, and he feels much more relaxed than he otherwise would about working with his women clients.

If this issue is a problem for you, there is no magic solution. Simply be honest with yourself, and exercise your will and creativity to avoid confronting your clients with sexual energy that will create problems in your professional life.

Avoiding allegations of impropriety

Although only about one in five U.S. massage practitioners is a man, male massage practitioners are the subject of more than half of the allegations of improper conduct. An allegation of this type, even if eventually proven to be untrue, can nonetheless be terribly traumatizing, embarrassing, and costly.

A male massage therapist must be very clear and very careful to ensure that he will not be the subject of an allegation of improper conduct. Clear communication with clients will help. Having clear intention to work solely in a therapeutic way will help. Having strong and well-defined boundaries will help.

Male therapists should pay close attention to the advice in Chapter 9 (Sex and Massage), Chapter 11 (Working with Survivors of Childhood Sexual or Physical Abuse), and Chapter 13 (Ethics and Boundaries). Together, the awarenesses and recommendations in these chapters will give you a framework for practicing in a scrupulously ethical way that will greatly reduce any possible confusion on the part of you or your clients, and will be your best "insurance" against allegations of impropriety.

11 Working with Survivors of Childhood Sexual or Physical Abuse

Recent years have seen a dramatic increase in society's awareness of childhood abuse as a prevalent social problem. Those who have been abused as children may or may not remember being abused. They may have been abused sexually or non-sexually, and may or may not have begun the journey of healing the effects of that abuse.

As a massage practitioner, chances are you will come in contact with a number of clients who experienced childhood abuse. There are no definite figures about the extent of the problem, but some studies have estimated that 20 to 30 percent of females and 10 to 15 percent of males in the U.S. and Canada are sexually abused before reaching age 18.

Some of these individuals become massage clients, and they may or may not have a conscious awareness of the abuse they endured. If they come to a massage practitioner without any awareness of their childhood trauma, treatment by an unprepared massage therapist can result in the client having extreme reactions that include terror, convulsions and withdrawal. The purpose of this chapter is to learn about these potential clients, their sensitivities and vulnerabilities, and the precautions and procedures that will assist you in avoiding re-injuring such clients.

Most massage clients are women, so the female pronoun is used throughout this chapter. Also, most childhood abuse is sexual in nature, but many clients have also experienced non-sexual abuse as children.

I wish to thank Mary Ann DiRoberts, who provided substantial assistance in the preparation of this chapter, and also Diana Lonsdale and Anya Seerveld, both of whom provided useful information.

Childhood abuse and the damage that results

Children have natural mechanisms to deal with stress, but extremely strong experiences can overwhelm these mechanisms. Sexual or physical abuse is too much for the child to deal with, and it can prevent the normal integration of the psyche as the child matures.

One aspect of this process is numbness, or dissociation. Minor dissociation is a natural part of life for most people, taking the form of spacing out, daydreaming, or similar behaviors. However, more significant dissociation can result in a state in which the person is not aware of the physical sensations of the body, or is not consciously present in the experience of the body. In extreme cases, multiple personalities are created and the person lives a life as different personalities who may not even know each other.

Psychologically, childhood abuse destroys the child's sense of safety and trust, and drastically violates the child's boundaries. The child may grow into an adult who has difficulty trusting and is confused about boundaries. One who experienced childhood sexual abuse may have guilt about the sensations she had during the abuse, feel shame or responsibility for the abuse, and have terror buried in her body from these childhood experiences. As an adult, she may feel like "damaged goods" and may believe that sex is all she is good for, or that she is not even good for that.

While you should not attempt to diagnose someone psychologically, certain traits can provide clues that childhood abuse *may* be an issue in someone's life. Signs to look for include depression, lack of emotion, extreme changes in emotion, feelings of being different or defective, dysfunctional relationships, irresponsible sexuality, anorexia, bulimia, obesity, childishness or excessive vulnerability, inability to take care of oneself, workaholism, compulsive rituals or other compulsive behaviors, and anxiety attacks.

It is important to remember that unless you are trained as a mental health professional, you should not attempt to be a psychotherapist for a person who experienced childhood abuse. In fact, unless you have specialized training in practicing massage with abuse survivors, you should consider declining to practice massage with such a client. Without the understanding and skills necessary to work with such clients, you may do more harm than good by giving a massage.

The intake interview

When initially interviewing a client, do *not* directly ask if she experienced childhood abuse. Asking this question violates the client's boundary; it requires her to either lie or disclose something she may not wish to share with a person she does not yet trust.

It is better to ask generally whether bodywork brings up feelings for her. You may tell her orally or in your printed information that you invite her to let you know if she is in psychotherapy. Rather than probing too deeply, carefully listen and watch for signs that may alert you to a history of abuse.

During the massage

The abused child has been dis-empowered, has had trust violated, and has not had boundaries honored. When massaging this adult client, be careful to empower her and to operate with clear boundaries. Be scrupulous about giving control of the session to the client. Be clear about your permission to touch in specific places or in specific ways. Check in often with your client to be sure she is comfortable with the session and is present in her body. To feel safe is the primary need for a client who has been abused, and a lack of safety can cause such a client to dissociate even before being touched.

Even a client who is not an abuse survivor will appreciate being empowered, respected, and given control. Since you likely will not know that a particular client is a survivor, consider these guidelines with all clients.

It is especially important to check in often during the massage with a client who has a history of abuse or who shows any indications of such a history. When your touch triggers an emotional response or a memory of abuse, this client may be unable to tell you what is happening. The abusive experience often includes training in "not telling," and when a memory of that experience is triggered, the training to be silent may prevent the client from letting you know what is happening.

If a client recalls a portion of the abusive treatment during a massage session, it can be extremely upsetting for the client and a difficult situation for the massage therapist. A "flashback" can feel to the client like a flood of terrifying feelings. She may dissociate from current time and reality and be completely immersed in an experience of the childhood events. She may shake with terror, convulse, go into tetany, curl up in a ball, or shout at the perpetrator.

If you as a therapist find yourself with a client having such an experience, remember that this person is re-experiencing a terrible event from her past. If you can, talk to her in simple language, telling her where she is and what is happening in the present moment. Suggest that she open her eyes and describe the room you are in, or make eye contact with you, or change her position to sitting or lying on her side.

If she tells you about her experience, let her know you understand what she tells you by rephrasing it in your own words. Maintain boundaries and give her control over what happens, and assure her that you will stay with her and keep her safe as long as she needs you. After the experience has passed, she may still need your support and attention. Help her make specific plans for the rest of the day, and encourage her to use whatever support is available in her life. If the client is not in psychotherapy, this would be a good time to make a referral to a qualified practitioner.

Because flashback experiences can be so very unsettling, it is advisable to assure that a client with a history of childhood abuse has a psychotherapist if she is going to work with you doing massage. Because of the likelihood that your work will bring up such an intense experience, the client should have the services of a professional who can help process such an event if it occurs. If you intend to specialize in working with clients with histories of childhood abuse, you should have additional training in this area, be in supervision, and have done your own psychotherapy.

One survivor's experiences with massage

The following is excerpted from an article that appeared in The Journal of Soft Tissue Manipulation. Written by Tess Edwards, it describes the experiences of a woman who experienced ritual satanic abuse as a child, and became a massage therapy client as an adult.

Her descriptions of various massage experiences and suggestions for therapists have great value. As you will see from reading the following, Tess is a client who dissociates during massage. Her massage therapist practices safe touch work, which requires specific training to do.

I wish to express my gratitude to the Journal of Soft Tissue Manipulation for permission to reproduce this essay.

One trauma survivor's experience of massage
by Tess Edwards

I believe strongly in the importance of massage for survivors of child abuse. I feel very lucky that I am one of the few survivors I know who can both afford and tolerate a weekly massage.

In my search for healing, I saw an applied kinesiologist who told me that my trauma has settled mostly in the muscle and skeletal systems instead of the organs, as is more common. So for me, I believe that massage is crucial to the healing process because the toxic effect of the trauma is lodged in my muscles. Even when the toxic effect of abuse is primarily in the organs, I believe that massage is essential to the healing process—not only because safe touch is an important and unusual experience for most survivors, but also because trauma is held in the body.

Dancers talk about muscle memory—that is how they learn the intricate moves they must make on stage. We all have muscle memory. I have never been comfortable placing my arms above my head—I have never been able to paint a ceiling or hang curtains without going into a state of panic. Similarly, I usually postpone washing my hair for as long as possible. I always called myself lazy, stupid or other nasty names because I could not do these tasks. And I never understood that this had any meaning.

I now understand that many of my worst life experiences took place while my hands were tied above my head for long periods of time. I still have trouble with this. In fact, as the memories surface, difficulty with these tasks has increased. Now even in aquabics class I have tears rolling down my face when I try to do the above-the-head arm exercises. This is typical. As the memory surfaces, the symptoms intensify.

I've always thought that massage would help me, but it has been a long battle to allow myself to afford it and to learn how to tolerate it. For three or four years, I got massage treatments about three times a year. For the most part, I don't think they helped me at all because I simply left my body during them. Touch of this type is really a re-enactment of the original abuse and in fact gives me even further to go in my healing journey. In one case, the massage I received was truly a re-enactment of the abuse and for months undermined the healing work I was doing.

One massage therapist really upset me when she was giving me her new-age philosophy about how we all choose our lives—have choice even about abuse in childhood. One of the hardest things to recover from is the guilt and shame that every survivor I've met feels about the abuse. Hearing their stories, I have noted that in most cases, the abuser blames the victim: "You're too sexy." "You make me do it." "You love it." "You know you want it."

"You're making me evil" was what my father used to say to me and he even taught one of my personalities to beg him for intercourse at an early age. So for my massage therapist to tell me that I chose either to come back in this life as a victim of child abuse, or that I as a child had some choice in the matter, pushes all my shame and guilt buttons. If I'm lucky, this makes me very angry. If I'm not, I feel despair.

My biggest difficulty with massage, although it took me a long time to realize it, was that any touch was triggering. Two years ago, a group of four survivors of sexual abuse started a self-facilitated group based on giving and receiving safe touch. In our weekly five-hour sessions, we would ask for what we wanted that night — anything from getting a back rub, to being rocked while we sang lullabies, to massaging just a hand, to building a protective igloo with pillows, to brushing hair. Any activity involving touch that the survivor could accept that evening.

During these sessions two of us began retrieving new memories of abuse while in the group. Instead of being a group for safe touch, the group became, temporarily, a group for memory retrieval. The memory work triggered by the touch was so intense for the other two members of the group that they asked us to stop. We then formed a group specifically for memory retrieval, which has been going on for over a year now and from which I have benefited enormously. Another survivor I know began the process of retrieving memory when she began to receive massage. This is why I feel that massage is so very important and so very tricky for survivors.

Currently, I see a massage therapist once a week, and it is helping enormously. Three nights ago, I had a dream that my body turned from metal into flesh. Last Sunday in my memory retrieval group, I was able to feel and express many more of the feelings that I felt as a child than I have before.

The massage is still hard sometimes. We're still trying to develop a system so that I can ask her to stop. We haven't found a good way yet because when I need her to stop, I'm in a child part who was trained not to speak; stopping wasn't an option, no matter how desperately she wanted to. It's hard for my massage therapist to help when I go there because the signs are subtle to non-existent. This is partly because I received tons of training on how to pretend everything was alright.

I think my massage therapist is learning my body enough to notice when I hold my breath or, more often, when my flesh just feels dead or uninhabited. I don't know how she does it. She checks with me a lot, which for me is great because it can sometimes give me permission to say that I am in trouble.

I have learned to set some boundaries. We do not work on my bum. I allowed her to work on my upper legs once and got so badly triggered that I was unable to say so until a week later. During that week, I wandered around in flashbacks. My inner thighs are now off limits.

My massage therapist tells me a lot of things about my body which are very useful to me because I've spent most of my life outside of it. She is helping me to learn about my body, making it easier to reside there.

There are a number of things I feel that a massage therapist should do when working with me. I am sharing these ideas so that other massage therapists might learn about how to help someone who has been abused.

- First and foremost, I am more important than your technique. If I can't lie face down, I need you to accommodate me. Maybe massage me while I'm on my side, even if it means you can't give me what you feel is your best work. Give me what is best for me, not your best work.

If I leave my body, you can make my circulation shoot around better, but that's it. For me, the purpose of massage is to get more into my body, not leave it more. If I'm not present, I'm not getting what I need. I need to learn to feel pleasure in my body. Pleasure is something that has never been safe for me.

- Be creative. If I can't tolerate lying down, you could have me sit on a chair with my arms on the table and do just my head and neck. If I need to keep my clothes on, figure out how you can help me with my clothes on. Encourage me to bring my teddy bear if I am terrified.

- Help me to feel safe and comfortable. I love to be rocked and so do my inner kids. I love to be warm and adore my massage therapist's heating pad and the warm blankets she covers me with.

- Find out what you need from me in order to help me. Find out my other support systems. You can't be all things for me. You're not my therapist and you're not responsible for my healing or the bad things that happened to me. If you sense that my support structure is weak, be careful if you trigger memories that you can't take me through.

- Respect me and my process. I know best about me, just as you know best about you.

- One of the skills I value the most in my massage therapist is her understanding of emotional release. It is wonderful to know that she can handle anger, grief or terror as they come up and work with them, instead of being terrified by them. She has a big bucket with a pillow on it for resting my hands on when I am on my front or hitting if I need to release some anger.

- Learn to detect the difference between re-enactment and release. Re-enactment and release can look the same but have an opposite impact on the survivor. Both re-enactment and release can cause the survivor to show physical symptoms of grief, fear or anger. However, in re-enactment, the survivor is lengthening the work she has to do. She has yet one more incident of feeling powerless and victimized to recover from. In release, she is letting go of some of the abuse and actively reclaiming her life.

Being placed in a re-enactment can help enormously if I am ready for it and I choose it. I went to my massage therapist once after a particularly nasty memory where my hands were tied. I specifically asked her if she could work on my wrists and as she did, it felt as though hundreds of wrist restraints fell off as I cried. The relief was wonderful.

- Learn about triggers: what they are, how they work and how to cope with them.

- Please refer me if you are uncomfortable working with me. Don't sabotage my courageous act of attempting to find safe touch and learning to re-inhabit my body.

To me, my healing process involves recalling my life and integrating the sensory information that I blocked or dissociated from my awareness. This includes my emotions, my spirituality and the events, sights, sounds, smells, tastes, textures that I have been unable to allow into conscious awareness. I want to experience my life as a whole.

One of the most useful parts of healing is massage. To be touched without sex, without violence, is a first for me and a great gift. To learn that it is safe to allow someone into my space is incredible. To begin to release the trauma is a relief.

IV

Business, Practical and Legal Information for the Practitioner

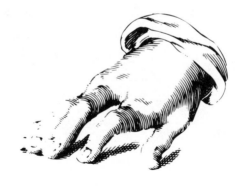

12 Business Basics and Practice Pointers

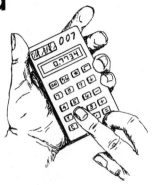

Practicing massage means operating in the business world. If you have no significant experience doing business, certain expectations of the business world may not be familiar to you. The purpose of this chapter is to give you enough information to avoid pitfalls and facilitate your success.

The subjects covered in this chapter are Steps You Can Take Toward Professionalism, What to Expect From Clients, and Pricing Your Services.

A. Steps You Can Take Toward Professionalism

1. Communicate Clearly and Keep Agreements

The business world operates by mutual agreement. In order to run smoothly, agreements must be unambiguous, and both parties must be able to rely on the other to keep the agreement.

In practice, this means you and your client should have no confusion about where or when appointments are to take place, how long they are for, how much they cost, and what sort of therapy the client is expecting you to provide. Keeping your agreement means arriving on time to all appointments with all the equipment you will need.

If an appointment is tentative, make sure both of you know when you will speak again to make it definite. If there are any questions in your mind about an agreement, speak to the client about them. The chances are that your client also has questions.

2. Present a Well-Groomed Image at Work and After Work

Most massage therapists understand the need to present a professional image at work. Your physical appearance announces who you are, and if you are proud of your work the image you present should convey that pride.

As a community member, you will see and be seen by your clients after working hours at unexpected times. Your appearance and your actions at these times will also have an effect on your clients' perceptions of you. While you need not constantly look over your shoulder, keep in mind that anything you do in public reflects on your professional character. If you have a wild side, you might want to keep it indoors.

3. Answer Your Phone in a Businesslike Manner

Even if you have separate office and home phone numbers, you should answer both your home and office phones in a polite way. You never know who is calling with what opportunity, and it is a shame to spoil an opportunity by creating a poor first impression.

4. Return Phone Calls Promptly

Make a point of returning your phone calls as soon as you can. Keeping people waiting for a return call will train them to expect you to be hard to reach; they may think twice about calling you next time. You also run the risk that the person who is trying to reach you will find someone else to meet her needs, and you will have missed an opportunity.

5. Make Cleanliness a Priority

Massage clients are very sensitive to the issue of cleanliness. If they find you or your office unclean, they will not tell *you*, but they will tell others.

Since massage is such a personal service, clients will want to be sure the linens are fresh, the carpet is clean, and your clothing and body are clean. If in doubt, go overboard, as some clients have a very critical eye when it comes to hygiene.

6. Avoid Talking Too Much During a Massage

If your client wants to talk, let her talk. It's her massage and her hour. However, do not use the massage as a time to talk about yourself, your problems and your opinions. If your client is being quiet, then you should be quiet as well, unless your conversation concerns an issue related to the massage session.

Several of my clients have told me they left their previous massage therapist because he or she would not keep quiet during a massage. Notice that they did not tell the talkative therapist—they told their new therapist.

7. Watch the Details of Client Comfort

Show concern for your clients' experience. Their perception of their entire experience with you is important, not just the result of your hands working their muscles.

On a physical level, make sure your clients are warm enough. Be aware of any modesty issues. Avoid getting oil in their hair, and offer to towel off excess oil. Avoid causing any pain during the massage, unless you and your client both agree that aggressively working a body part is the best thing to do.

On the level of emotions and boundary issues, make sure you honor the right of your clients to reveal or not reveal facts about themselves, to have portions of their body worked or not worked, and in general to be in charge of their session. Don't let your desire to give override the client's wishes about what to receive.

8. Finish on Time

Clients are often on a busy schedule. You may want to do that extra five or ten minutes, but your client may feel it's more important to be on time for her next meeting. If you want to go past the agreed ending time, get the client's permission beforehand.

9. Get to Know the Other Therapists in Your Area

Become acquainted with as many massage therapists, fitness trainers, physical therapists, bodyworkers, chiropractors, acupuncturists, psychotherapists and medical doctors as you can. The more people who know you, the more opportunity there is for them to assist you in your professional growth.

Remember that you are becoming a service professional. Allow yourself to assume membership in the community of those who are serving others' health needs. Knowing a large number of health professionals gives you a broad perspective on the field, and on the level of activity in your community. Be as involved in the total picture as you can.

10. Foster Your Own Personal and Professional Growth

As one therapist told me "There are massage therapists, and there are massage therapists, but the ones who make it are the ones who are working on themselves."

Examine what it is you offer your clients—what benefits your work gives them, and what kinds of difficulties your work helps them get through. Chances are, you are offering your clients help with the kinds of issues you also face in your life.

Acknowledge that you are also a client. Practice what you preach. Nurture your own growth through finding therapists and healers and teachers who help you grow. In the process, you will also learn new techniques that you can incorporate in your bodywork. The process of growth has no end.

B. What to Expect from Clients

1. Cancellations

Clients will cancel; plans change. It is an unavoidable fact of life. You can create a cancellation policy to protect yourself, so long as you communicate it to your clients. One fair cancellation policy is to require 24 hours advance notice, and to charge a penalty (such as $25) for canceling on shorter notice. A sign on your desk or office wall, where it can be seen by your clients, is adequate to communicate your policy.

Consider a "one-miss" policy; each client gets to cancel or miss one appointment without penalty, and is then told that your standard procedure will be enforced for all subsequent times. You may also want to consider a "percentage" policy; a client can cancel or miss once after ten or more consecutive appointments.

Whatever policy you choose should be fair to you and fair to your clients. You must be able to manage your time so that your practice supports your life. At the same time, your clients' lives may be complicated and they may have to deal with emergencies and unexpected events. Try to create a policy that balances your need for a predictable schedule with clients' needs for flexibility in extraordinary situations.

2. Great Expectations

One lesson I have learned over and over is not to place any importance on statements by clients like "I'm going to get a massage every week" or "I've got half a dozen friends who have been looking for someone like you." If I had the fee I would have charged all the people who told me they were coming in for a massage, I'd be considering retirement by now...

I'm sure they mean it when they say it, but the fact is people talk about getting massage much more than they actually follow through. Once you are an established therapist, these "great expectations" are not of great importance. However, if you are seeing four clients a week and needing the rent money, it can be harder to keep this sort of thing in perspective.

3. No-shows

Some clients make an appointment, do not cancel, and do not show up. This is about as frustrating a situation as you can get practicing massage, and there is very little you can do about it.

The great majority of no-shows are clients who have never been to see you before, and who learned about you either through the yellow pages or a newspaper ad. One way to control the problem is to require that all people making appointments give you first and last name and a phone number where they can be reached to confirm the appointment.

If you call the number and they never heard of the person, don't be surprised if he does not show up. If you call the number, and they sound shocked that the person is getting a massage, don't be surprised if he never arrives. With experience, you will learn to evaluate the likelihood of the person showing up for the appointment based on your experience in calling to confirm.

When a first-time client fails to cancel or to show up, let that person go. This is a person you will not hear from again, and it will not do you any good to try to track him down. Put your energy into those who want and need your services.

The decision what to do when a regular client fails to cancel or to show up for an appointment is more difficult. It helps to have an announced cancellation policy, but if you do not you will need to decide whether to charge your client for the missed appointment or simply reschedule.

4. Angels

Once in a blue moon, you will get a client who takes it upon herself to be your fan club, publicity agent, networker and marketing strategist. Say a prayer of thanks.

An angel is someone who thinks so much of you and your work that she is inspired to do anything she can to help you succeed. This person will be thinking about you and talking about your work many times a day. Some are able to do more than others, but all act out of a feeling of love and caring.

My angel is one of my less affluent clients, and as a gesture of my appreciation, I have never raised his rate from the low introductory rate I was offering when he first became my client several years ago.

5. *Constructive Critics*

Most clients will not let you know that you caused them pain, or that they were too cold or too hot, or annoyed about something in your massage room. Although they will not tell you, such unspoken dissatisfactions cause many clients not to return for another massage.

That is why you should be grateful for the very few clients who ask you not to do a certain stroke, or complain about the temperature, or ask you to change this or that about your massage or the surroundings. In all likelihood, these clients speak for many others as well.

One such client of mine is a chef with a very acute sense of smell. One day while I was seated and working on his face and head, he asked me to please breathe to the side. Apparently, he was able to identify just what I had eaten several hours ago.

Until this time, I had not realized that I have a tendency to breathe through my mouth, and to exhale onto my clients' faces. Most clients probably did not notice any breath odor, but they probably did feel my breath on their faces. Either way, I no longer breathe on people's faces. Unless my constructive critic had spoken up, I would never have realized what I was doing.

C. Pricing Your Services

Pricing your services can be a difficult issue. This discussion is meant to give you guidance in what to consider in order to find the most appropriate price for your services.

Several factors enter into a decision about pricing. The factors to consider are the "going rate" in your community, your expenses involved in providing the treatment, the price you feel comfortable charging, and the effect your price will have on your clients' ability to come to you.

1. *The "Going Rate"*

This refers to the customary charge for your kind of services in your area. The "going rate" for a one hour massage may be as low as $30 in some areas, and as high as $90 in other areas. Usually, there is a variation of $5 or $10 between the low and high ends of the "going rate." In my area, for example, the price for a one-hour massage ranges from $55 to $65.

Consider that the "going rate" is the rate charged by established professionals who have a clientele. A time-honored custom among newly-trained professionals is to slightly undercut the going rate when they are first attracting a clientele. To the cost-conscious consumer, the lower fee is an incentive to try this therapist. In addition, the lower fee is an acknowledgement that a newly-trained professional is still learning, and has not yet acquired fully mature skills.

If you choose a rate *far* below the going rate, for example $15 per hour, people will become suspicious that you are not really a trained therapist, and it may actually be harder for you to attract clients than if you charged a fee nearer the going rate.

As your skills and reputation grow, you will naturally raise your rates to a level that reflects your growth. Your clients will adjust to your new rates without much difficulty, especially since your new rates will be in line with the rates established therapists are charging. While some clients may find it hard to accept a rate increase after becoming accustomed to a lower price, most clients who know and like you will not leave you when your rates rise to the "going rate."

2. A Price You Are Comfortable With

For you to be comfortable with the fee you charge for your services means at least two different things. It means, first, that you are comfortable asking your client to pay your fee—you believe your service is as valuable as the money you receive for it. This touches on issues of self-worth. Your fee should be one that you can ask for and receive without mixed feelings.

Second, being comfortable with your fee means that it creates an income for you that meets your needs. You should feel that it compensates you for what you have given in your therapy session, and that it provides you with the means to have the material things you need to keep your life and practice going. If you feel you are not being nourished in your professional life, you may find yourself resentful and unenthusiastic about your work.

3. Effect of Pricing Decisions on Clients

One massage client told me "If massage costs $40, I'll come in twice a month. If it costs $60, I'll come in once in six months." I suspect this client speaks for many others.

Massage clients are generally quite cost-conscious. Many people would like to have massage on a regular basis, but feel they cannot afford it. Compared to items like a bag of groceries, a movie ticket or a tank of gasoline, massage is an expensive item to fit into a budget.

Even the wealthy are often quite cost-conscious. Many wealthy individuals either do not believe they have enough money, or resent people trying to charge them a premium because they are wealthy. They will shop for the best price, and reject a therapist who charges what they consider too high a price. This may not apply to a celebrity clientele, or the enormously wealthy, but the run-of-the-mill millionaire often watches prices very closely.

Therefore, your pricing decision may well affect the amount of business you get, the ease with which you generate new business, and the frequency of your repeat business.

4. Working on a "Sliding Scale"

Sometimes it is not possible to meet all the goals mentioned above with one set fee. In some cases, you may need to make exceptions to your price or work on a "sliding scale." This means that you charge some clients a lower fee because that is all they can afford.

Some clients refuse to pay a reduced fee as a matter of pride. Others may ask you directly for a reduced fee. If you are comfortable working at a reduced fee for those with a financial need, there is nothing wrong with doing so. Charge a fee they can afford and you can comfortably accept. Do not price your work so low that the client no longer places a value on it, or that you become resentful of the imbalance in the relationship.

My normal fee is $65. For clients with financial hardship, I will reduce my fee as low as $40. If I worked for less than $40 I would feel taken advantage of. However, for someone who cannot afford $40, whom I feel really needs my services, I will work without charge.

5. Discounts for Series Purchase

A common device therapists use is to offer a discount to clients who purchase several massages in advance. For example, if the cost of one massage is $60, a therapist may sell a series of five massages for $250 ($50 per massage).

This benefits both parties. The client saves $50, and the therapist has the use of the money in advance for any necessary expenditures. The client has the option of giving one or more of the series massages to a friend, which brings potential new clients to the office.

To offer a series, you can have a coupon printed up and sell the coupon. It may have five places to punch holes, or five numbers to cross off, or any system you prefer for keeping track of when the massages are used up. You can also create a system without coupons, by keeping track in a record book.

6. Other Discount Arrangements

Create any discount arrangement that serves a business purpose. This can include discounts for those who refer new clients, or promotions in which you give a free massage to someone who buys two gift certificates, or any other such idea that makes sense to you. One discount I offer is $15 off the second massage in one week for any client.

Sometimes it is appropriate to offer a discount to a client for becoming a "regular." Take the example of Ray, one of my early clients. Ray came for massage an average of once a month. Sometimes he would come more often, sometimes less often.

At the end of a massage, I asked Ray if he would come in regularly if the price were lower. He said he would, and we discussed possible agreements.

We decided that he would like to come twice a month, and could afford to do so if he paid $30 per visit instead of the $40 I was then charging. This seemed advantageous to both of us, and we agreed to adopt this plan. Ray began coming in twice a month. He enjoyed receiving more massages and I appreciated the added business and income.

I would not make this offer to most of my clients. It felt right to do so with Ray, in part because Ray did not know any of my other clients, so I knew I would not be presented with multiple requests for the same arrangement. I offer this as an example of the creative marketing you can come up with to fit a particular situation.

7. Barter for Goods or Services

Bartering—exchanging your service for the product or services of another—can be a means of gaining clients who would not otherwise receive massage. It can also be a good way for you to receive valuable goods or services without a cash outlay. In addition, clients with whom you barter may refer cash clients to you.

Barter can be done on an equal basis—one hour for one hour. It can also be done on an unequal basis. For example, if you barter with your physician, you may have to give more massage time than you receive from your doctor. On the other hand, if you barter for house-cleaning, you may receive more house-cleaning time than you give in massage service. One starting-point for negotiations is to compare the hourly rate for your services and the services you are bartering for, and adjust your barter arrangement accordingly.

Massage therapists who use barter find they can receive some great products and services through barter. Following is a list of services and items therapists have reported bartering for:

> Accounting services, advertising banner, airline tickets, auto repair, Barbie clothes, bodywork & massage, candles, chiropractic, computer equipment, contact lenses & eye exams, decorated cake, dentistry, dinners, electrical work, facials, gluten-free bread, graphic design, hair styling/haircuts, house cleaning, landscaping, legal services, linens for the office, manicures, medical services, office shelves, office sign, opera tickets, pedicures, prayers, printing services, psychic readings, sewing, stained glass, sweet corn, swing, teddy bears, trip to Cancun, voice coaching, waxing, wedding flowers & wedding cake, wristwatch.

You should be aware that the IRS treats barter as a taxable transaction. You are required to include the fair market value of the goods or services you receive as "income" when you file your year-end tax return, and pay taxes on it. It is true that the lack of a paper record of the transaction makes it difficult for the IRS to prove, but their policy is to prosecute those who do not report barter transactions when they can. In 1997, the pop artist Peter Max pled guilty to tax fraud, partly as a result of having bartered his artwork in partial payment for several homes without paying the proper taxes.

Another concern about barter is the issue of dual relationships. If you do emotional-based work, structural work, or work that involves any aspect of psychotherapy, barter may be an inappropriate way to interact with your clients because of boundary issues in the therapeutic relationship. Most psychologists will not barter for massage for this reason. Ethical issues about bartering for massage services are explored more fully in the next chapter.

13 Ethics and Boundaries

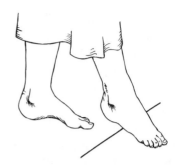

In simplest terms, having ethics means doing the right thing, or acting morally. In ordinary relationships, this means such things as telling the truth, being honest in business and keeping your promises.

In a professional relationship with patients or clients, you have a stricter standard of ethical conduct as a result of your professional relationship with your clients. For example, psychiatrists and psychologists encourage patients to share their secrets; therefore they have a special duty to protect their client's secrets. Lawyers encourage clients to entrust financial affairs to them; therefore they have a special obligation to be careful with clients' funds. All professions have special ethical rules and obligations based on the nature of their relationship with clients or patients, and the special kind of trust the professional requires to do their work.

As a massage therapist, the extent of your ethical obligations depends on the type of work you do. The more vulnerable your clients become, the higher your ethical obligations. The more your work requires clients to trust you in order for the work to succeed, the higher your ethical obligations.

If your work involves encouraging clients to access emotions, or if you work at a deep level with clients' bodies or psyches, your ethical obligations are stricter than someone who does only chair massage or relaxation massage.

The Fundamentals of Ethics for Bodyworkers

What are the basic ethical requirements for a massage practitioner? The most essential ethical obligations can be summarized in the following three categories: (1) confidentiality, (2) integrity in your business practices, and (3) respect for boundaries. Let's look at each of these items individually.

Confidentiality

In some professions, the law creates a formal guarantee of confidentiality—lawyers, doctors, priests, and psychiatrists have a *legal* obligation, not just an ethical obligation, to protect any communications between themselves and their clients, patients, or parishioners.

As a massage therapist or bodyworker, you do not have the same legal obligation of confidentiality, but you do have an ethical one. Your clients should never have to worry that anything about their relationship with you will ever embarrass or injure them.

That means that all discussions with your clients should be considered confidential and should not be repeated. The details of a client's personal life should never be repeated outside the office. Even repeating the facts in a story without naming the person can be risky, as the person you tell the story to may have enough information to "put two and two together" and figure out the identity of the person in your story.

Consider the idea that confidentiality might even extend to the question of whether a certain person is a client or not. Is it possible that any of your clients would not want a certain person to know they are a massage client? Perhaps you have a high-profile client whose privacy is extremely important to him or her? Perhaps you have a client who comes from a social group in which massage is not accepted and has chosen not to let her friends or associates know she receives massage. This is a "gray area" in a practitioner's ethics, but give some thought to this question, and you will see how important it is to safeguard your clients' confidences in general.

Integrity in Your Business Practices

In Chapter 12, we discussed the basics of business for a massage practitioner, including such topics as being on time and keeping agreements. Some of these topics overlap with ethics.

One important part of integrity for a massage practitioner is making sure that your clients understand in advance what service you are providing and what compensation you expect. If you give a "one-hour" session, does that mean you schedule appointments on the hour—including time for intake, undressing, and dressing—or does it mean you have a session lasting one hour on the table? This should be discussed in advance so there is no chance for confusion to arise.

If your gift certificates have an expiration date, explain that when you sell them and let the purchaser know the reason. If you have a cancellation policy that requires full or partial payment for a missed appointment, make sure your clients understand the policy clearly before you enforce it.

The key elements of business integrity are standing by your word and clarifying the terms of your agreements. Practice these two traits and clients will be better able to relax about the business aspects of your relationship and focus on receiving the healing and nurturance you are there to provide them with.

Boundaries

Sometimes part of a massage education is learning to become intuitive and "merge" with your clients at some level.

Another aspect of your work as a massage therapist is to recognize and enforce the separation between yourself and your clients. Protecting the "sovereignty" of your clients will help them feel safe in their relationship with you. Protecting your own "sovereignty" will help you to focus your full healing abilities on your clients without distraction or confusion over personal issues.

In short, boundaries ensure that, as a massage practitioner:

- your clients are safe

- you are comfortable

- you are not distracted in your role as therapist

The term "boundaries" may not be familiar to you. The word boundary usually means the border, or edge, or limit of something. In the context of a massage practice, "boundary" refers to the separation between you and your client; respect for the separateness of the two of you and for the areas within each of you that should remain off limits to the other. In this chapter we are discussing boundaries both for you and your clients; each of you needs to be able to set limits.

The Primary Boundary Is the Client's Right to Set Limits on Touch

The first and foremost "boundary" in a massage relationship is that the client is in control of where and how to be touched.

In other words, whatever the client asks you not to do must be scrupulously honored. This may be something as simple as not getting oil on her hair, or not touching her feet, or any other request the client may make. In addition, touching any body areas that could be considered sensitive or inappropriate should not be done without first specifically asking the client.

You create safety for the client by establishing that boundary between the client and yourself, so that the client knows her privacy and safety will be respected.

The primary boundary of inappropriate touch means of course that any sexual contact during a massage is unethical. However, it means much more than that. It means that any unwelcome contact during a massage is unethical. Some clients may be uncomfortable with massage on their chest, abdomen, buttocks, inner thigh or upper leg.

As the therapist, it is your ethical obligation to make sure that you understand the client's wishes about being touched. You should ask about any possibly sensitive or questionable areas before massaging them.

Beyond the Primary Boundary

Touch is not the only subject that raises boundary issues for a massage therapist. Let's look at some examples of day-to-day activities in the life of a massage practitioner that can also raise the issues of boundaries:

- Do you allow clients to phone you at home? If so, what times of day are OK and what times of day are not?

- Do you work in a home office? If so, does it have a separate entrance or do clients walk through your home to get to the office? Do you allow pets into your office? Are the sounds of your home audible during sessions? Do clients encounter other family members as they enter or leave?

- How much do you tell your clients about your personal life? Do you volunteer information about yourself or only answer their questions, or not answer any personal questions at all?

- Do you socialize with your clients?

- Do you barter with your clients?

Dual Relationship

Socializing or bartering with your clients creates a "dual relationship". The term "dual relationship" refers to the situation where you have a therapist/client relationship, and you enter into another, different relationship with the same client. The second relationship may be a social or romantic relationship, or it may be an employer/employee relationship, where the client works for you in a barter arrangement.

A number of ethical concerns need to be addressed regarding dual relationships to assure you do not endanger your basic therapist/client relationship when you also engage in another kind of relationship with a client.

The major risk in dual relationships is that your therapist/client relationship will be compromised by some aspect of the new relationship. For example, assume you trade massage services for lawn mowing services. You agree that each hour of your services will be compensated by two hours of lawn mowing.

What if you feel your grass needs to be cut on Thursday, but your client is not available to do it until Sunday? What if the client does not mow to your satisfaction, missing an edge now and then, or leaving too many clippings on the lawn? What if you sense the client is working slowly and you feel you are not receiving full value in return for your services?

Any of these could cause you to feel resentful, or to feel like you should hold back and not give your finest work to the client because you are not being properly compensated in the barter relationship. Anything that causes you to hesitate in giving your best work creates a problem in your therapeutic relationship with your client.

On the other hand, what if your client feels taken advantage of because she is spending more time mowing than you are massaging? What if the client feels your standards about how she performs her lawn cutting are too high and she resents you telling her how to perform the work? These feelings can easily carry over to the massage relationship and make the client uneasy about continuing as your client.

I used the example of lawn mowing, but similar problems could creep in for any kind of barter relationship—if you trade for hair cutting, accounting services, house cleaning, or any other kind of service, there is always the possibility that the way the service is performed will create an issue for you or for your client, which will affect your therapist/client relationship.

Barter for goods is less of an ethical problem, because goods can be objectively valued, but even so you still need to be careful of ethical issues. If you and your client decide in advance on the value of your service and the value of the item you are bartering for, you might avoid conflicts.

But what if you "really" feel you should give only three massages for an item, whereas the client wants four? If you agree to four massages instead of three, will you skimp on the time or hold back to make the deal seem fair to you? If not, will you feel resentful about the arrangement? Such a feeling could hinder your work and unconsciously create a situation where your therapist/client relationship is compromised.

Your client also may have difficulties with the barter relationship — she could feel that she is not receiving your "best" professional services, or that the terms of the exchange are not fair to her.

Power Imbalance in the Therapeutic Relationship

To complicate matters further, there is a natural tendency in a therapist/client relationships for the therapist to be "in charge". After all, you set the fee, you direct the activities during the session, you are the "performer" and the client receives your work. Because the relationship has you as the "expert", there is a tendency for the client not to speak up when troublesome feelings creep in, or to defer to your judgment or authority within the context of the massage relationship.

Therefore, if a client with whom you are bartering has some discomfort about the way the barter transaction is going, she may not feel free to express these feelings, and these unresolved feelings can become an irritation to the client and damage the working relationship you both have with each other.

Romance and Dating

Another kind of dual relationship is the social or romantic relationship with a massage client. We all know that social and romantic relationships can have their ups and downs, and can get complicated. Combining social or romantic relationships with a therapeutic relationship can create confusion and even turmoil in the therapeutic relationship.

To avoid difficulties, I recommend that if you are interested in dating a client or seeing a client socially, you first refer that person to another therapist and stop your therapist/client relationship. There is no ethical barrier about dating an ex-client. This does not involve a dual relationship and it does not raise any ethical questions (unless your work is psychotherapeutic in nature).

Find Your Individual Answers to Ethical Questions

Not all massage practitioners need to set up exactly the same boundaries. The need for boundaries depends in part on the kind of massage work you do, and in part on your personality and the way you relate to your clients.

For example, are you naturally a very open person, sharing your life with friends and acquaintances alike, comfortable opening up without first forming a close personal bond? Or are you more reserved, needing to feel comfort and trust before revealing the feelings and ideas that are important to you, reserving such communications for close and trusted friends? Your personal style may dictate how open you are with your clients and how much of your life you will allow them to share without risking your comfort zone.

With these considerations in mind, make policies that are appropriate for you as to:

- The times at which you will take calls at home
- The extent to which you socialize with clients, either individually or in group situations
- Whether to barter your sessions for goods or services
- What kind and how much personal information you tell your clients

Do you work with vacationers, or on-site clients, or other people whom you probably will not see on a regular basis? Or do you work with people in distress, those experiencing emotional problems, survivors of touch trauma, or those who are seeking more than just massage, but some form of healing?

The kind of work you do dictates the level of trust your clients need and deserve, and should guide you in establishing boundaries that make your therapy room a safe place for your clients to become vulnerable and receive your deepest work without risk.

Consider whether it is appropriate for you to:

- restrict or eliminate dual relationships with clients
- research or study the issues of transference and counter-transference
- engage a supervisor who can oversee and guide your professional conduct

It may seem contradictory, but many therapists have found that limiting their relationships with clients improves their work. By having clear boundaries, both parties are able to keep their focus on the therapy and not be distracted. Clients can remain clients longer and can receive your best work.

Supervision

A common practice among psychotherapists is to hire an experienced colleague to provide supervision. Supervision involves meeting on a regular basis to discuss with your supervisor the work you are doing with your clients. It is a time to bring up any difficult, confusing, or unclear elements of the relationships with your clients, and receive objective evaluation and guidance.

If you are doing relaxation massage, you probably do not need supervision. If you are doing medical massage, you likewise probably do not need supervision. However, if you are regularly working with survivors of abuse, or touch trauma, supervision may be an important part of your professional life. Work such as this, which can evoke strong and unpredictable feelings in the client, requires a degree of attention and skill that may not be natural to you unless you have had specific training in working with clients such as these.

Even with less sensitive clients, supervision may be helpful to a practitioner in developing communication skills that allow clients to be heard more fully about how they need the therapeutic relationship to change. This type of supervision is akin to coaching, in which a more experienced practitioner can show you opportunities you may be missing to listen more carefully to your clients' needs and provide your clients with a more comfortable and effective relationship. This can have a very positive effect on your practice, improving the effectiveness of your work and helping with client retention.

Transference and Counter-transference

These are terms psychologists use to discuss aspects of the therapist/patient relationship. Transference refers to the client bringing feelings into the relationship from experiences earlier in life, and experiencing those feelings about the therapist. For example, a client's feelings about a father or mother may unconsciously be "transferred" to the therapist, and the client's relationship with the therapist can be colored by these feelings.

Counter-transference is when the therapist brings feelings to the relationship which become "transferred" to the client, such as identifying with the client, or trying to "fix" the client instead of providing the client with the tools to solve her own problems.

Dr. Ben Benjamin, head of Muscular Therapy Institute in Cambridge, Massachusetts, has written:

> Normal personal boundaries and cultural taboos of touch are automatically transgressed in massage. For this reason, massage is a relationship in which therapists need to be cognizant of transference and counter transference, boundaries, abuse, and therapeutic dynamics.

To a certain extent, the simple act of touch, especially coupled with disrobing, creates the possibility for feelings to arise and cloud the relationship between the client and the therapist. Because massage inherently transgresses boundaries, perhaps all massage practitioners should undertake supervision to improve their professional relationships and provide the best possible care to their clients. However, supervision would probably be regarded as an unnecessary refinement by most practitioners of pure relaxation massage.

However, anyone who works more deeply than the basic levels of muscle, fascia and physiology should seriously consider supervision, or at least a study of transference, counter transference, abuse and therapeutic dynamics. Once you enter the realm of emotions and the psyche, you can find yourself swimming in deep waters before you know your way around.

If your work is intended to provide healing, or emotional or psychological growth, you should invest in some study of the therapeutic relationship so you have a better understanding of the predictable issues that will arise both for you and for your clients as you do this work.

If you wish to further explore the issues discussed in this chapter, you may want to read *The Educated Heart*, by Nina McIntosh, Decatur Bainbridge Press 1999 ($22.95). This book is a detailed instructional guide about ethics for bodyworkers by a certified Rolfer. It is written from the perspective of one whose work is intended to be deeper than relaxation massage, and if your work is of that type, it contains many insights and awarenesses that may be useful to you in your practice.

14 Staying Healthy in a Demanding Field

Every successful massage therapist I have spoken to has had to deal with some kind of physical or psychological problem that resulted from doing the work.

The most common physical problems are wrist injuries, back strain, neck and shoulder pain, and nodules (ganglia) in the fingers. In addition, some therapists suffer depression, some take on pain in places where their clients have it, and some "burn out" from the stresses involved in a massage practice.

There are practical ways you can avoid these problems. Successful therapists offered these tips from their experience:

Body Mechanics

Watch your body mechanics. Don't bend over when you work. Keep your spine straight and bend your knees. Let your force come from your hara, your abdominal center. Use the minimum number of muscles necessary for any particular motion. Make your body mechanics your first priority, even above the quality of work you do on your clients.

Exercise

Do yoga, tai chi, aikido, stretching, jogging, swimming, aerobics or some other exercise to improve your own bodily well-being. This helps not only to keep your body in good condition, but also to reduce the effects of stress.

Introspection

Involve yourself in psychotherapy, or meditation, and have a support group you can turn to in times of need. This will help you release your emotions, help you stay healthy, and promote your own growth.

Diet

Eat a balanced diet and drink plenty of water. You depend on your body as you would on a professional tool. You put good gasoline in your car, and keep the oil changed. Treat your body at least as well.

Attitude

Learn to let go. Life in the business world will bring you ups and downs, rewards and frustrations. Learn how to let go of the painful aspects. Letting go is not the same as denial or repressing your feelings. Accept people and situations as they are, let your emotions flow, and move on.

Receive Massage

Get massage on a regular basis. Three reasons: it promotes your overall health and well-being; you will learn techniques and awarenesses from receiving massage that will make you a better massage therapist; your credibility with your clients will be better if you "practice what you preach."

Specifics of Body Maintenance

Keep your wrists straight as much as possible while you work. Stretch your wrists before and after working. Use open fist or elbows to do deep work instead of fingers or thumbs.

If a nodule appears in a finger, try not to use that finger in your work for a week or two; apply pressure with the other fingers of that hand, but raise the finger with the nodule slightly so it is not used. If the nodule persists, work it with transverse friction to break it up. Consult a physician if the nodule will not recede.

Use a paraffin bath for sore hands, ice forearms or use liniment if inflamed.

The Sense of Isolation

In many ways, massage is a solitary occupation. That may seem strange, since massage cannot take place unless two people are together at the same time and place. However, in most settings, a massage practitioner typically has little verbal communication with clients during the session. This can lead to a feeling of loneliness for the practitioner.

Those who practice chair massage may feel less of this effect, since conversation is more common during chair massage than table massage. However, in a clinic or office setting where you are practicing relaxation or therapeutic massage, most practitioners do not start conversations unless the client does, and usually limit conversation to topics related to the treatment or the client's concerns.

Some practitioners find that keeping a keen focus on the client's needs and the importance of each session helps to avoid a sense of isolation. Others find that entering a meditative state while working helps. Also important is to set aside quality time for yourself after work, whether that is social interactions, self-guided time, hobbies or, as is discussed below, vacations and days off.

Vacations and Days Off

After working intensely to make your practice a busy one, you may find that success, when it finally comes, is a shock to your system. If you find yourself very busy, make time to take care of yourself physically and emotionally.

Sometimes it is difficult to switch from the "I need all the clients I can get" consciousness to that of "I need to take time for myself." In the beginning, you do not have enough clients, and you are doing everything you can think of to get more. The time will arrive, however, when the clients will be coming. Allow yourself at that point to step back from your practice and make sure you are not wearing yourself out trying to achieve more "success" than you can stand.

Don't Lose Your Sense of Humor

Sometimes we can take our work so seriously that we lose our spontaneity or suppress our individuality. Charlotte M. Versagi, a professional journalist and massage therapist, wrote an essay that first appeared in Massage Magazine exploring this important aspect of staying healthy in a demanding field. "How Enya Stole My Sense of Humor" is about the art of balancing your professional demeanor with the need to be who you really are.

How Enya Stole My Sense of Humor—And How I Got It Back Again
By Charlotte M. Versagi

Somewhere in this process of becoming a massage therapist, I've lost my sense of humor. In the past, I listened to Broadway soundtracks; I whistled while I worked, said hello to strangers on elevators, smiled at my plants. Somehow, as I became focused on healing, I became morose.

We're not talking clinical depression here, folks; I'm getting out of bed in the morning and dressing myself. But I've lost part of myself—my joy—and as much as I love my profession, I'm quite sure it's a direct result of my immersion into this healing business.

I think this is how it happened: I'm a career changer, so when I started massage therapy school I worked full-time and attended school full-time. I hunkered down, determined to learn it all and prove to myself I hadn't lost the ability to succeed in academics. For two straight years I lost all social skills while I merely worked and studied.

I then became keenly aware of the beautiful responsibility of actually putting my hands on complete strangers who were naked under sheets on my table. *Wow*, I thought. *Awesome. Better take this seriously.* So again, I hunkered down, and studied energy work and the chakras so I could combine my spiritual knowledge with bodywork. Made me very successful, but again, very serious.

Then the music. Got to have that new-age sound. So instead of remembering the words to the *Mickey Mouse Club* theme song, I repeatedly listed to the music of dead, chanting monks or deader saintly nuns. Enya and Yanni were as light as I allowed myself to get.

People were leaving my table calm, all right. Feeling as if they had been given a haven, a safe place from the world. My candles, my hands and my music were really doing the job. And I became progressively more serious. No more hellos on the elevator; after all, I was looking for auras. No more singing Broadway musicals while I cleaned house. Tina Turner gathered dust.

Then one day I realized I had lost joy. I thought I was supposed to be a certain kind of person in order to be a massage therapist—calm, quiet, gentle, wise, somehow deeper and more perceptive than the rest. OK, fine, I may be some of those things—but I am also an Italian-American woman who occasionally raises a little hell; someone who has been known to stop traffic on a busy street just for the fun of it. And that's what I had lost—the fun of it.

It's time to loosen up, to rediscover my joy. But how? Baby steps.

Last night I dusted off Tina Turner and Gershwin. I blasted them so loud I thought my neighbors would come knocking. I ate a chocolate donut—taking the dreadful risk of upsetting my chakras—gasp! I dragged out all my rhinestone jewelry and put every piece on a purple sweatshirt and sat in my apartment, grinning. I packed up all my white cotton uniforms and made a note to purchase colorful, lively professional garb.

And today, when I saw a client who has multiple sclerosis—and who loves Broadway shows, I played Gershwin during the massage. You should have seen his smile. And the energy we exchanged during that massage—Wow! He left the table with a lift in his step I hadn't seen before

No, I'm not tossing all my Enya—but she's no longer the reigning queen.

I'm a complicated, joyful human being. My clients deserve better than a tightly wrapped massage therapist with a preconceived, canned concept of what it's like to be a healer.

With all due reverence to my beloved profession, I nailed a favorite picture of myself on my office wall—right next to my Reiki certificate. It's a picture of me at 3 years old. I'm running straight at the camera, hair flying, coat wide open, and a smile on my face that could warm the world. That picture is going to remind me to keep singing musicals and to give that smile to the world. Preconceived ideas of healers be damned—my hair's too busy flyin'!

15 Laundry and Linens

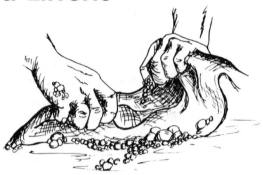

If you do Swedish massage, the issue of laundry is one you will face throughout your career. Unless you work in a setting where your employer takes care of laundry, you will have to make certain decisions about how to supply yourself with fresh linens to practice your trade.

Hire a Laundry Service vs. Do It Yourself

Depending on the laundry service you choose and what type of draping you use, having your laundry done for you can cost between $1 and $2.50 per client. Doing it yourself will bring the cost down dramatically, to between 10 cents and 50 cents per client.

If you hire a service, you will have to choose between furnishing your own linens and using theirs. If you use theirs, the cost will be higher. If you furnish your own, you will need twice as many as if you did your own wash, because at any given time, half your sheets and towels will be at the laundry.

Hiring a service makes the most sense in these situations:

1. You do not have a washer and dryer in your home or office. Trips to the laundromat can be very wearing when you are taking several loads per week.

2. You have a busy massage practice. If you are seeing lots of clients, then you are making enough money to afford paying a service to launder for you. If you have a busy practice, you probably do not have the time or energy to be dealing with the large amount of laundry your practice generates.

Choosing a Laundry Service

If you decide to use a laundry service, shop around. The prices charged by different services will vary quite a bit, as will the quality of their service.

Things to consider in hiring a service:

1. They may require you to use their sheets and towels, or they may be willing to sell you sheets and towels at wholesale prices.

2. If you use their linens, be sure this company will supply sheets and towels you will like. See and feel samples before making an agreement.

3. Some massage oils can be difficult to remove from linens unless the company has the proper chemicals. Be sure they have experience with massage therapists and they understand how to get these linens clean.

4. If you use a service, and they deliver a load of sheets and towels which are unsuitable in some way, you will be stuck with them unless the company is willing to make a special trip to remedy the problem. Find out how willing the company is to make sure problems will be taken care of and your needs will be met.

Drop-off at a Laundromat

Another choice is to use your local laundromat as a cleaning service. Most laundromats offer the option of having their staff wash your clothes for a fixed price, usually 50 to 75 cents per pound. You may have to supply special detergent to make sure the oil residues are fully removed. (See page 126) However, having a laundromat launder your linens may be a cost-effective "in-between" solution that is cheaper than a service but easier than doing your own laundry.

Finding Suppliers of Sheets and Towels

Buying a few linens at a time

If your practice is a casual one, meaning that you work on just a few clients a week, you will need a relatively small amount of linens, and should therefore purchase sheets and towels in the same way you do for personal use.

One option to consider is buying twin sheet sets. These include one fitted sheet, one flat sheet and one pillowcase, and sometimes can be found on sale for not much more than the cost of a single sheet. The fitted sheet on the table covered by the matching flat sheet creates a pleasant appearance.

Some therapists are quite particular about the linens they use, and this can be a very sensible attitude. The sheets and towels come in contact with a client's body, and you may want to create a luxurious impression by using colorful linens with a lush texture.

Buying in quantity

If you are most interested in presenting a clean (white) image, and keeping your costs to a minimum, consider purchasing sheets and towels through business channels. This is a decision to make when you begin to establish yourself in the field. It is not unlike a carpenter buying a set of tools—think toward the future and invest in a supply of sheets and towels you will be able to use for years to come.

Most companies that sell sheets and towels commercially are in the habit of selling at least 50 dozen at a time. The difficulty lies in finding a vendor who supplies linens commercially and is also willing to sell by the dozen. These are rare, but they do exist.

You will get some help looking in the yellow pages under "laundries." If your community has a Business-to-Business yellow pages, check under "linens." Occasionally, a commercial or institutional laundry will sell you one or two dozen odd or surplus sheets. These companies have large clients, and need to buy sheets by the gross for their own purposes. If they are willing to deal with you, you may be able to get a couple of dozen sheets from them at a discount price.

If you cannot locate any such businesses in your area, consider contacting someone who may have the connections you do not have. Your local hospital may be a wholesale purchaser of sheets and towels, and if you get in touch with the purchasing agent, she or he may be willing to resell a few dozen to you.

Choosing Sheets and Towels

Sheets

Whether you do your own laundry or use a service, you will still need to decide what size and quality sheets and towels to use. The thicker and more luxurious the linens, the more they will cost to buy and the more they will cost to launder.

Composition of sheets.   The quality and comfort of sheets is determined by the "thread count." This is the number of threads used in a square inch of the fabric the sheet is made of. A higher thread count means a softer sheet. A thread count of 180 or higher usually signifies a good quality sheet. A thread count of 250 or more signifies a very luxurious sheet.

Also consider the fabric composition. The higher the percentage of cotton, the softer the sheet; the higher the percentage of polyester, the coarser the sheet.

Size of sheets.   Keeping the size small helps a great deal in keeping the cost down at laundry time. Sheets come in a great variety of sizes, and the actual size of the sheets you receive may be a few inches smaller than the stated measurements.

The normal size of a massage table is between 72″ × 26″ and 72″ × 30″. Two standard sheet sizes to consider are 72″ × 42″ and 75″ × 54″.

The actual size of the sheets you buy will be slightly smaller than the size stated on the package. This is partly because the stated size is "before hemming," and partly because it is accepted practice in the industry to have minor variations in sheet sizes. Therefore, a sheet that is called 72″ long will actually be a few inches shorter than that, and will not quite cover the length of a massage table.

A 72″ × 42″ sheet is ideal for a table that has a face hole; it will cover the rest of the table and overlap a bit on all sides. It is also a good size to drape over a client, as it will cover most people from the neck down. A 75″ × 54″ sheet will cover the entire massage table, and will drape a few inches farther over the sides.

For a better looking image, you can leave a larger sheet draped over the table, concealing the legs. For each client, change the 72″ × 42″ or 75″ × 54″ sheet.

These smaller sheets are convenient to handle in laundry, and will take up a minimum of space in your washing machine. In fact, well over a dozen 72″ × 42″ sheets will fit into a normal washing machine at a time.

As you shop for sheets, you may hear a confusing mix of terms used to describe sheets—terms like "draw sheet," "twin sheet," "standard," and other terms. These names have general meanings, but they do not convey accurate information about the size of the sheets you will actually be buying. Keep in mind actual measurements only. Decide what size will be best for your style of draping and the image you want to create, and then shop with these requirements in mind.

Towels

The same considerations apply to towels as apply to sheets. The larger and more luxurious a towel is, the costlier it will be to purchase and launder. Keeping the size down is a big help.

Many standard sizes are available to fit almost any need. The size I find most convenient is 20″ × 40″. This is the size of a small bath towel. I find it meets my needs for draping very well, while taking up a minimum of space in the cabinet and the washer.

The quality of towels is measured in "pounds per dozen." This means, simply, how much does a dozen of these towels weigh? For a given size towel, the "pounds per dozen" figure will give you an idea of how thick and fluffy the towel is.

For the size I use, 20″ × 40″, a normal weight might be 6 or 7 pounds per dozen. I use a towel that weighs 8.5 pounds per dozen, because I want a soft and hefty feel to my towels. Towels like these are available for around $2.50 each, plus shipping, when purchased wholesale. A wholesale order is usually 16 dozen towels. I purchased 16 dozen of these towels, and had no trouble selling my extras to local massage therapists, leaving me with a large supply of towels at a low cost.

If you are doing comparison shopping, remember that increasing thickness increases "pounds per dozen," and increasing size also increases "pounds per dozen." It helps to decide on the size you want, and then compare the different towels of that size based on the "pounds per dozen" figure. So long as you are comparing towels of the same size, the "pounds per dozen" figure will give you a good measure of the thickness of the towel.

Tips for Do-It-Yourself Launderers

Doing your own laundry has advantages. First, you are in control of how many clean sheets and towels you have, and you know you will not run out unexpectedly, or have to rely on someone else to get your needs met.

Second, it is much cheaper to do your own laundry. Even factoring in the cost of a washer and dryer, in the long run doing your own laundry will probably cost only 10% to 20% as much as hiring a service.

Have the machines at your place

The most important consideration, if you plan to do your own laundry, is to have your own washer and dryer, in your home or in your office—whichever will be most convenient to your practice.

When your washer and dryer are convenient to use, you can throw in a load and be busy working, reading or relaxing. Throwing in a load becomes a routine activity and not a tedious chore, as it is when you have to leave your home or office to go to a laundromat. In addition, if the washer and dryer are for the exclusive use of your business, their cost can be deducted for income tax purposes (see Chapter 19).

Water dispersible oils

Most oil manufacturers now sell water-dispersible oils that reduce to oil buildup in sheets and towels. With water-dispersible oils, the oil removal process is now needed much less frequently than it was before this innovation. However, even with these "improved" products, oil will still accumulate in your linens, and you may need to purchase a product to remove oil residues.

Jojoba oil and fractionated coconut oil

Practitioners recommend pure jojoba oil as a non-staining oil that reduces or elimi-nates oil buildup in sheets.

Another non-staining oil is fractionated coconut oil, which has the greasy com-ponents removed by a high-pressure process. If you purchase fractionated coconut oil, find a supplier you can trust, as some practitioners have reported quality issues with distributors of this product.

Beating oil residues

The following common products are all recommended by practitioners as success-fully removing oil residues from linens:

Additives
½ cup baking soda added to each load
one cup vinegar plus ½ to one cup borax added to each load
one cup powdered bleach plus one cup borax added to each load
2 to 3 tablespoons of Dawn dishwashing liquid added to each load
Biz non-chlorine bleach (follow instructions on box)

Pre-soaks
Citra-Solv – soak linens for 1 to 24 hours before laundering
Simple Green – soak linens for 1 to 24 hours before laundering

In addition to these "home remedies," several different products are marketed specifically to massage therapists for removing old residues from massage linens: Fresh Again, Oil Be Gone, Sunfresh Soap, Pure Pro Orange, and Totally Clean and Fresh. You can purchase these products from the following suppliers:

Fresh Again is available from:

Biotone
4757 Old Cliffs Rd.
San Diego, CA 92120
1-800-445-6457
(619) 582-0027
www.biotone.com

Oil Be Gone is available from:

> **Golden Ratio Bodyworks**
> P.O. Box 440
> Emigrant, MT 59027
> 1-800-796-0612
> www.goldenratio.com

Sunfresh Soap is available from:

> **The Body Shop**
> 2051 Hilltop Dr., suite A-5
> Redding, CA 96002
> (530) 221-1031

Pure Pro Orange is available from:

> **Pure Pro** at 1-800-900-7873

Totally Clean and Fresh is available from:

> **Order Desk** at 1-800-541-8904

Hints for success with Fresh Again

Fresh Again is the oil removal product I tried first. I have been happy with it, so I have stayed with it. Through experience, I have learned the following:

You do not need to use Fresh Again each time you wash. Use it to treat your sheets and towels when you notice a buildup of oil. You will notice either a rough texture, or the odor of cooked oil when the linens get hot in the dryer.

Shake well before pouring to mix the detergent fully. Use the hottest water you can. Use a larger amount of detergent for heavy oil stains. For persistent stains, soak the linens in hot wash water overnight and complete the wash in the morning.

If you have stubborn oil stains, you can use about ⅓ cup Fresh Again to one or two gallons of water, and boil the linen in this mixture at a low boil for about five minutes. A remarkable amount of oil comes out of a soiled linen with this process.

16 Professional Associations

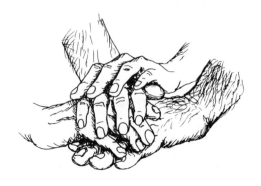

This chapter describes the major professional associations for practitioners of massage. The largest of these organizations are American Massage Therapy Association, Associated Bodywork and Massage Professionals, and IMA Group. These three associations are profiled first.

For many practitioners, the primary motivation for joining a professional association is to obtain liability insurance, also called malpractice insurance. If liability insurance is the only benefit of membership you are looking for, you have the option of purchasing such insurance without joining any association. Insurance is available for $109.92 to $125.28 per year through Massage Magazine (1-800-872-1282 or **www.massagemag.com**), or for $175 per year through Healthcare Providers Services Organization (1-800-982-9491 or **www.hpso.com**).

However, the major professional associations offer more than just insurance. Each of the "big three" professional associations has a referral program for its members, and provides all members with practice-building materials. In addition, AMTA provides a bi-monthly magazine, a newsletter, chapters in all 50 states, and the opportunity to vote in association elections. ABMP provides a bi-monthly magazine and pre-paid legal consultation services.

Each of the associations has a different view of the issue of state regulation of massage. AMTA promotes standardized educational requirements and seeks to set the standard for massage education in the United States. ABMP has no official position for or against massage legislation, but tries to work for laws based upon consensus among the practitioners that will be affected by the laws. IMA Group has not been active in the legislative arena, but maintains divisions for many non-massage modalities such as movement, reiki, estheticians, and many others.

As is discussed in Chapter 3, politics often plays a major role in the interactions between these associations. Some people have strong feelings about the conflicting approaches of the associations, and sometimes have strong opinions about one or more of these associations. Your choice of which association to join may be a practical one, or it may be an emotional one. Below are some of the facts and figures you can use to help you make your choice.

Association Profiles

General Membership Organizations

American Massage Therapy Association ® (AMTA®)

820 Davis St., Suite 100
Evanston, IL 60201-4444
(847) 864-0123
www.amtamassage.org

The AMTA is the oldest professional association for massage. It was founded in Chicago in 1943.

Requirements for membership:

> *Associate Memberships* is available to massage students and recent graduates, and to massage therapists who were trained outside the United States. Associates may belong to the organization for up to three years while they pursue the requirements of Professional Active Membership. ($169 per year plus chapter fee of $0 to $30.)

> *Professional Active Membership* is available to practitioners who are certified by NCTMB, or licensed by states that meet AMTA's 500-hour curriculum requirement, or who have graduated from a COMTA-approved school or have previously been Active or Professional AMTA members. ($235 per year plus chapter fee of $0 to $30.)

All members receive professional and general liability insurance, optional health, life, business and disability insurance at group rates, member discounts on catalog products, listing in AMTA's *Membership Registry*, voice at AMTA meetings, *Massage Therapy Journal* and *HANDS ON Newsletter*, right to use ATMA logo in promotional materials, and the right to participate in state chapters and on state and national committees.

Professional Active members also receive inclusion in the free therapist locator service, voting privileges at meetings, the right to serve as officer of the organization, and pin and patch.

AMTA's Commission on Massage Therapy Accreditation (COMTA) accredits massage therapy training programs. As of publication, the following schools were accredited by COMTA:

AK: University of Alaska, Anchorage

AR: Arizona School of Massage Therapy
     Desert Institute of the Healing Arts

CA: Mueller College of Holistic Studies

CT: Connecticut Center for Massage Therapy

DC: Potomac Massage Training Institute

FL: Core Institute
      Educating Hands School of Massage
      Florida College of Natural Health
      Florida School of Massage
      Sarasota School of Massage Therapy

GA: Atlanta School of Massage

IL: Chicago School of Massage Therapy
      Kishwaukee College

IN: Alexandria School of Scientific Therapeutics

IA: Carlson College of Massage Therapy

ME: Downeast School of Massage
      New Hampshire Institute for Therapeutic Arts

MD: The Baltimore School of Massage

MI: Ann Arbor Institute of Massage Therapy

MS: Mississippi School of Therapeutic Massage

NV: Nevada School of Massage Therapy

NH: New Hampshire Institute for Therapeutic Arts

NJ: Academy of Massage Therapy
      Healing Hands Institute for Massage Therapy
      Institute for Therapeutic Massage
      Somerset School of Massage Therapy

NC: Body Therapy Institute

OR: East-West College of the Healing Arts

PA: Career Training Academy
      Pennsylvania Institute of Massage Therapy
      Pennsylvania School of Muscle Therapy

TN: Tennessee Institute of Healing Arts

TX: Lauterstein-Conway Massage School

UT: Utah College of Massage Therapy

VA: Cayce / Reilly School of Massotherapy
      Virginia School of Massage

WA: Ashmead College
      Brenneke School of Massage
      Brian Utting School of Massage

WI: Lakeside School of Massage Therapy

COMTA can be contacted at (847) 869-5039, ext. 140 or at **www.comta.org**.
AMTA has created the AMTA Foundation, a tax-exempt public charity which funds massage therapy related research, community outreach, educational scholarships and conferences (see Chapter 20).

Each year the association sponsors one national conference and one national convention. Chapters exist in all 50 states, the District of Columbia, and the Virgin Islands, and some chapters have regional meetings.

Of the professional associations for massage, AMTA is the most active in the legislative arena. AMTA helps chapters and members to promote legislation which it believes will assist the profession, and it funds selected efforts to keep or change laws governing massage. Some individuals within the AMTA work to have laws passed that require attendance at an AMTA-approved school, and some states have passed laws requiring AMTA-approved schooling, but the advocacy of such laws is not official AMTA policy.

Associated Bodywork And Massage Professionals (ABMP)

28677 Buffalo Park Road
Evergreen, CO 80439-7347
1-800-458-2267 or (303) 674-8478
www.abmp.com

ABMP was founded in 1987. It attempts to be an effective, efficient, non-bureaucratic networking and services organization.

Requirements for membership:

Membership at the *Certified* or *Professional* level requires a practitioner to be licensed by a state that licenses massage, *or* be currently a registered or certified member of an approved association, *or* obtain a passing score on a recognized certification exam, *or* demonstrate at least 50 hours massage training plus a nursing or physical therapy degree.

Certified level requires 16 hours of continuing education every two years. Cost of membership: *Certified* $229 per year; *Professional* $199 per year

Membership at the *Practitioner* level is available to those in non-licensed states with at least 100 hours training from an approved program. Cost of *Practitioner* level membership is $199 per year.

Membership at the *Student* level costs $39 per year

Membership at the *Supporting* level costs $60 per year

Members at the Certified, Professional or Practitioner level all receive professional liability insurance including yoga instruction coverage (Certified has higher liability limit), referral service, regulatory interaction, pin, decal and certificate, subscription to *Massage & Bodywork*, membership newsletter, Massage & Bodywork Yellow Pages and Successful Business Handbook. Members are also eligible for group rates on business insurance and disability insurance. Members who join for longer than one year receive a discount on the second year dues.

ABMP sponsors IMSTAC, the International Massage & Somatic Therapies Accrediting Council, which accredits massage schools. As of publication time, the following schools had been accredited by IMSTAC:

AZ: Rainstar University

CO: Colorado School of Healing Arts

GA: Academy of Somatic Healing Arts
     Atlanta School of Massage
     Lake Lanier School of Massage

IL: Northern Prairie School of Therapeutic Massage
     Central Illinois School of Massage Therapy

IA: Carlson College of Massage Therapy

ME: Polarity Realization Institute

MA: Polarity Realization Institute
     Healing Touch Institute

MI: Kalamazoo Center of Healing Arts

MN: Minneapolis School of Massage and Bodywork
     Sister Rosalind Gefre Schools

MO: Massage Therapy Training Institute

NM: New Mexico School of Natural Therapeutics

PA: Career Training Academy
     East-West School of Massage Therapy
     Pennsylvania Institute of Massage Therapy
     Pennsylvania School of Muscle Therapy

TX: New Beginning School of Massage

ABMP sponsors research by Touch Research Institute and the Stanford Myofascial Institute.

ABMP attempts to foster a favorable legal climate for its membership, and has worked on a state-by-state basis to amend or defeat laws it considers biased.

International Massage Association (IMA Group)

P.O. Drawer 421
Warrenton, VA 20188
(540) 351-0800
www.imagroup.com

IMA was founded in 1994. Its mission statement includes the goals of taking massage mainstream, uniting all natural health care professionals and gaining respect for their professions, providing members with liability insurance at the lowest possible cost, and giving members marketing tools to help their practices grow.

Requirements for membership: 100 hours of approved training for practicing members.

Practicing membership costs $129 per year and includes liability insurance.
Associate membership costs $79 per year.
Student membership costs $50 per year.

Benefits of membership include free internet referral service, opportunity to establish merchant accounts to accept credit cards, opportunity for mortgage financing for home or office, and debt consolidation loans.

The IMA Group links the International Massage Association to its other divisions for movement therapies, aromatherapy, reflexology, yoga, caricaturists, colonic educators, kinesiology, personal trainers, aerobics instructors, and dance teachers.

In addition, the IMA Group sponsors the IMA Group Education Foundation, which provides massage training to single mothers, and the IMA Group Research Foundation, which benefits Touch Research Institute.

IMA hosts two annual conventions in Washington, D.C.; one for members and one for school owners.

In 2001, the IMA Group launched Touch Research Associates (TRA), a professional organization that offers the same benefits as IMA Group. However, a portion of the costs of membership in TRA is donated to Touch Research Institute (see page 171). Annual membership in TRA costs $179.00 or $249.00 depending on the level of professional insurance chosen.

International Myomassethics Federation (IMF)

1720 Willow Creek Circle, Ste. 517
Eugene, OR 97402
(800) 433-4IMF

IMF is an organization of professionals whose goal is to incorporate a wide range of accepted massage and bodywork techniques to promote health and well-being. It is run by the members and the officers are volunteers. IMF hires an executive director to run its daily operations. Its motto is: IMF is the "Organization with a Heart."

Requirements for membership:

Myomassologist: Minimum of 500 hours education from a state licensed or approved school of Myomassology or Massage Therapy, or equivalent. Continuing education requirement applies.

Certified Myomassologist: Successful completion of any recognized state, national or international massage or bodywork examination. Continuing education requirement applies.

Student Member: Currently enrolled in a state licensed or approved school of myomassology or massage therapy, or equivalent. Limit: two years.

Cost of membership is $65 per year in states without affiliate organization, and is determined by the affiliate in those states that have affiliates (currently Illinois, Michigan, Wisconsin and Ontario).

Benefits of membership include fellowship and networking, volunteer service recognition, discount on continuing education at conventions and affiliate conferences, product discounts, quarterly newsletter and professional massage journal, listing in IMF's International Directory, discounts on liability insurance through IMA Group or ABMP, available group medical and dental insurance, 800 number for home office resource information, certificate, patch and pin.

Specialized Membership Organizations

Medical Massage: American Manual Medicine Association

2040 Raybrook, SE, Ste. 104
Grand Rapids, MI 49546
(888) 375-7245
www.americanmedicalmassage.com

The American Manual Medicine Association was created to promote medical massage therapy as an allied health care profession and to differentiate it from other forms of massage. This goal is achieved through professional standards, education, and testing.

The association offers two levels of certification, a basic level of medical massage certification, and an advanced "board certified" level. Each level requires passing a different certification exam.

Membership is open to massage therapists with 600 hours of education including anatomy, physiology and pathology. Annual membership costs $175.00 and includes insurance.

The AMMA approves the following schools as offering training in medical massage:

AZ: Southwest Institute of Healing Arts
West Valley Massage College

CA: Advanced School of Massage Therapy
Alive & Well! Institute of Conscious Bodywork
Calistoga Massage Therapy School
The Institute of Professional Practical Therapy
Mueller College of Holistic Studies
Phillips School Of Massage

CO: Cottonwood School Of Massage Therapy
Massage Therapy Institute of Colorado

CT: Galen Institute

FL: Coastal School of Massage Therapy, Inc.
Core Institute
Florida College of Natural Health

GA: Georgia Institute of Therapeutic Massage

HI: Hawaiian Islands School of Body Therapies
Maui Academy of the Healing Arts
Maui School of Therapeutic Massage

ID: The American Institute of Clinical Massage, Ltd

IL: LifePath School of Massage Therapy
National University of Health Sciences

IN: Regional College Of Massage Therapy, Inc.
Vibrant Life Resources School of Wholistic Health

IA: Institute of Therapeutic Massage & Wellness

LA: Blue Cliff School of Therapeutic Massage
LA Institute of Massage Therapy

MI: Blue Heron Academy of the Arts and Sciences
Michigan School of Myomassology

MT: Asten Center of Natural Therapeutics

NJ: Academy of Natural Health Sciences
Body Mind & Spirit Learning Alliance
Institute for Therapeutic Massage, Inc.
JSG School of Massage Therapy

NM: BodyDynamics School Of Massage Therapy
The Medicine Wheel

NY: New York Institute of Massage
Onondaga School of Therapeutic Massage

NC: Therapeutic Massage Training Institute

SC: Charleston School of Massage

TN: Tennessee School of Massage

TX: Asten Center of Natural Therapeutics
Massage Institute
Sterling Health Center

VA: Cayce/Reilly School of Massotherapy
Virginia Academy of Massage Therapy

WA: BodyMind Academy
Spectrum Center School of Massage

WI: Blue Sky Educational Foundation

The above schools can all be located in the State-by-State directory beginning on page 237. AMMA's website lists several additional approved schools.

American Oriental Bodywork Therapy Association (AOBTA)

1010 Haddonfield-Berlin Rd., Ste. 408
Voorhees, NJ 08043
(856) 782-1616
www.aobta.org

The AOBTA is a non-profit membership organization for practitioners of oriental bodywork that was formed in 1989. It maintains a "Council of Schools and Programs" (COSP) which approves curricula that meet AOBTA educational standards. As of publication time, 17 schools and programs had been accepted into the Council.

Requirements for membership:

> *Certified Practitioner* level: 500 hours training, at COSP-approved school or taught by AOBTA-certified instructor. Application fee $30, dues $100 per year.

Associate level: 150 hours training, taught by AOBTA-certified instructor or qualified certified practitioner. Application fee $30, dues $75 per year.

Student level: Must be studying with AOBTA-certified instructor or practitioner. Application fee $10, annual dues $30.

Benefits of membership include the Organization's protection of the interests and rights and professional standards of Oriental Bodywork Therapy, high quality educational opportunities, legislative support and action-oriented representation, *Pulse* quarterly newsletter, member discount for advertising, optional insurance (professional liability, group health, disability), annual membership directory, practitioner referral service.

American Polarity Therapy Association (APTA)

P.O. Box 19858
Boulder, CO 80308
(303) 545-2080
www.polaritytherapy.org

Established in 1985, The American Polarity Therapy Association sets standards in Polarity Therapy practice and ethics, promotes public awareness, and cooperates with public agencies and other professional groups.

APTA approves polarity training programs, and as of publication date, there were 29 approved programs in the United States.

The association hosts an annual conference, publishes a membership directory, and produces Energy, a quarterly newsletter.

Membership costs $60 per year. Student membership is $40.

American Holistic Nurses' Association (AHNA)

P.O. Box 2130
Flagstaff, AZ 86003
(800) 278-2462
www.ahna.org

An organization founded in 1981 to promote the inclusion of alternative healing modalities into the practice of nursing. Membership is open to nurses, and costs $100.00 per year, or $50.00 for supporting members, students and seniors.

National Association of Nurse Massage Therapists (NANMT)

2203 Woodridge Court
Grand Island, NE 68801
(800) 262-4017
www.nanmt.org

The NANMT was formed in 1987. The NANMT is committed to bringing an increased awareness and acceptance of touch therapy to the mainstream medical and hospital community. It supports gaining insurance reimbursement for massage services, and also supports research into the health benefits of massage.

Active membership costs $75 per year, senior and student memberships cost $50, corporate membership costs $125, and supporting membership costs $75. Benefits of membership include NANMT's bulletin and quarterly publication, listing in annual directory, copy of directory, discounts, CEUs and use of NANMT seal on promotional material.

Nursing Touch & Massage Therapy Association, International (NTMTA)

1438 Shortcut, Ste. E
Slidell, LA 70458
(504) 893-8002
http://members.aol.com/ntmta/

A recently formed association for nurse-massage therapists. Active membership costs $100 per year, supporting membership costs $80, student and senior memberships cost $70.

Hospital-Based Massage Network

Hospital Based Massage Network
612 S. College Ave., Ste. 1
Fort Collins, CO 80524
(970) 407-9232
www.hbmn.com

A resource to promote and support the establishment of massage therapy in hospitals nationwide. The organization produces a regular newsletter, and provides a network of consultants and organizations that can be contacted for assistance with developing a hospital-based massage program (see page 32).

Volunteer Opportunities for Massage Practitioners

www.volunteeringmassage.org

It can be difficult to find information about volunteering your services as a massage practitioner. This website publicizes volunteer opportunities in the San Francisco area, and offers links to many resources about working with the infirm, the elderly or the dying.

Bodywork Modality Organizations

For additional specialized membership organizations see the Bodywork Directory that starts on page 217, as many individual forms of bodywork have guiding organizations that are catalogued under the particular bodywork modality listing.

State and Local Organizations

Many states and regions have their own massage and bodywork associations. Since these are usually volunteer organizations, the contact information changes frequently as officers serve their terms of office and move on. The best sources of up-to-date information for state and local associations are massage schools and practitioners in your local area.

17 Insurance

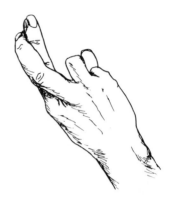

This chapter is about the types of insurance you can buy to protect yourself against certain risks. This chapter does not discuss having your work paid for by your clients' insurance, which is covered in Chapter 21.

Why Buy Insurance?

Insurance is risk protection. If you have no insurance, you bear all of life's financial risks alone.

The kinds of risks insurance covers are illustrated by the following examples:

- If you are sued by a client and lose, you are responsible to pay the amount awarded to your client by the court.

- If a client slips and falls in your office, you might be required to pay for that injury.

- If you are sued by a client for any reason, you will have to pay your own legal fees for defending the suit.

- If your office burns down or is vandalized, you absorb the loss.

- If you are injured and cannot work for a period of time, you will have no assistance in meeting your financial obligations.

- If you fall ill and need medical attention, you will have to pay the full amount of the medical expenses.

Each of the examples above illustrates one type of risk for which the self-employed bodyworker can purchase insurance. Each kind of insurance is profiled in the next part of this chapter.

Kinds of Insurance Available to the Professional Bodyworker

Professional Liability Insurance

This insurance defends you against claims by clients that you harmed them in the course of performing your professional services. The insurance company will provide a legal defense against a claim, and will pay any judgment against you, up to the policy limit.

These policies cover practically all claims of harm to a client during a massage. The major exception is for allegations of sexual misconduct by a practitioner. The insurance carrier used by ABMP provides a legal defense when a member is sued by a client for sexual misconduct, but will not pay a judgment if the practitioner is found guilty. The insurance carriers used by AMTA and IMA do not provide a defense to a charge of sexual misconduct, nor will they pay a judgment based on sexual misconduct.

Professional liability insurance has become very expensive in other professions. Lawyers and doctors pay very large annual premiums for this type of coverage because of the large number of lawsuits that are filed and the large judgments that result. However, the average doctor is about 60 times more likely to be sued for malpractice than the average massage therapist—and the average amount paid to settle a malpractice suit against a doctor is about 35 times as much as the average to settle a malpractice suit against a massage therapist. Since the risk of harm to clients by massage practitioners is so low, professional liability insurance for massage is quite inexpensive.

Sources of Professional Insurance

Professional liability insurance is a benefit of membership in the AMTA, ABMP and IMA. The associations purchase group insurance policies, and their per-member cost is very low. Discounted professional liability insurance is also available at an additional charge to members of the AOBTA, Rolf Institute, American Polarity Therapy Association, Trager Institute and Feldenkrais Guild.

Professional liability insurance is also available without joining an association. Insurance can be purchased for $109.92 to $125.28 per year through Massage Magazine (1-800-872-1282 or **www.massagemag.com**), or for $175 per year through Healthcare Providers Services Organization (1-800-982-9491 or **www.hpso.com**).

Types of Professional Insurance

Two general types of professional liability insurance are sold: "claims-made" insurance and "occurrence form" insurance.

A claims-made policy covers you for claims that are made while the policy is in force. "Claim" refers to the announcement by the client of their complaint against you. With this type of policy, you are covered if it was in force when the claim was filed.

An occurrence form policy covers you for incidents that "occur" while your policy is in force. The act occurs at the moment you allegedly caused harm to the client. With this type of policy, you are covered if it was in force when the alleged misconduct occurred.

The difference between these two types of policy comes up if you discontinue your insurance—for example, if you stop practicing massage. Say you began practicing in 1995 and purchased professional liability insurance at that time. On January 1, 2005, you retire from the practice of massage and discontinue your insurance coverage. A client comes forth on February 1, 2005 and claims you injured her during a massage you gave her in 2003.

An occurrence form policy would cover you in this case, because the alleged injury *occurred* while the policy was in force. A claims-made policy would not cover you, because the *claim* was made after your insurance had lapsed. For your protection, you should obtain "occurrence" form insurance, so that you are covered no matter when the client decides to bring a claim. Fortunately, all of the major professional associations for massage offer "occurrence form" policies.

The need for professional insurance

If you plan to have a significant career in the massage or bodywork field, professional liability insurance is virtually a necessity. While you may think you do not need such insurance because you have no significant possessions to lose anyway, consider the broader question of how being uninsured might restrict your career.

Spa owners, chiropractors and other massage employers will usually not hire an uninsured massage therapist. If the therapist is uninsured, then any client with a claim against the therapist would likely sue the employer, who does have insurance. An uninsured therapist is seen as an unnecessary risk and most employers therefore will not hire an uninsured practitioner.

Business Liability Insurance

Business Liability, or premises liability insurance, is "slip and fall" coverage. It protects you against suits that result from injuries people sustain on your business premises. The cause of these injuries might be icy steps, loose carpet, or any other cause of accidental injury.

Legally, you are liable for these injuries only if you do not keep your office in a reasonably safe condition for your clients. The legalities of how safe you need to keep it vary slightly from place to place. However, as a practical matter, any injury to a client is a potential problem, even if you are not ultimately legally responsible for it. If the client sues, you still will have to bear the expense of lawyer's fees to defend the action.

Business liability insurance covers both attorneys' fees to defend an action and any recovery that is ultimately awarded. It is included in the cost of membership in some professional associations (check with the association), and can be purchased on the open market through insurance agents and insurance companies.

If you practice in a home office, you can try to get a rider for your homeowner's policy to cover business liability. Some companies will issue these and others will not. You may need to change insurance carriers after setting up a home office because some companies will discontinue your coverage if they learn you operate a business in a home office. If available, a rider for your home office should cost between $100 and $250 per year.

Business Insurance

Business insurance covers your business equipment and premises against losses such as fire and theft. These policies usually cover the replacement cost of your equipment and supplies, and perhaps even petty cash in the office. Many will also cover lost income while your office is closed and the cost of renting temporary office space if your office is destroyed. Policies are generally available through major insurance companies and independent agents. Prices usually range from $250 to $500 per year.

Disability Insurance or Business Interruption Insurance

In the event you are unable to work due to accident or illness, disability insurance provides you with continued income. You usually must be disabled for several weeks (or several months) before the policy will pay you a weekly income, and you can usually collect payments under the policy up to a maximum of one year.

Disability insurance is not cheap; a policy to provide you with $300 to $400 per week in the event of disability may cost around $1,000 per year to purchase. It has also become increasingly difficult to find a company willing to write a disability insurance policy, especially for women. Decide whether or not to buy such insurance based on how strong your need is to be sure of continued income.

Medical Insurance / Group Medical Insurance

Policies for medical insurance are available in many forms, from bare-bones to deluxe. The costs of such insurance range from high to exorbitant.

The least expensive coverage is referred to as "catastrophic illness insurance." This insurance will pay for most of the expense of a hospital stay, after a deductible of, for example, $2000. This is protection against being turned away from a hospital when you need care, and against being placed into bankruptcy by an illness. Such insurance may cost $500 to $2,000 per year, depending on your age and place of residence. It is not available in all states. It can be combined with a "medical savings account" which is a tax-saving way of putting money aside for routine medical expenses.

The most expensive coverage is major medical, which will cover a wide range of treatments, procedures and medications. The cost of this type of coverage has been rising dramatically for a number of years, much faster than the rate of inflation, and seems to just continue to become more and more expensive.

In-between are a wide range of compromise plans with varying price tags. AMTA and ABMP offer members opportunities to purchase discounted group health policies. Many other groups offer their members group health insurance of one sort or another. One good source is the local chamber of commerce or other non-profit civic group.

You can also check with National Association for the Self-Employed (1-800-232-6273 or www.nase.org) and the Home Office Association of America (212-588-9097 or 1-800-809-4622 or www.hoaa.com). Other options are Costco (1-800-974-0500 or www.costco.com), farmers' cooperative organizations, and any organization that bands together large numbers of consumers to improve their bargaining power.

One more idea to consider is that most colleges and universities offer very cheap medical insurance to students—both full-time and part-time students. Consider enrolling for one or two classes at a local college and purchasing discounted student health insurance. You may be able to purchase insurance *and* college courses substantially cheaper than you could purchase just insurance outside the university setting.

18 Laws You Should Know About and State Regulation of Massage

The first section of this chapter, "Laws you should know about", summarizes basic laws and legal principles. This section will provide you with background information you should understand before entering the business world as a massage practitioner.

For example, you will learn about the different functions of local, state and federal governments; zoning laws that relate to massage offices; types of businesses you can form for your practice, and rules that govern contractual relationships such as leases and employment contracts.

The second section, "State Laws Regulating Massage", has a directory of the licensing laws in the 30 states (plus the District of Columbia) that regulate the practice of massage, including contact information for all of the regulatory boards. In addition, there is information about related laws and legislative activity in some states that do not have state-wide massage regulation, such as California, Colorado, Georgia, Michigan and Minnesota.

A quick-review chart summarizing all 31 state laws regulating massage is on page 154.

Laws you should know about

Federal, State, County and Local governments. Most Americans live under the authority of four different governments. Each one has its own areas of major influence, in terms of what it offers you and what it requires of you.

The *Federal* government requires you to pay federal taxes on all the money you earn. The federal government also authorizes certain organizations to accredit massage schools, paving the way for the granting of financial aid for massage education. (See pages 241–242 for further information on financial aid.)

State governments sometimes enact laws regulating the practice of massage in the state. These laws are described in the second part of this chapter, and summarized on page 154. State governments sometimes require the payment of income taxes on the money you earn.

County governments occasionally pass laws concerning the practice of massage in the county. Such laws apply only in unincorporated areas of the county — that is, in areas which are not within the borders of a town or city that has a municipal government. The county government may also take over zoning and health requirements in unincorporated areas within the county, and has the power to levy some taxes.

County governments also keep records of business names ("assumed names" or "fictitious names") and issue certificates to businesses allowing them to use business names.

City (or township or village) governments, also called *municipal* governments, regulate zoning, parking, health concerns, and the operation of businesses within the city limits. They have the power to decide what businesses can and cannot operate in the city, and what locations within the city are permissible locations for different types of businesses. Some cities have regulations for the practice of massage within the city limits, and some even prohibit the practice of massage. Many cities also have some form of municipal taxation.

If there is ever a conflict between the laws of different governments, the power structure works as follows: Federal law always has priority; state laws have priority over county and local laws; municipal laws control within the borders of the city, town or village; in unincorporated areas of the county, county law applies unless it is in conflict with state or Federal law.

County and Municipal Professional Licensing Laws. As mentioned above, laws specifically regulating the practice of massage can be enacted by state, county or local governments. In many areas, no regulatory law applies to the practice of massage, as neither the state, county nor city has enacted one.

Many local laws regulating the practice of massage require the applicant for a massage license to submit items like fingerprints, recent photo, recent employment history, references, and physician's certificate that he or she has no communicable disease. In addition, some have educational requirements.

Some representative municipal educational requirements are listed below: Ames, IA 750 hours at AMTA-approved school; Cedar Rapids, IA 500 hours; Colorado Springs, CO 1000 hours; Davenport, IA 500 hours over a period of at least one year; Des Moines, IA 1000 hours; Las Vegas, NV 500 hours; Pueblo, CO 70 hours; St. Louis, MO 70 hours; St. Paul, MN, 40 hours; Tempe, AZ 600 hours; Tucson, AZ 1000 hours (500 in-class hours), Newport Beach, CA 500 hours plus background check, dress code, $342 annual fee (see also the list of California municipal laws on pages 148–149).

As you can see, the range of 40 hours to 1000 hours is quite a broad one, and this reflects the situation within the nation as a whole concerning massage licensing.

Other Local Requirements. If your local government has a law regulating massage establishments, the law may have requirements for bathrooms, lighting, signs and other specifics. If there is no such law, consider contacting the health department, fire department and the police department to see if there are any requirements you should know about before committing to a particular office space.

Sometimes local laws require large licensing fees, background checks, fingerprinting, or medical examinations. Some locations have severe zoning restrictions, dress codes for massage therapists, or other restrictive ordinances. Before establishing an office in a particular location it is prudent to investigate the local laws affecting massage businesses.

Business License. Business licenses are usually required by city governments. Occasionally a county requires a business license, and the state of Alaska requires such a license. It is used by the city government to keep track of who is performing what business activity, to generate money for the municipal treasury, and to make sure that zoning laws are being followed. The license fee may be a fixed annual fee, or it may be a percentage of your annual income.

Zoning Laws. Most cities have a special map of the city that divides every location into one of several zones (see Sample Zoning Map, page 69). A key explains the meaning of each zone. The zones create different kinds of neighborhoods — business areas, residential areas, industrial areas, and areas of mixed usage.

When you open a massage or bodywork practice, you will need to be sure you are locating your office in an area that is zoned for your type of business. You may find there is a dispute about the type of business you have — some zoning agencies classify massage as a profession, others consider it a health service, others call it a personal service, and others classify it as adult entertainment. The zoning board's classification decision can affect permissible locations for your office.

While most states leave zoning issues to the local governments, Florida has a state-wide ban on home offices in residential zones. Other states, such as Vermont, take the opposite approach and have state-wide laws specifically protecting the right to operate a home-based business. The Home Office Association of America, **www.hoaa.com**, advocates for greater freedom for home offices in zoning laws.

Local Taxes. Some local governments charge businesses a tax on business property. That means that they decide the value of the business property you own, and tax you a fixed percentage of that value each year. Some local governments also charge a sewer tax, which may be based on water usage or number of plumbing units.

Fictitious Name (or Assumed Name) Statement. If you use a made-up name for your business that does not include your own name, you should register that name with the county government. There is a fee, usually around $20, and you may be required to search through the county's record books to make sure that no one has already taken the name you are choosing. You may also be required to advertise the name in the legal classifieds of your local newspaper. Registering your fictitious name is a requirement for opening a checking account in the name of the business.

Taxpayer Identification Number. If you are a sole proprietor (see below) and do not have any employees, you can use your social security number on all tax documents. If you have employees, or if you incorporate or form a partnership, you will need to apply for a taxpayer identification number. Obtain form SS-4 from the Internal Revenue Service. For information on how to get the form, see the end of Chapter 19.

Business identity. In the eyes of the law, there are several possible "identities" for your business. The main ones are corporation, partnership and sole proprietor.

Corporations have a separate legal identity apart from the shareholders and employees. They can have tax advantages in some sophisticated situations, but if you are a self-employed bodyworker, it is not an advantage to incorporate.

Partnership is a special legal relationship in which the two or more partners can speak and act for each other. A promise by one binds the other, so if your partner makes a business deal and then fails to follow through, you can be held responsible for it. Partners usually share the partnership income, without regard to who actually did the work that generated the money.

Sole Proprietor means you, and you alone, run your business. In legal terms, there is no difference between you and your business. Your business is treated legally just as it is in fact—as an extension of your life and a part of yourself.

Practically every bodyworker operates as a sole proprietor, and unless you have some good reason not to, you should too. Becoming a corporation or a partnership will not benefit you unless you are involved in some complicated or sophisticated business dealings. If you become involved in a group practice, the group may choose to incorporate. This is something the group will decide in consultation with a lawyer or accountant.

Contractual relationship. A contract can be oral or written. It is simply an exchange of promises in which each party agrees to do or give something of value to the other party. Once made, a contract is legally enforceable until it is ended by the parties who made it.

Written contracts are easier to enforce, because the exact terms of the agreement are on paper for all to see. Oral contracts can also be enforced, but the specifics must be proven by testimony about the agreement.

Even something as simple as opening a checking account involves making a contract. The bank agrees to hold your money and give it to you or the people you write checks to, according to certain rules the bank establishes. You agree to pay a set fee per check written, or keep a minimum monthly balance, and to pay prescribed penalties for writing checks that your account cannot cover.

As a massage therapist, contracts you are likely to enter into include agreements to work for others or to have others work for you, rental agreements for office space, contracts with the phone company for business phone service, and contracts for performance of services like printing, laundry and cleaning.

Does a law regulating "massage" include "bodywork"?

As state regulation of massage practitioners becomes more and more common in the United States, practitioners of various forms of bodywork may find themselves required to obtain massage licenses to practice, even though their work is very different from massage.

Licensing laws are enacted by legislators, and implemented by Boards or Commissions, such as the Board of Massage. When a state law specifies which forms of bodywork are included in its regulation and which are excluded, there is no room for confusion and no need for the Board to make an interpretation. However, most of the massage laws in the 30 states regulating massages give only a "definition" of massage, leaving it up to the Board to determine which therapies fit under that definition.

In Florida, the Board of Massage has ruled that Reiki practitioners must be licensed as massage therapists. Under this ruling, one who works only with Reiki energy must devote thousands of dollars and many months to learning all the subjects necessary for the practice of Swedish massage.

Following is a sampling of some of the current rulings and controversies about the licensing of bodywork practitioners in states that license massage therapists.

Maryland enacted in 2000 an exemption from massage licensing for therapies directed at the "energetic field of the human body." Therefore, practitioners of Reiki, polarity, and other energy-based forms of bodywork do not have to obtain massage licenses.

Mississippi's licensing law *includes* "shiatsu, acupressure, oriental, eastern or Asian massage, spa, rub, and therapeutic touch" and *excludes* "allied modalities that are certified by a nationally accredited organization recognized by the board."

New York includes shiatsu, polarity, reflexology, Alexander, Trager, and other bodywork modalities in massage regulation, by ruling of the Board, but exempts Reiki.

North Carolina exempts Trager, Reiki, Healing Touch, Bowen, Jin Shin, Polarity, Therapeutic Touch, Body Mind Centering, Feldenkrais and Alexander from its massage licensing law.

North Dakota exempts reflexology from massage licensing but includes Reiki as massage.

Tennessee's Board originally ruled that reflexology should be regulated as massage, but reflexologists subsequently obtained an exemption from the law.

Utah's Department of Occupational and Professional Licensing previously regulated Reiki as massage, but reviewed their position 2002 and ruled that Reiki is a "spiritual healing art" and therefore not subject to the massage licensing laws.

As the field of massage and bodywork continues to evolve, some forms of bodywork will establish strong independent certifications that may allow them to be regulated independently from massage. At the moment, there are no generalities that give any useful guidance on this topic. It is a question that is addressed state by state, and even within states, a specific bodywork modality may be regulated as massage one year but not the next.

If you belong to a professional organization for the form of bodywork you practice, that organization is probably the best source for current information about licensing issues. Another source for such information is any of the massage schools in the state in which you practice.

The unique status of animal massage

The regulation of animal massage may become the next political battleground, as there are indications that veterinarians may be attempting to exert control over the field through legislation.

In the last few years, the American Veterinary Medicine Association has sponsored legislative efforts in many states aimed at restricting animal massage to veterinarians or those under direct supervision of a veterinarian.

In 1996, when Maryland adopted massage licensing, a lobbyist for the state veterinary association worked to ensure that massage therapists would be authorized to work on human patients only.

In 1997, a Maine law added massage therapy (and other complementary therapies) to the veterinary practice act, which made veterinarians the only practitioners authorized to perform animal massage.

New Hampshire has a bill pending that limits alternative therapies to veterinarians, and there may be a movement toward enacting such legislation in both New York and Texas.

Individuals and grass-roots organizations are attempting to take countermeasures.

At the time of publication, a bill was pending in New Jersey that would give animal owners the right to choose their own service providers so long as diagnosis and surgery were not involved.

In 2001, Washington state passed a law recognizing animal massage as a professional service, and establishing the right of non-veterinarians to practice animal massage with a 100-hour credential.

A practitioner who wishes to practice massage in a given state should contact the state veterinary board to make inquiry. Another source of information is the International Alliance for Animal Therapy and Healing (**www.iaath.com**).

The most common animal massage is equine sports massage, since sports massage for high-performance horses is in demand and is well-paid work. For further information and resources about equine sports massage, see page 223.

State Laws Regulating Massage as of May, 2002

State laws regulating the practice of massage are described below, along with contact information for the boards that license or otherwise regulate massage practitioners.

Moving from state to state

Moving from state to state is complicated by the fact that the various state educational requirements range from 300 hours (Texas) to 1,000 hours (Nebraska and New York), and Maryland requires 500 hours plus 60 college credits. However, one recent trend that has made it easier to move from state to state is the *National Certification Exam*.

The *National Certification Exam* is now either required or accepted in 26 of the 30 states that regulate massage, plus the District of Columbia. Once you pass the *National Certification Exam* in any location, your passing test score will satisfy the written test requirement in all 26 of those states.

Remember, though, that individual states have other licensing requirements that must be met to qualify for a license, such as hours of education, required courses, practical exam, health certificate, fees, and continuing education requirements.

These are not listed in this book. For these details you should visit the State Board's website, or contact the Board directly to obtain guidance about your exact situation.

Obtaining updated information on state licensing laws

Information of this nature necessarily goes out of date, since legislation regarding massage is continually evolving. Fortunately, there are sources you can turn to that will provide periodic updates to this information.

For up-to-date information on massage laws, a good resource is *Massage Magazine*, which prints a summary of current licensing laws near the back of each issue. Another good source is any of the massage schools located in the state you are interested in. In addition, numerous websites maintain updated information about nationwide licensing laws, including this book's website. The site's home page **www.CareerAtYourFingertips.com** has a link to "State Laws Regulating Massage" which is updated whenever significant changes in massage laws take place.

For quick and easy reference, all of the current state licensing laws are summarized in the State Licensing Chart on page 154.

Alabama

State licensing, 650 hours required from an institution approved by the Board, *National Certification Exam*

> **Alabama Massage Licensing Board**
> **660 Adams Ave., Suite 301**
> **Montgomery, AL 36104**
> **(334) 269-9990**

Arkansas

State licensing, 500 hours required. Reciprocity is on a case-by-case basis and requires education in an accredited school

> **Arkansas Massage Board**
> **P.O. Box 20739**
> **Hot Springs, AR 71903**
> **(501) 623-0444**

California

California does not have statewide massage regulation. Massage schools are regulated by the Bureau of Consumer Affairs, and licensing of massage practitioners is done only by city and county governments.

A State of California law (Chapter 6, sections 51030 through 51034) gives authority to cities and counties to regulate massage. The law states what aspects of the practice may and may not be regulated. Section 51034 states that local laws may not restrict the practice of massage to same-sex massage only.

Some southern California jurisdictions exempt "Holistic Health Practitioners" from their massage regulation laws. This type of local law originated in San Diego and has been adopted in several other locations. A Holistic Health Practitioner is usually defined as someone with demonstrable training and experience in massage.

The following table of municipal and county licensing requirements was originally compiled in 1991, and has been only partially updated since then. While most of this information is still accurate, it is the nature of such information that it slowly goes out of date. Nonetheless, this table provides a useful picture of the diverse massage licensing laws in California.

Aside from the educational requirements listed below, many towns and cities have some practical requirements for a person who wants to practice massage. For example, some towns prohibit "outcall" massage, or house calls, and some regulate it separately and require a special outcall massage license.

The amount charged for business or professional licenses varies tremendously from place to place, from a few dollars to over two thousand dollars. Some towns require a business license but no professional credentials. Some regulate massage as "adult entertainment". Some prohibit the practice of massage altogether. The world-renowned massage program at Esalen Institute in Big Sur still functions by authorization of the local sheriff's department.

For updated information about local laws, inquire at the town hall or city hall for municipal laws, or the county government building in the county seat for county laws.

1,000 hours (6): Orange, San Clemente, Santa Paula, Thousand Oaks, Tustin, Vista

600 hours (3): Fontana, Rialto, San Bernardino

500 hours (6): Alameda County (NCE), Brea, Cupertino, Emeryville (NCE), Newport Beach, Palm Desert, Seal Beach

225 hours (1): Marina

200 hours (42): Alhambra, Auburn, Bakersfield, Big Bear Lake, Camarillo, Carlsbad, Carson, Chula Vista, Covina, Cudahy, Cypress, El Segundo, Fairfield, Glendale, Grover City, Hayward, Hercules, Highland, Imperial, Imperial Beach, Kern County, Laguna Beach, Loma Linda, Los Alamitos, Huntington Park, Marysville, Montebello, Ontario, Orange County, Placentia, Ridgecrest, San Bernardino County, San Buenaventura, Santa Barbara, Signal Hill, Solano Beach, Torrance, Twentynine Palms, Union City, Ventura County, West Sacramento, Yuba County.

180 hours (7): Atwater, Ceres, Dublin, Livingston, Merced, Modesto, Turlock

100 hours (20): Corona, Desert Hot Springs, Dublin, El Dorado County, Escondido, Fresno, Gardena, Hollister, La Mesa, Livermore, Merced County, Monterey, Monterey County, Novato, Palm Springs, Redlands, San Francisco, San Leandro, San Luis Obispo, Santa Monica.

70 hours (20): Alameda, Burlingame, Colma, Contra Costa County, Daly City, Half Moon Bay, Lakewood, Livermore Manteca, Milpitas, Pacifica, Palo Alto, Portola Valley, Richmond, San Mateo County, San Pablo, San Ramon, Santa Clara, Santa Clara County, Saratoga, Selma.

Any approved or recognized school (37): Adelanto, Arroyo Grande, Azuza, Beaumont, Belmont, Beverly Hills, Cloverdale, Encinitas, Eureka, Foster City, Fullerton, Glendora, Healdsburg, Imperial County, Lemon Grove, Millbrae, Napa, Oceanside, Oxnard, Pacific Grove, Pleasanton, Poway, Rancho Mirage, Sacramento County, San Bruno, San Diego County, San Marcos, San Mateo, Santa Rosa, Santee, Simi Valley, South Lake Tahoe, Stockton, West Covina, West Hollywood, Westmoreland, Whittier.

No educational requirement but other requirements (12): Anaheim, Bell Gardens, Burbank, Commerce, Culver City, Hemet, Long Beach, Los Angeles, Manhattan Beach, Riverside, Riverside County, San Ramon, Santa Fe Springs.

Colorado

In 1989, representatives of AMTA and ABMP, school owners, and several unaffiliated massage therapists came together to form a coalition to represent massage practitioners on licensing issues. These efforts resulted in a law defining "Massage Therapist" as a graduate of a state-approved school with at least 500 hours of education. One who meets this definition is exempted from the "massage parlor" law.

Massage regulation in Colorado is done by city and county governments, and approximately 15 county and municipal governments have laws regulating the practice of massage. At present, there is no plan to pursue state regulation of massage or bodywork.

Connecticut

State licensing, 500 hours at a school approved by COMTA *and* by an accrediting agency recognized by the U.S. Department of Education. Reciprocity is available if school is on CT's approved list—contact the department. *National Certification Exam*

> Ct. Dept. of Public Health
> Massage Therapy Licensure
> 150 Washington St.
> Hartford, CT 06106
> (860) 509-7570
> www.ct-clic.com/detail.asp?code=1730

Delaware

Massage Therapist: 500 hours, *National Certification Exam*

Certified Technician: 100 hours

> Delaware of Massage and Bodywork
> Cannon Building, Ste. 203
> 861 Silver Lake Blvd.
> Dover, DE 19904
> (302) 739-4522, ext. 205
> www.http://www.professionallicensing.state.de.us/boards/massagebodyworks/index.shtml

Only licensed massage and bodywork therapists may work by prescription of physicians. Certified technicians may work in any other massage setting. To practice massage in Delaware, one must be either licensed or certified.

District of Columbia

State Licensing, 500 hours, *National Certification Exam*

> Board of Massage Therapy
> 941 N. Capitol St. NE #7243
> Washington, DC 20002
> (202) 442-4320 or 442-4764
> http://obc.dc.gov/services/profiles_m.shtm#massage

Florida

State licensing, 500 hours required, *National Certification Exam*. Reciprocity (called Endorsement in Florida) for graduates of a school or apprenticeship approved by the Board.

Florida Department of Health
Board of Massage Therapy
4052 Bald Cypress Way, Bin #C06
Tallahassee, FL 32399
(850) 245-4161
http://www9.myflorida.com/mqa/massage/ma_home.html

Semi-official rumors have persisted that the requirement for licensing would be increased to 700 or 750 hours at some future date. However, as of press time for this Edition, there was no official confirmation of such a change.

Georgia

Bills to regulate the practice of massage have been introduced in Georgia in 1992, 1995, and 1997. None of these passed the legislature. The process of attempting to create massage legislation has brought out varying opinions from practitioners within the state. The state AMTA chapter's president wrote in 1998 that he believed the process of voicing conflicting concerns and ideas would result in eventually enacting a unified law representing the different modalities of the massage therapy profession.

Hawaii

State licensing, 570 hours required; or apprenticeship of 150 in-class hours and 420 hours practical.

Educational institution must be approved or licensed by a state department of education or approved by an accredited community college, college or university or approved by the AMTA or approved by the Rolf Institute.

Dept. of Commerce & Consumer Affairs
State Board of Massage
P.O. Box 3469 / 1010 Richards Street
Honolulu, HI 96801
(808) 586-3000
http://www.state.hi.us/dcca/pvl/areas_massage.html

Illinois

A Bill to license the practice of massage was introduced in the legislature in 2001, and it was approved by the House of Representatives in 2002. The new law creates a 500-hour licensing requirement and a competency exam, effective January 1, 2004. At publication time, the bill was awaiting the Governor's signature. Progress reports

and the text of the proposed law can be viewed at: **www.amta-il.org**

Iowa

State licensing, 500 hours, *National Certification Exam*

Iowa Department of Public Health
Massage Therapy Board
321 E. 12th St.
Lucas State Office Building
Des Moines, IA 50319
(515) 281-6959
http://www.idph.state.ia.us/licensure/massage_therapy_index.html

Louisiana

State licensing, 500 hours, *National Certification Exam* (optional)

Louisiana Board of Massage Therapy
P.O. Box 1279
Zachary, LA 70791
(225) 658-8941   www.lsbmt.org

National Certification Exam may be used to substitute for the written portion of State Exam.

Maine

State Licensing, 500 hours from a Department-approved school (no exam) or *National Certification Exam* in lieu of approved education

Maine Department of Professional and Financial Regulation, Division of Licensing and Enforcement — Massage Therapists
State House Station #35
Augusta, ME 04333
(207) 624-8603
http://www.state.me.us/pfr/olr/categories/cat26.htm

Maine's law does not prohibit the practice of massage by non-licensed persons, but it prohibits the use of the terms "massage therapist" or "massage practitioner" by unlicensed persons.

Maryland

State Certification / State Registration, 500 hours massage education and 60 college credit hours, *National Certification Exam*

Maryland Board of Chiropractic Examiners
4201 Patterson Avenue
Baltimore, MD 21215
(410) 764-4738   www.mdmassage.org

Maryland was a battleground between the professions of Physical Therapy and Massage in the 1990s. The Physical Therapy Board made a serious attempt to prohibit the practice of massage by anyone except physical therapists during the 1990s. This battle raged in Maryland for about a decade, and it ended with the enactment of massage licensing legislation in 1998.

Effective 2002, Maryland adopted a two-tier licensing scheme. Certified Massage Therapists (CMTs) must have 500 hours of education, NCE and 60 college credit hours (in any subjects). CMTs may give and receive referrals from other health-care practitioners and may practice in health-care settings, such as hospitals, medical offices, clinics and nursing homes.

Registered Massage Practitioners (RMPs) must have 500 hours training and pass the NCE, but are not required to have 60 college credits. RMPs may practice in spas, health clubs, or private practices. RMPs cannot practice in health-care settings and cannot receive or give referrals to health-care practitioners.

Michigan

A statewide massage licensure law was adopted in 1974 and modified in 1980, but it is legally defective and has never been implemented. Even though there is a licensing law "on the books," there is no license available in Michigan to those who practice massage or bodywork.

Minnesota

In 1999, a bill to license massage was defeated in the Minnesota legislature. The bill had the backing of the local AMTA chapter and many of the state's massage schools, but was opposed by an independent coalition of massage therapists who mounted a campaign in the state legislature to defeat the bill.

Then, in 2000, Minnesota sent shock waves throughout legislative circles by enacting the first of its kind "Freedom of Access" act for alternative health care. Rather than establishing requirements for *licensure* of alternative medical practitioners, the legislature chose to protect consumers by requiring practitioners to *disclose* certain facts to their clients.

Under the Minnesota freedom of access law, practitioners are required to (1) tell their clients that the state has not established educational requirements for unlicensed practitioners, (2) reveal their academic and professional credentials, (3) inform clients of their right to confidentiality and right to choice of services, and (4) advise clients about the procedure for filing complaints.

This law gives consumers the right to know what services are being provided and what qualifications the provider has. This is "true free-market capitalism" applied to alternative health care.

The law applies to any unlicensed health care modality and it specifically mentions massage, as well as acupressure, naturopathy, aromatherapy, ayurveda, craniosacral therapy, energetic healing, homeopathy, meditation, and other therapies involving foods, supplements, and applications of heat, cold, water, touch and light.

The Minnesota act is being studied by many other states, and similar bills are currently in process or being drafted in California, Florida, Georgia, Iowa, Kansas, Oklahoma, New Jersey, New York, and Rhode Island. A number of other states have citizen groups pursuing similar legislation.

Mississippi

State Registration, 700 hours, *National Certification Exam*

State Board of Massage
P.O. Box 12489
Jackson, MS 39326
(601) 957-7074   www.msbmt.state.ms.us

Missouri

State Licensing, 500 hours, *National Certification Exam*

Division of Professional Registration
Massage Therapy Board
P.O. Box 1335
Jefferson City, MO 65102
(573) 522-6277   www.ecodev.state.mo.us/pr

Nebraska

State licensing, 1000 hours, *National Certification Exam*, Reciprocity for those attending a school approved by the Board, or upon review of school transcript.

Department of Health, Credentialing Division
301 Centennial Mall South
P.O. Box 94986
Lincoln, NE 68509
(402) 471-2117
www.hhs.state.ne.us/crl/massrulesregs.htm

New Hampshire

State licensing, 750 hours, *National Certification Exam*

NH Dept. of Health and Human Services
Bureau of Health Facilities Administration
6 Hazen Drive
Concord, NH 03301
(603) 271-4594   http://www.nhes.state.nh.us/
elmi/licertoccs/massa01.htm

New Jersey

State Licensing, 500 hours, *National Certification Exam*

> **Board of Nursing**
> **PO Box 45010**
> **Newark, NJ 07101**
> **(973) 504-6430**
> **http://www.state.nj.us/lps/ca/nursing/mass.htm**

New Mexico

State licensing, 650 hours (may be 300 hours plus 350 hours Alternative Qualifying Experience) *National Certification Exam* plus Jurisprudence Exam. Reciprocity on a case-by-case basis (referred to as "by credentials")

> **New Mexico Board of Massage Therapy**
> **P.O. Box 25101**
> **Santa Fe, NM 87504**
> **(505) 476-7090**
> **http://www.rld.state.nm.us/b&c/massage/index.htm**

New York

State licensing, 1,000 hours, *National Certification Exam*. Reciprocity is case-by-case and requires proof of practice for two years

> **New York State Education Department**
> **State Board for Massage Therapy**
> **Cultural Education Center, Room 3041**
> **Albany, NY 12230**
> **(518) 474-3817 (general info)**
> **(518) 474-3866 (practice issues and applications)**
> **http://www.op.nysed.gov/massage.htm**

North Carolina

State Licensing, 500 hours from a school approved by the Board, *National Certification Exam*

Board of Massage & Bodywork Therapy

> **P.O. Box 2539**
> **Raleigh, NC 27602**
> **(919) 546-0050   www.bmbt.org**

North Dakota

State certificate of registration, 750 hours, state exam. Requires attendance at COMTA-approved school

> **North Dakota Massage Board**
> **P.O. Box 701**
> **Dickinson, ND 58601**
> **(701) 225-3906 (Phil Reisenauer)**
> **http://www.governor.state.nd.us/boards/boards-query.asp?Board_ID=67**

Ohio

State licensing, 600 hours (during at least 12 months), state exam. Reciprocity is on a case-by-case basis, but an exam is still required.

> **Ohio State Medical Board**
> **77 South High St., 17th floor**
> **Columbus, OH 43266**
> **(614) 466-3934**
> **http://www.state.oh.us./med/limbrch.htm**

In Ohio, a massage license is required for use of the title "licensed massage therapist". A massage license is required to practice therapeutic massage, but is not required to practice relaxation massage. Unlicensed practitioners probably cannot receive reimbursement from insurance companies.

Oregon

State licensing, 500 hours, *National Certification Exam*

> **Oregon Board of Massage Technicians**
> **3218 Pringle Rd. SE, Suite 250**
> **Salem, OR 97302**
> **(503) 365-8657   www.oregonmassage.org/**

Rhode Island

State licensing, 500 hours at a COMTA-approved school, *National Certification Exam*

> **Rhode Island Department of Health**
> **Room 104, Cannon Building**
> **Three Capitol Hill**
> **Providence, RI 02908**
> **(401) 222-2827 ext. 112**
> **http://www.healthri.org/hsr/professions/massage.htm**

South Carolina

State licensing, 500 hours, *National Certification Exam*

> **Division of Professional Licensing**
> **110 Center View / P.O. Box 11329**
> **Columbia, SC 29210**
> **(803) 896-4830**
> **http://www.llr.state.sc.us/POL/MassageTherapy/**

Tennessee

State Licensing, 500 hours from State-accredited school (no exam) or *National Certification Exam* in lieu of accredited schooling

> **Board of Massage Therapy**
> **First Floor, Cordell Hull Building**
> **425 5th Ave North,**
> **Nashville, TN 37247-1010**
> **(615) 532-5080   http://www2.state.tn.us/health/Boards/Massage/index.htm**

Students who attend a school on the state's list of accredited schools do not need to take a written test. Anyone who has passed the *National Certification Exam* and submits proof of passing may be licensed, regardless of what school they attended. In addition, those licensed in states with equivalent educational requirements may be admitted by reciprocity.

Texas

State registration, 250 hours plus 50 hours internship, state exam

**Texas Massage Therapy Registration
Texas Department of Health
1100 W. 49th St.
Austin, TX 78756
(512) 834-6616
www.tdh.state.tx.us/hcqs/plc/massage.htm**

Registration is required to practice massage in Texas.

Utah

State licensing, Board-approved massage education or apprenticeship of 1000 hours, state exam or *National Certification Exam.* Reciprocity is available to licensed out-of-state therapists whether or not their training was at board-approved school.

**Utah Department of Commerce
Division of Occupational and Professional Licensing
Herbert M. Wells Building
160 East 300 South
P.O. Box 45805
Salt Lake City, UT 84145
(801) 530-6628
http://www.dopl.utah.gov/licensing/massage.html**

Virginia

State certification, 500 hours, *National Certification Exam.* Certification required for the use of the term "therapeutic massage" or "certified massage therapist"

**Virginia Board of Nursing
6606 West Broad St., 4th floor
Richmond, VA 23230
(804) 662-9909
www.dhp.state.va.us/nursing/nursing_laws_regs.htm**

Washington

State licensing, 500 hours, *National Certification Exam*

**Washington Department of Health
Massage Licensing Program
P.O. Box 47867
Olympia, WA 98504
(360) 236-4866
http://www.doh.wa.gov/Massage/**

West Virginia

State licensing, 500 hours from a massage therapy school approved in its home state (no exam) or *National Certification Exam* in lieu of approved education

**Massage Therapy Licensure Board
200 Davis Street, #1
Princeton, WV 24740
(304) 487-1400   www.state.wv.us/massage**

As originally enacted, the law required attendance at a COMTA-approved school (even though there were none in the state). Before long, a coalition of members of all the major massage associations worked together to amend the law to its current form.

Wisconsin

State licensing, 600 hours, *National Certification Exam*

**Department of Regulation and Licensing
1400 E. Washington Ave. / P.O. Box 8935
Madison, WI 53708
(608) 266-0145, ext. 111   http://
www.drl.state.wi.us/Regulation/applicant_
information/dod2000.html**

State Licensing Chart as of July, 2002

State	Education Required	NCE	Year Begun	Number licensed
Alabama	650 hours	yes	1996	1,114
Arkansas	500 hours	yes	1951	1,474
Connecticut	500 hours COMTA	yes	1993	1,842
Delaware	500 (therapist) 100 (technician)	yes	1993	544
Dist. of Columbia	500 hours	yes	1999	255
Florida	500 hours / 700 hours	yes	1943	18,517
Hawaii	570 hours or 150 plus 420 apprenticeship	no	1947	3,922
Illinois	500 hours		2004	
Iowa	500 hours	yes	1992	1,107
Louisiana	500 hours	yes	1992	1,502
Maine	500 hours	yes*	1991	1,081
Maryland	500 hours / 60 credits	yes	1998	1,637
Mississippi	700 hours	yes	2001	
Missouri	500 hours	yes	1998	
Nebraska	1000 hours	yes	1958	720
New Hampshire	750 hours	yes	1980	1,125
New Jersey	500 hours	yes	1999	
New Mexico	650 hours or 300 plus 350 experience	yes	1991	3,850
New York	1,000 hours	yes	1967	10,041
North Carolina	500 hours Board-approved	yes	1999	2,656
North Dakota	750 COMTA	no	1959	479
Ohio	600 hours	no	1916	5,607
Oregon	500	yes	1999	3,400
Rhode Island	500 hours COMTA	yes	1980	645
South Carolina	500 hours	yes	1997	1,537
Tennessee	500 hours	yes*	1995	2,080
Texas	300	no	1985	18,579
Utah	Board-approved or 1,000 apprenticeship	yes	1981	3,516
Virginia	500 hours	yes	1996	2,514
Washington	500 hours	yes	1976	9,146
West Virginia	500 hours	yes*	1998	700
Wisconsin	600 hours	yes	1999	1,479

*In Maine, Tennessee, and West Virginia, NCE is optional; it is accepted as an alternative to education at a state-approved school.

19 Income Taxes

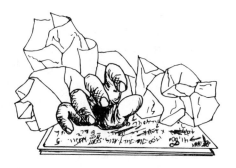

This chapter cannot give you all the information and advice you will need to prepare your income tax return. Instead, this chapter will:

1. Familiarize you with all of the key facts and ideas you need to understand Federal income tax;

2. Explain what records you should keep for tax purposes, why you need them and how to keep them;

3. Guide you to all the resources you will need to do your own taxes, or to hire a professional to do your taxes for you.

The Big Picture

The following discussion gives you the basis of the federal tax laws that determine how much money you give the government at the end of the year.

This information is presented in condensed form, and on the first reading it may seem difficult to understand. This is only because the words are strange, not because the ideas are difficult.

Really try to "get" this big picture in your mind. Everything else in this chapter relates to this overall picture.

Some of the statements in this "big picture" would need additional explanation to be 100% accurate, so just use this information to understand the concepts at this point.

1. Employment income only

If you are an employee, and have no income from self-employment, your taxes will be very simple. You employer will give you a W-2 form showing income and withholding, and the forms the IRS sends you to fill out your taxes should be sufficient.

2. Self-employment income

Almost all massage therapists and bodyworkers are at least partially self-employed. When you are self-employed, your business activity is reported on a separate IRS form, called Schedule C (see pages 158–159). In reporting your business activity on your Schedule C, you add up all of the money you received during the year in your business, and you subtract your business deductions. (What you can subtract as business deductions will be discussed later).

If the money you *received* is a larger amount than your allowable *deductions*, you have a *profit*. We will call this your "business profit." You have to pay a percentage of your business profit as self-employment tax, and you also have to pay a percentage of your business profit as income tax.

3. Self-employment tax

Business profit is subject to a "self-employment tax" as well as income tax. This is the self-employed person's equivalent of Social Security Tax. This tax rate for 2001 was 15.3 percent on self-employment profit up to $80,400.

4. Income tax

Business profit is also subject to income tax, which is separate from self-employment tax. In 2001, Income tax rates were between 10% and 39.1%, depending on your income and your marital and family status. As a rough rule of thumb for planning purposes, you may want to estimate that about 15% of your income will be taken as income taxes.

Your income from non-business sources is called "Personal Income". Examples are interest and dividend income. Personal income is subject to the income tax only, *not* the self-employment tax.

If you have been following along this far, see if the following chart makes it a little clearer for you:

Business earnings	Personal income
minus	*minus*
Business deductions	Personal deductions
equals	*equals*
Business profit	Personal income
Pay self-employment tax on business profit (approximately 15%)	Pay income tax on personal income (approximately 15%)
and	
Pay Income tax on business profit (approximately 15%)	

Notice that you pay both self-employment tax and income tax on your business profit, or a total of about 30% of your earnings. Personal (non-business) income is subject only to the income tax of about 15%.

Deductions are Beautiful

Once you grasp the overall picture of how taxes are figured, it becomes apparent that business deductions and personal deductions put money in your pocket. Since they reduce the total amount subject to taxes, they reduce the total taxes you have to pay.

Business deductions are especially helpful, since they reduce both the self-employment tax and the income tax.

If you earn $40,000.00 in business income and have no deductions, your overall tax burden would be about $12,000.00 (approximately $6,000.00 for social security tax and $6,000.00 for income tax).

However, if you earn $40,000.00 in business income and have $10,000.00 in deductions, you pay taxes on $30,000.00 ($40,000.00 minus deductions of $10,000.00), and you overall tax burden would be about $9,000.00 (approximately $4,500.00 for social security tax and $4,500.00 for income tax). Your $10,000.00 in deductions would save you about $3,000.00 in taxes.

In other words, since your overall tax rate is about 30%, whenever you can "deduct" a business expense, you save about 30% of the cost of that item in the form of reduced taxes.

Personal deductions reduce only the income tax. Personal deductions include items such as charitable contributions, certain medical expenses, and the like.

Business deductions are discussed in some detail below. Become familiar with this information so that you have a clear understanding of what is deductible, and what records you need to keep to support your deductions.

You will list your deductions on "Schedule C" which is the form self-employed persons file with their income tax returns. If your total deductions for the year were $2,500.00 or less, you may be able to use Schedule C-EZ (see page 159). Otherwise, you must use the slightly more complicated Schedule C.

What Can I Deduct?

In general, if it's a business expense, it's deductible. The expense must be for something "appropriate and helpful in developing and maintaining your trade or business" and the cost must be reasonable. This allows for a broad range of business deductions.

The following list demonstrates the most common deductible items.

- Business use of your automobile

- Office rental expense

- Massage table and other equipment for treatment room

- Music system and music for treatment room

- Painting or repair costs for office

- Advertising

- Long-distance business phone calls

SCHEDULE C
(Form 1040)

Department of the Treasury
Internal Revenue Service (99)

Profit or Loss From Business
(Sole Proprietorship)

▶ Partnerships, joint ventures, etc., must file Form 1065 or Form 1065-B.
▶ Attach to Form 1040 or Form 1041. ▶ See Instructions for Schedule C (Form 1040).

OMB No. 1545-0074

2001

Attachment
Sequence No. **09**

Name of proprietor

Social security number (SSN)

A Principal business or profession, including product or service (see page C-1 of the instructions)

B Enter code from pages C-7 & 8 ▶

C Business name. If no separate business name, leave blank.

D Employer ID number (EIN), if any

E Business address (including suite or room no.) ▶ ....
City, town or post office, state, and ZIP code

F Accounting method: (1) ☐ Cash (2) ☐ Accrual (3) ☐ Other (specify) ▶ ....

G Did you "materially participate" in the operation of this business during 2001? If "No," see page C-2 for limit on losses ☐ Yes ☐ No

H If you started or acquired this business during 2001, check here .... ▶ ☐

Part I   **Income**

1	Gross receipts or sales. **Caution.** If this income was reported to you on Form W-2 and the "Statutory employee" box on that form was checked, see page C-2 and check here ▶ ☐	1
2	Returns and allowances	2
3	Subtract line 2 from line 1	3
4	Cost of goods sold (from line 42 on page 2)	4
5	**Gross profit.** Subtract line 4 from line 3	5
6	Other income, including Federal and state gasoline or fuel tax credit or refund (see page C-3) . . .	6
7	**Gross income.** Add lines 5 and 6 . . . . ▶	7

Part II   **Expenses.** Enter expenses for business use of your home **only** on line 30.

8	Advertising	8	19	Pension and profit-sharing plans	19
9	Bad debts from sales or services (see page C-3) .	9	20	Rent or lease (see page C-4):	
			a	Vehicles, machinery, and equipment .	20a
10	Car and truck expenses (see page C-3) . . .	10	b	Other business property . .	20b
11	Commissions and fees . .	11	21	Repairs and maintenance . .	21
12	Depletion	12	22	Supplies (not included in Part III) .	22
13	Depreciation and section 179 expense deduction (not included in Part III) (see page C-3) . .	13	23	Taxes and licenses . . .	23
			24	Travel, meals, and entertainment:	
			a	Travel	24a
14	Employee benefit programs (other than on line 19) . .	14	b	Meals and entertainment	
15	Insurance (other than health) .	15	c	Enter nondeductible amount included on line 24b (see page C-5)	
16	Interest:				
a	Mortgage (paid to banks, etc.) .	16a	d	Subtract line 24c from line 24b	24d
b	Other	16b	25	Utilities	25
17	Legal and professional services	17	26	Wages (less employment credits) .	26
18	Office expense	18	27	Other expenses (from line 48 on page 2) . .	27
28	**Total expenses** before expenses for business use of home. Add lines 8 through 27 in columns . . . ▶				28

29	Tentative profit (loss). Subtract line 28 from line 7 . . . . .
30	Expenses for business use of your home. Attach **Form 8829** . . . . .
31	**Net profit or (loss).** Subtract line 30 from line 29.
	• If a profit, enter on **Form 1040, line 12,** and **also** on Schedule SE, line 2 (statutory employees, see page C-5). Estates and trusts, enter on Form 1041, line 3.
	• If a loss, you **must** go to line 32.
32	If you have a loss, check the box that describes your investment in this activity.
	• If you checked 32a, enter the loss on **Form 1040, line 12,** and **also** on Schedule SE, line 2 (statutory employees, see page C-5). Estates and trusts, enter on Form 1041, line 3.
	• If you checked 32b, you **must** attach **Form 6198.**

For Paperwork Reduction Act Notice, see Form 1040 instructions.

**IRS form 1040
Schedule C,
page 1**

Schedule C (Form 1040) 2001   Page **2**

Part III   **Cost of Goods Sold** (see page C-6)

33	Method(s) used to value closing inventory: a ☐ Cost b ☐ Lower of cost or market c ☐ Other (attach explanation)
34	Was there any change in determining quantities, costs, or valuations between opening and closing inventory? If "Yes," attach explanation . . . . ☐ Yes ☐ No
35	Inventory at beginning of year. If different from last year's closing inventory, attach explanation . . . 35
36	Purchases less cost of items withdrawn for personal use 36
37	Cost of labor. Do not include any amounts paid to yourself 37
38	Materials and supplies 38
39	Other costs 39
40	Add lines 35 through 39 40
41	Inventory at end of year 41
42	**Cost of goods sold.** Subtract line 41 from line 40. Enter the result here and on page 1, line 4 . . . 42

Part IV   **Information on Your Vehicle.** Complete this part **only** if you are claiming car or truck expenses on line 10 and are not required to file Form 4562 for this business. See the instructions for line 13 on page C-3 to find out if you must file.

43 When did you place your vehicle in service for business purposes? (month, day, year) ▶ ....../....../......

44 Of the total number of miles you drove your vehicle during 2001, enter the number of miles you used your vehicle for:

a Business .... b Commuting .... c Other ....

45	Do you (or your spouse) have another vehicle available for personal use?	☐ Yes ☐ No
46	Was your vehicle available for personal use during off-duty hours?	☐ Yes ☐ No
47a	Do you have evidence to support your deduction?	☐ Yes ☐ No
b	If "Yes," is the evidence written?	☐ Yes ☐ No

Part V   **Other Expenses.** List below business expenses not included on lines 8–26 or line 30.

....
....
....
....
....
....
....
....

48	**Total other expenses.** Enter here and on page 1, line 27 48

Schedule C (Form 1040) 2001

**IRS form 1040
Schedule C,
page 2**

| SCHEDULE C-EZ
(Form 1040)

Department of the Treasury
Internal Revenue Service (99) | **Net Profit From Business**
(Sole Proprietorship)
▶ Partnerships, joint ventures, etc., must file Form 1065 or 1065-B.
▶ Attach to Form 1040 or 1041. ▶ See instructions on back. | OMB No. 1545-0074
20**01**
Attachment
Sequence No. **09A** |

Name of proprietor | Social security number (SSN)

Part I General Information

You May Use Schedule C-EZ Instead of Schedule C Only If You:

- Had business expenses of $2,500 or less.
- Use the cash method of accounting.
- Did not have an inventory at any time during the year.
- Did not have a net loss from your business.
- Had only one business as a sole proprietor.

And You:

- Had no employees during the year.
- Are not required to file **Form 4562,** Depreciation and Amortization, for this business. See the instructions for Schedule C, line 13, on page C-3 to find out if you must file.
- Do not deduct expenses for business use of your home.
- Do not have prior year unallowed passive activity losses from this business.

A Principal business or profession, including product or service   **B** Enter code from pages C-7 & 8 ▶

C Business name. If no separate business name, leave blank.   **D** Employer ID number (EIN), if any

E Business address (including suite or room no.). Address not required if same as on Form 1040, page 1.

City, town or post office, state, and ZIP code

Part II Figure Your Net Profit

1 **Gross receipts. Caution.** If this income was reported to you on Form W-2 and the "Statutory employee" box on that form was checked, see **Statutory Employees** in the instructions for Schedule C, line 1, on page C-2 and check here . . . . ▶ ☐   **1**

2 **Total expenses.** If more than $2,500, you **must** use Schedule C. See instructions **2**

3 **Net profit.** Subtract line 2 from line 1. If less than zero, you **must** use Schedule C. Enter on **Form 1040, line 12,** and **also** on **Schedule SE, line 2.** (Statutory employees **do not** report this amount on Schedule SE, line 2. Estates and trusts, enter on Form 1041, line 3.) **3**

Part III Information on Your Vehicle. Complete this part **only** if you are claiming car or truck expenses on line 2.

4 When did you place your vehicle in service for business purposes? (month, day, year) ▶ .... / .... / ....

5 Of the total number of miles you drove your vehicle during 2001, enter the number of miles you used your vehicle for:

a Business ....   b Commuting ....   c Other ....

6 Do you (or your spouse) have another vehicle available for personal use? . . . . ☐ **Yes** ☐ **No**

7 Was your vehicle available for personal use during off-duty hours? . . . . ☐ **Yes** ☐ **No**

8a Do you have evidence to support your deduction? . . . . ☐ **Yes** ☐ **No**

b If "Yes," is the evidence written? . . . . ☐ **Yes** ☐ **No**

For Paperwork Reduction Act Notice, see Form 1040 instructions.   Cat. No. 14374D   Schedule C-EZ (Form 1040) 2001

IRS form 1040 Schedule C–EZ

- Business travel expenses (cost of lodging plus 80% of cost of meals)

- Entertainment expenses (50% is deductible)

- Gifts to clients (up to $25 per client per year)

- Professional convention fees (and travel expenses)

- Continuing education expenses, including books

- Professional association dues

- Licensing fees

- Laundry expenses

- Your appointment book

- Business cards and any other business printing jobs

- Costs of oil and other supplies

Education

You can deduct the cost of education, plus travel and meals expenses, if the education maintains or improves your professional skills, or is required by law for keeping your professional status.

Educational expenses are *not* deductible for training in a new field, or to meet minimum professional requirements, because that is considered a "start-up" cost, and start-up costs are not deductible. The only exception to that is the new "HOPE" Credit or Lifetime Education Credit, which are available only if you attend a degree-granting institution. Your accountant can tell you if these apply to you.

Once you are a practicing massage therapist, the expenses of continuing education are deductible, even if they are for education that "improves" your professional skills. Therefore, you can probably deduct even a major educational expense, as long as you are already a practicing massage therapist.

This is one advantage of taking a small amount of training and practicing massage on the side (in states where this is permissible) before making a commitment to a more serious educational program.

Gifts

You can deduct the cost of gifts you give as part of doing business, up to a maximum of $25 worth of gifts to any one individual in one year. If there is a question whether something is a gift or entertainment (such as football tickets) it will be considered entertainment.

Handicap Accessibility Costs

If you have a disabled client, the cost of making your office disabled accessible is subsidized by a special tax credit.

Assume, for example, that you spend $5,000.00 on ramps and a hydraulic lift table for handicapped access. First you deduct $250.00 (the current amount specified by the law), leaving $4,750.00 that qualifies for a credit. Then you multiply that amount by 50% because the law gives you a credit for 50% of the allowable expenses. Therefore, you get a tax credit of $2,375.00 (50% of $4,750.00). Unlike a deduction, this $2,375.00 *credit* reduces your income taxes by $2,375.00 – as if you had already paid that amount to the IRS.

Now your out-of-pocket expense for making your office accessible is only $2,625.00 (the $5,000.00 you spent minus the $2,375.00 the government gave you back as a tax credit) and this $2,625.00 expense qualifies as a business deduction, further reducing your taxes.

Home office expenses

Rent and other costs for an office in your home are deductible if:

1. You use a part of your home as your principal place of business, *or*

2. You use a part of your home as a place to meet and deal with clients in the normal course of your practice, *or*

3. You use a separate building in your business, such as a cottage or detached garage *or*

4. You use a part of your home as a place to do necessary activities such as billing and phone calls, and you do not have any outside office available to you to do these tasks.

To qualify as a home office, the room or part of your house needs to be used "regularly" and "exclusively" in your practice. That means you have to use it for your business on a regular basis—not just on rare occasions. It also means you cannot use it for any other purpose, such as a den or guest bedroom.

Additionally, your home office must qualify under number 1, number 2 number 3, or number 4, above. Most home offices for massage therapists qualify under number 2. You give massages to clients there, so obviously, you meet and deal with clients there in the normal course of your practice. You qualify for the home office deduction.

The same applies if your office is in a separate building on your property. (An office in a separate building is deductible even if you only do your bookwork there, as long as you use it only for business). And if you have another business, such as selling products to your clients, the office where you store your inventory or where you do your bookkeeping for that business also qualifies as a home office under number 1, as long as you use it exclusively for business.

If you qualify for a home office deduction, you can deduct a proportionate share of all household expenses. Such expenses include real estate taxes, mortgage interest, rent, utility bills, insurance, repairs, security systems and depreciation. *Not* included are repairs or improvements that increase the value of a home you own.

To determine the percentage of your home expenses that is deductible as a business expense, calculate the total square footage of your home, and the square footage of your home office. Divide the square footage of the office by the total square footage of the home, and you will get a decimal, for example .23. You then multiply your home expenses (or your rent if you are a renter) by .23 (or whatever number applies) to find the amount of your deduction for your home office.

If the rooms in your home are roughly the same size, and you use one room as an office, you can use a fraction instead of doing the square-foot computation. For example, if you have six equal-sized rooms and use one as an office, deduct one sixth of your household expenses (or rent) as your home office expense.

The home office deduction cannot be larger than the amount of business income generated in the home office. In other words, the deduction cannot be used to create a business loss, only to offset income that you actually earned using that office.

Meal and Entertainment Expense

If you purchase meals or entertainment as a means of conducting business, you can deduct 50% of the cost of the meals and entertainment, including tips (as long as the costs are reasonable). You can also deduct 100% of your automobile costs for driving to the meal or entertainment. An example of meal and entertainment expense would be taking a chiropractor to lunch to discuss the possibility of cross-referrals.

Rent and other office expenses

Rental payments for your business office are fully deductible, as are other costs such as heat, electricity, insurance and the like.

Self-employed health insurance

In 2002, you could deduct 70% of the premiums you paid for health insurance if you were self-employed. In 2003, it increased to 100%.

Self-employment tax

You can deduct one-half of your self-employment tax from your gross income when you figure your income tax.

Start-up costs

If you are already a practicing massage therapist, and open a new office, or expand an exiting office, the costs involved in doing so are ordinary and necessary business expenses, and are fully deductible.

However, when you first begin your business as a massage therapist, the costs involved in starting your business are "start-up costs" and these are *not* deductible.

This issue generally will not arise for a massage therapist or bodyworker, since opening an office without prior professional experience is not usually a realistic approach. It does, however, become an issue when you want to deduct education expenses. Continuing education is deductible, but your initial educational expense is a non-deductible "start-up" cost.

Travel

When you travel away from home for business, most of your expenses are deductible. Travel away from home means going for more than just a day's work, and must include going away long enough to need sleep or rest before coming home.

Deductible items

When traveling away from home on business, your deductible expenses include airplane, rail or bus tickets, automobile expenses, taxi fares, baggage costs, meals, lodging costs, cleaning and laundry expenses, telephone, fax, internet access costs, tips, and other similar expenses related to travel.

Travel receipts

Keep receipts during your trip. If you travel by car, keep an envelope in the glove compartment, and put all receipts in the envelope. When you get home, staple them together and put them in the place where you collect all business receipts. At the end of the year, they will be together and easy to handle when you are totaling your deductions.

Optional methods for deducting meal costs when traveling

Meals can be deducted two ways — (1) you may deduct amount you actually spend or (2) you may deduct the "standard meal allowance" which varies between $30 and $46 per day, depending on location. For detailed information on the standard meal allowance, request Publication 463 free from the IRS (see page 169).

When using the standard meal allowance, you do not need to produce receipts for your meals. For all other expenses, however, you need to have receipts to document your travel expenditures.

Mixed business and personal travel

If a trip is mainly business but partly personal, you can deduct the round trip travel expenses to get to your business destination, and the meals, lodging and incidental expenses that relate to the business portion of your trip. Any personal side trips, or expenses on days that were vacation days, are not tax-deductible.

If your trip was primarily for vacation and partly for business, no part of the expense is tax-deductible.

Business use vs. Personal use

If a particular expense has aspects of business and personal activity mixed together, remember that the test is whether it is "appropriate and helpful in promoting your business." If it meets this test, the fact that it also helps you personally is irrelevant; it is still deductible.

Some activities are personal and not business-related. For example, if you go to a bar on Saturday night hoping to meet someone who will become a bodywork client, you will not convince the IRS that your expenses are business-related.

However, if you go to the hardware store to get a wing nut to repair your massage table, that is a business trip, and it remains a business trip even if you also pick up a surge protector for your home computer while you are there.

If you pay attention to all the things you do for your business, you will see that much of your lifestyle actually is deductible. The cost of professional books, phone calls, entertainment, uniforms, and business laundry are all deductible expenses. You can also deduct the cost of traveling to shop for items for the business and to do errands for the business. You are entitled to proper business deductions, so plan for them, document them and take them.

Documenting deductions

The key to documenting deductions is keeping receipts, canceled checks, and in the case of automobile mileage, a log of business miles driven in your car.

What is documentation?

The IRS can demand a paper record of any transaction you are claiming as a deduction. If you pay a bill for a business expense, keep the bill. When you get your canceled checks from your bank, save the ones that relate to business expenses.

Where to keep your documents

Create a space in your office or your home where you regularly keep a whole year's bills, receipts and canceled checks. It can be a drawer, a filing cabinet, a sturdy box, or any space that you can regularly keep these records. At the end of the year, you will take them out and organize them so they can be totaled and figured into your tax return.

What to document

Keep all records of money spent on goods or services that relate to your business. These are items listed above under the heading "What Can I Deduct?", and any other items which are related to the operation of your business.

At the end of the year

When you go through your year's receipts and canceled checks, gather them into categories of deductions. This will make it easier for you or your accountant to make a final presentation of your business activity on your schedule C.

Schedule C contains a partial list of business deductions. These include: advertising, bad debts, car and truck expenses, depreciation, insurance, legal and professional services, office expenses, supplies, travel, meals, and entertainment. In addition, the form provides space for other categories than the ones listed.

Use this list as a basis for organizing your receipts. Other categories you might use for organization purposes are printing and photocopying, telephone expense, and gifts to clients. Receipts which do not fit into any other category can be labeled "miscellaneous."

Business use of your car

Are you a commuter?

Business use of your car is deductible, with one important exception: Commuting expense is not deductible. For tax purposes, commuting means traveling between your home and your main or regular place of work. The trip to your work and the trip home again are both considered non-deductible commuting. The IRS enforces this prohibition against deducting commuting expenses strongly and completely.

Perhaps you have no regular place of work; you may do house calls, or you may work in several different locations doing massage. In such a case, you are not a commuter. However, if you work principally in one office, that is your main or regular place of work, and the miles you drive to and from that place are not deductible… unless you have a valid home office.

If you have an office in your home, then travel between your home and your workplace is not commuting, but business travel. The idea is that going from office to office is business travel, but going from home to office is commuting. With a home office, you get to decide whether it is your home or your office you are leaving from.

If you have a home office, step into your home office just before you leave on any other business trip. Then you are going from one place of business to another. When you return, step into your home office before doing anything else. Thus your return trip is from one office to another. In this way, none of your business driving is considered commuting. While this may sound a little shady, it is apparently entirely legal, at least at the present moment.

It is possible the IRS would question this deduction if you were audited. If you wish to be more conservative, then deduct mileage expenses only on days when you see clients in your home office. If you are actually working in your home office on a particular day, there can be no question that travel from that office to some other business destination is business travel.

Two methods of computing automobile deduction

You may choose either of two methods to compute your deduction for business use of your car.

The methods are to use the standard deduction (34.5 cents in tax year 2001) for each mile driven for business, or to calculate actual expenses of operating your car for the year and to figure mathematically the amount of your deduction.

If you have a car that is not very expensive and costs little to operate, such as a Honda Civic, you will come out ahead using the 34.5 cents per mile computation. If you have an expensive new car or one that required lots of expensive repairs this year, you may come out ahead using the actual computation method.

The standard per mile method is quite simple to use, and the actual cost method can become quite involved. I use the per mile method on my tax return, because I don't enjoy keeping all the records necessary to use the actual cost method. Even if I am paying a few dollars more in taxes, for me it is worth it to simplify my record-keeping.

A brief explanation of both methods follows.

Standard deduction method—34.5 cents per mile (tax year 2001)

Keep a daily log of the use of your car. You should record business and personal use.

The best kind of record to keep is a list of the starting and ending odometer mileage for each business trip. This type of record shows each business trip individually. It is also acceptable to list only the destination and the number of miles driven for each trip.

At the end of the year, total all the business miles and multiply the total by .345 to get the deduction for business use of your car.

Example: Your total business miles turn out to be 3,000.

$$3000$$
$$\times\ .345$$
$$\$\ 1,035$$

Your deduction for business use of your car is $1,035.00. This figure is included on your Schedule C as your mileage deduction.

Actual cost method

Keep itemized records of all expenses related to operating your car. These include gasoline, oil, tires, lubrication, repairs and maintenance, insurance, license and registration fees and automobile club membership dues.

These actual costs will be added up at the end of the year. Another actual cost that can be included is the depreciation in value of your car during the year. The IRS has guidelines for computing depreciation.

Keep a log of business and personal miles, since you will need to figure the percentage of business use. At the end of the year, divide the year's total business miles by the year's total miles to arrive at the percentage of business use. Multiply the total of actual expenses by percentage of business use to determine your deduction.

For example, your total costs of operating your car for the year were $1,758. In addition, your depreciation allowance was $3,500. The total of these figures is $5,258.

If your business use of the car was 20% of the year's total use, your calculation would be:

$$5258$$
$$\times\ .20$$
$$\$1,051.60$$

Your deduction for business use of your car is $1,051.60. This figure is included on your Schedule C as your mileage deduction.

Depreciation

Depreciation is one of the most complex concepts facing someone trying to understand income taxes. Fortunately, you can get along just fine without ever conquering this particular challenge.

In a nutshell, depreciation refers to spreading out the cost of a large expense over a period of years, and deducting part of the expense each year. This usually applies to heavy equipment which costs a great deal and lasts for many years. During each tax year, the owner takes a portion of the total cost as a deduction. A small business person, such as a massage therapist, usually does not have to worry about depreciation, unless you purchase something with a large value that will last many years. The rules for spreading out the deduction over many years get extremely complicated and difficult to apply.

The government has given small businesses the option of avoiding the whole problem, by using what is called a "section 179 deduction". By using this option, you can deduct the entire cost of business items up to $25,000 entirely during the year you purchase the deductible item. Therefore, even if you purchase ten massage tables this year, you can take the whole deduction as a business expense during the year in which you spend the money. Consult a professional tax preparer if you are planning to use this type of deduction.

In some cases, there can be tax advantages to using depreciation instead of taking the whole deduction in one year. For example, if you make a large expenditure this year, and earn very little, the expenditure would be "wasted" if you took the whole deduction this year, because you would pay no taxes whether or not you take the deduction. Next year, when you have more income, you would like to be able to use part of the deduction to reduce you income taxes.

If you think that using depreciation could help you, send for IRS publication 946, How to Depreciate Property, or buy *Small-Time Operator*. See pages 168–169 for information on obtaining these items.

Estimated tax payments

If you will owe at least $1,000 in tax next year, you are required to pay estimated tax payments four times a year, on April 15, June 15, September 15 and January 15. You can also be penalized if you make your estimated tax payments late.

Estimated taxes are paid on IRS form 1040-ES, and the form includes a worksheet for you to use to calculate the amount of your estimated tax payments. It is based on the previous year's income, and if you follow the instructions in the worksheet, you are guaranteed not to be assessed a penalty for underpayment. To avoid penalties, you must pay either 90% of the tax you owed in the previous year, or 100% of the tax you owe for the current year.

Consider this: Your estimated tax payments are based on last year's income. If you make exactly the same income this year, your estimated payments will exactly pay your tax bill. However, what if you make more this year than last year? Your estimated tax payments cover the amount you earned last year, but on April 15, you will owe tax on any amount more than that. If you had a really good year, this additional amount could be several thousand dollars.

Consider also that April 15 is the date you must pay your first estimated tax payment for the coming year. In addition to paying the excess tax for last year, you must now make the first installment on next year's taxes. This "double whammy" can make April 15 a very expensive day for the self-employed bodyworker. Remember this if your practice is increasing, and find the discipline to put some money away all year so you will have enough to pay your taxes in April.

Hiring an accountant

Accountants are not cheap, but often they can pay for themselves in tax savings they find that you might miss. If you are motivated to do your own taxes, there is no reason you cannot do so. The resources listed below will give you all the information you need. With some time and study, you can learn what you need to know.

However, it can get complex, and unless you enjoy this sort of thing, consider hiring professional help. Non-CPA tax preparers may know just as much as an accountant, and may charge a little less.

Ask other therapists for recommendations for an accountant. When they recommend someone, ask why they like him or her, or why they think he is a good accountant. If the reasons they give refer to things that matter to you in an accountant, consider using that person.

Consider finding an accountant who will trade accounting services for massage. Use the yellow pages, and call accountants. Explain that you are just getting established, have a simple return, and would like to find an accountant who appreciates massage. You may catch someone in the proper mood to make an arrangement to trade services.

Consider, also, hiring an accountant to get you started with bookkeeping and tax systems you can understand, so that you can do your own taxes in future years. An accountant may be able to explain everything you need to know, and set you up with forms you will be able to use in future years.

If you hire an accountant or tax preparer, keep your records clear and organized. If possible, keep them in categories that will make it easy to sort out at tax time. This will make the accountant's job easier, and may encourage him to keep his fees reasonable.

How long to keep tax records

Keep your records and receipts for four years after filing. You could be audited up to that time and told to prove the accuracy of your income and deductions.

Keep your actual tax returns "forever"—or as long as you can. After four years, the government will not demand to see all your receipts and records to defend your returns, but you should always have your tax returns available to prove what you filed in case there is ever a controversy about your taxes.

Getting further information

If you want help doing your own taxes, there are several good resources you can turn to.

1. One is a book, written by an accountant, for the purpose of helping small business owners take care of bookkeeping and taxes. It is well-organized, well written and inexpensive. It goes into more detail about depreciation, and a few other minor subjects, than this chapter, and has practical advice about book-keeping. The book is called *Small-Time Operator* and is available from:

   Bell Springs Publishing
   Box 640 Bell Springs Road
   Laytonville, CA 95454
   (707) 984-6746

2. Check out your local bookstore as tax season approaches. All major bookstores carry a selection of Do-It-Yourself tax guides. They are

usually several hundred pages, and cost around $15.00. They cover in detail any subject you would need to know about in order to do your tax return. When April 15 rolls around and you are up against a deadline, book like this can be a comforting resource to have with you.

3. The final source of information is the IRS, and its information is available at no charge. The IRS will send you booklets explaining various aspects of your taxes, and is also available to answer questions by phone.

IRS publications can be ordered by calling

1-800-829-3676 (1-800-TAX-FORM) or at www.irs.gov

The first publication to order is Tax Guide for Small Businesses, Publication 334. This contains the basics of record-keeping and taxes for small businesses, including filled-in sample forms.

The second publication to order is "Guide to Free Tax Services." This lists all the other IRS publications. Once you have this booklet, you can leaf through it to see what else is available and what you need.

Some of the subjects covered in these IRS publications are listed below. The IRS publication number is listed after each name. These can be ordered from the toll-free number listed above.

Travel, Entertainment and Gift Expense 463
Tax Withholding and Estimated Tax 505
Educational Expenses 508
Moving Expenses 521
Reporting Income from Tips 531
Self-Employment Tax 533
Business Expense 535
Retirement Plans for the Self-employed 560
Taxpayers Starting a Business 583
Business Use of Your Home 587
Alternative Minimum Tax for Individuals 909
Business Use of a Car 917
How to Depreciate Property 946

All of these publications provide good detail, and are written in clear and readable fashion. However, they are written by the IRS, and will not necessarily tip you off to the best ways of getting the most out of your deductions.

To reach an IRS representative by phone, check your local phone book blue pages under Federal Government, Internal Revenue Service. Major cities have local offices. To find your local office, visit www.irs.gov and use the "site map" link located at the top of the home page. From the site map, choose "contact my local office" If you do not have internet access, call the IRS toll-free at 1-800-829-1040.

20 Scientific Research on the Benefits of Massage

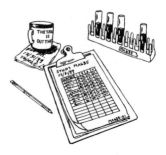

Although massage has been practiced for thousands of years, helping millions, perhaps billions of people, little scientific documentation of the health benefits of massage has existed until very recently. The massage profession was attempting to be taken seriously by the health care establishment with virtually no scientific evidence of the health benefits of massage.

All that has changed in the last ten years. Recent scientific research has produced verifiable data showing the efficacy of massage for a large variety of health problems. This documentation will be useful in promoting hospital-based massage, in securing reimbursement for massage from insurance companies, in gaining physician referrals and collaborations, and in convincing the general population of the benefits of massage as a health modality.

Three organizations currently involved in massage and bodywork research are the AMTA Foundation, the National Institutes of Health, and Touch Research Institute.

AMTA Foundation

The AMTA Foundation was created by AMTA in 1990. The Foundation awards grants to individuals or teams which promise to advance our understanding of specific therapeutic applications of massage, public perceptions of massage or attitudes toward massage, and the role of massage therapy in health care delivery. Information about the foundation is available on AMTA's website at **www.amtamassage.org**.

AMTA Foundation can be reached at:

AMTA Foundation
820 Davis Street, Suite 100
Evanston, IL 60201
(847) 864-0123

National Institutes of Health

Also sponsoring research in massage and bodywork is National Institutes of Health (NIH), a federal agency. Their research about massage is coordinated the National Center for Complementary and Alternative Medicine (NCCAM). Using federal grant money, the NCCAM reviews proposals for research and funds projects they believe are the most promising.

For basic information about NCCAM, contact:

NCCAM Clearinghouse
P.O. Box 7923, Gaithersburg, MD 20898
(888) 644-6226 or (301) 519-3153   www.nccam.nih.gov/nccam

General information about National Institutes of Health is available at www.nih.gov/health

Touch Research Institute

Of the three groups sponsoring or conducting massage research, by far the most studies are being conducted by Touch Research Institute. TRI was established in 1992 at the University of Miami School of Medicine. Under the direction of Tiffany Field, Ph.D., the institute has been conducting numerous studies to document the health benefits of massage. Some of their studies use licensed massage therapists, and others use college students or parents or grandparents who are given some training in how to give a massage.

Most of this chapter consists of a summary of the studies that have been conducted at TRI about the benefits of massage. Information about these studies and library references for all of them can be found at the Institute's website, www.miami.edu/touch-research.

Books About Scientific Research on Massage

Two recent books are available organizing and detailing scientific research on massage.

One is by the director of the Touch Research Institute, Tiffany Field. The book is titled *Touch Therapy* and is published by Churchill Livingstone. It sells for $32.95 and is available through all bookstores.

Another excellent volume of scientific research on massage is *Massage Therapy: The Evidence for Practice* by Grant Jewell Rich, published by Mosby. It is a well-organized and medically sound analysis of the current evidence for the efficacy of massage. It sells for $34.95 and is available through all bookstores.

Further information about both books is at www.harcourt-international.com

Both are written in the language of a medical researcher and present reviews of scientific data about massage in scientific terms. Either book could be something a massage practitioner might give or loan to a physician to convince him or her of the medical efficacy of massage, and may be useful to convince a mainstream physician to refer to massage practitioners.

Studies Conducted by Touch Research Institute

Adolescent and Child Psychiatric Patients

Adolescents and children who had been hospitalized for depression or adjustment disorder were given a 30-minute back massage each day for five days. Depression and anxiety were reduced and sleep increased compared to a control group who viewed relaxing videotapes.

72 children and adolescents aged 7 to 18 were studied. 52 received daily massage from psychology students who had massage training. The control group of 20 watched relaxing videotapes of pleasant sounds and images with psychology students while the subject group received massage. Observations, questionnaires, and measurements of pulse and saliva samples showed decreases in depression, anxiety, fidgeting and stress hormones (cortisol) immediately after treatment sessions. At the end of 5 days, depression levels were lower (though not in the control group) and nurses noted improved affect and cooperation. Massaged subjects also spent more of their bedtime sleeping and less time awake. The benefits of massage were greater for those subjects who were depressed.

Anorexia

Massage therapy reduced anxiety and stress, and resulted in decreased body dissatisfaction associated with anorexia.

Asthma

Asthmatic children were massaged by their parents and showed improvement.

The study compared massage with relaxation therapy, in both cases administered by parents who were taught the technique and performed it for 20 minutes at bedtime each day for 30 days. The 4 to 8 year-olds showed an immediate decrease in anxiety and stress hormones, and their peak air flow and other pulmonary functions improved over the course of the study. The 9 to 14 year-olds showed decreased anxiety and their attitude toward asthma improved during the study, but only one measure of pulmonary function improved.

Attention Deficit Hyperactivity Disorder

Adolescents with ADHD rated themselves as happier and were observed to fidget less after massage sessions. Also, teachers rated children receiving massage as less hyperactive and as spending more time on-task.

Autistic Children

After exposure to massage therapy, relatedness to teachers increased, and touch sensitivity, attention to sounds and off-task classroom behavior decreased.

Bulimic Adolescents

Massage decreased anxiety, depression and stress hormone levels in bulimic adolescent females, and improved body image and attitudes about their eating disorder.

Burn Patients

Massage with cocoa butter reduced anxiety, depression, pain and itching.

Burn patients were either massaged with cocoa butter for 30 minutes, two times per week for five weeks, or given standard medical treatment for burns. The massaged group reported less anxiety, depression, pain and itching immediately after the first and last therapy session, and their ratings on these measures improved over the five-week period.

Chair Massage enhances alertness & math computations, reduces depressed mood and job stress

Subjects were given chair massage for 15 minutes, twice a week for five weeks. The control group were asked to relax in the massage chair during the same period. Both groups had increased relaxation and reduced depression. The massaged group, however, also exhibited enhanced alertness (as shown by altered EEG levels), greater speed and accuracy on math computations, reduced anxiety levels, lower salivary cortisol levels, and lower job stress.

Children with Diabetes

Massage helped children with diabetes and their parents who gave the massages.

Parents of children with diabetes were taught massage or relaxation techniques. Children were massaged for 20 minutes at bedtime for 30 consecutive nights. Giving massage was found to decrease anxiety and depression in the parents, and receiving massage was found to reduce anxiety, fidgeting and depressed affect in the children. Over the course of the 30-day study, compliance for insulin and food regulation improved and blood glucose levels decreased from 159 to 118 (within the normal range).

Chronic Fatigue Syndrome

Immediately following massage therapy, depression, anxiety and stress hormones decreased. Following 10 days of massage, fatigue-related symptoms, particularly emotional stress and somatic symptoms, were reduced, as were depression, difficulty sleeping, and pain.

Cocaine-Exposed Premature Infants

Cocaine-exposed preterm neonates who received massage averaged 28% better weight gain than the control group and had better motor and stress scores on the Brazelton scale.

Babies were stroked and given passive movements for 15 minutes at a time, three times a day for ten days and were then compared to control group who were not massaged.

Cystic Fibrosis

Children receiving daily bedtime massages from their parents reported being less anxious, and their mood and peak air flow readings improved.

Dancers benefit from Massage

Massage Therapy improved range of motion, mood, balance and posture, and decreased stress hormone after receiving massage twice a week for one month.

Depressed Teenage Mothers

Massage was more effective than relaxation therapy to alleviate depression and anxiety in teenage mothers.

Dermatitis in Children

Massage improved affect and activity levels and all measures of skin conditions including less redness, lichenification, excoriation, and puritis. Parents' anxiety levels also decreased.

Diabetes in Children

Parents massaging their diabetic children for one month resulted in the children's glucose levels decreasing to the normal range, increased dietary compliance, and decreases in anxiety and depression for children and parents.

Fibromyalgia Patients

Fibromyalgia patients who received two 30-minute massages per week for five weeks had reduced anxiety and depression, less stiffness and fatigue, and fewer nights of difficult sleep.

One group received massage, one group received TENS (transcutaneous electrical stimulation) and one group received sham TENS (TENS equipment attached to subject but not activated). Massage therapy was most effective of the three, TENS was the next most effective, and even the sham TENS group had some improvement.

HIV-Positive Adults

Massage resulted in improvement of immune function for HIV-positive subjects.

Daily massage was given for one month. Significant increases in relaxation were noted, and significant decreases in anxiety. Also, significant increases were noted for Natural Killer Cell number, Natural Killer Cell Cytotoxicity, soluble CD8, and the cytotoxic subset of CD8 cells.

Infants Born to HIV-Positive Mothers

Neonates who received massage had greater weight gain and higher Brazelton scores than the control group.

Babies born to HIV-positive mothers were given three 15-minute massages per day for 10 days. The control group did not receive massage. The massaged group showed superior performance on almost every Brazelton newborn cluster score and had greater daily weight gain at the end of the treatment period, unlike the control group who showed declining performance.

Infants of Depressed Mothers

Massage was more effective than rocking to reduce stress, improve weight gain, promote sleep, and increase sociability and soothability.

Full-term 1 to 3 month old infants were either massaged or rocked for 15 minutes, two days per week for six weeks. Their mothers were all single adolescents of low socioeconomic status who suffered from depression. The massaged infants cried less, spent more time in active alert and active awake states, and had lower stress levels and lower stress hormone levels and their serotonin levels increased.

Infant Massage With Oil vs. Without Oil

Massage with oil was more effective than massage without oil.

Infants were separated into two groups, one which received massage with oil and one which received massage without oil. Both groups benefited, but the group massaged with oil were less active, showed fewer stress behaviors and head averting, and their stress hormone levels decreased more. Vagal activity also increased more with oil massage

Infants sleep better after massage

Massage was more effective than reading to children to promote sleep.

Parents in one group massaged infants and toddlers with sleeping problems for 15 minutes; parents in another group read bedtime stories to infants and toddlers with sleeping problems. The massaged infants showed fewer sleep delay behaviors and fell asleep more quickly by the end of the study.

Job Performance

Massaged workers showed indications of enhanced alertness; math problems were completed in less time with fewer errors after massage; anxiety and job stress levels were lower after one month of massage.

Job Stress

A 10-minute massage was as effective to reduce job stress as were 10-minute sessions of music relaxation, muscle relaxation with guided imagery, or social support group interaction.

Hospital workers were given one of the above brief treatments. Each group showed reduction in job stress as a result, and the reductions were approximately the same for all the methods tested.

Learning in Preschoolers

15-minute massages improved preschoolers' performance on block design and animal pegs subsets of the WPPSI.

Massage During Labor

Massage therapy during childbirth decreased anxiety and pain, and decreased the length of labor and decreased the need for medication.

Migraine Headaches

Massage therapy decreased the occurrence of headaches, sleep disturbances and distress symptoms.

Multiple Sclerosis

Massage therapy decreased depression and anxiety, and improved self-esteem, body image and social functioning.

Post-Traumatic Stress Disorder

Children who survived Hurricane Andrew received massage therapy, resulting in decreased anxiety, depression and stress hormone levels. In addition, their drawings became less depressed.

Pregnancy

Pregnant women who received massage had decreased anxiety and stress hormones during pregnancy, fewer complications and lower prematurity rates.

Premature Infants

Preterm infants who received massage averaged 47% better weight gain and averaged six days shorter hospital stay than the control group, resulting in savings of approximately $10,000.00 per infant.

Babies were stroked and given passive movement for 15 minutes at a time, three times per day for 10 days. The massaged infants were more alert, more mature, had better motor activity, and ranked higher on the Brazelton scale than the control group. These findings was replicated in a subsequent study which showed 21% greater weight gain, and discharge five days earlier than the control group.

A separate study found massaged preterm infants had 21% better weight gain per day and spent more time awake and active.

Psychiatric Patients

Child and adolescent psychiatric patients received five half-hour massages and showed improved sleep patterns, less depression, reduced anxiety and lower stress hormone, along with better clinical progress.

Sexual Abuse

Massage therapy reduced aversion to touch and decreased anxiety, depression and stress hormone levels.

Senior Citizens

Grandparent volunteers massaged infants for a 3-week period, and then received massages during a 3-week period. While giving massage, anxiety, depression and stress levels were decreased, and lifestyle, self-esteem and health improved. These effects were not as strong while receiving massage.

Sleep by Preschoolers

Massaged preschoolers fell asleep sooner, exhibited more restful nap times, had decreased activity levels and had better behavior ratings.

Women who have experienced sexual abuse

Massage was more effective than relaxation therapy for women who had experienced sexual abuse.

Massage was given by licensed massage therapists for 30 minutes twice a week for one month. A control group received relaxation therapy at the same time. Both groups experienced decreased anxiety and slightly decreased depression. The massage group also had decreased stress hormones (salivary cortisol) and less life event stress. The massage group did not experience a changed attitude toward touch, but the control group reported an increasingly negative attitude toward touch. The study suggests that a longer-term massage experience may be necessary to achieve change in attitude toward touch and significant change in depression.

Unpublished and Ongoing Studies

Additional completed studies awaiting publication demonstrate:

- Massage therapy reduces diastolic blood pressure and anxiety in patients with hypertension

- Massage improves premenstrual symptoms of anxiety, pain and water retention

- Massage relieves back pain and enhances range of motion

- Massage helps preschoolers be more on-task, less solitary, and less aggressive

- Massage therapy helps infants with cerebral palsy reduce spasticity, and improves posture, flexibility, motor function and social interaction

- Massage therapy helps infants with Down Syndrome to improve muscle tone and motor performance

- Ten massage sessions improve burn healing, including reduction in anxiety, anger, depression, pain and itching

- Massage therapy improves functioning in spinal cord injury patients

Studies that were in progress at the time of publication are expected to demonstrate:

- Massage may improve the interactions between caregivers and abused or neglected children

- Massage may be therapeutic for aggressive adolescents

- Massage may improve immunity in breast cancer patients as well as reducing anxiety and depression

- Massage may reduce colic in infants

- Massage may increase signs of alertness for children in coma

- Massage therapy may help children with muscular dystrophy by improving strength, range of motion and motor functioning

- Massage therapy may assist with treatment of Parkinson's Disease

- Massage may assist with treatment of prostate cancer

- Sports massage may enhance alertness and decrease anxiety.

The resources of the Institute are devoted to scientific studies and not public relations, so they request that all persons with inquiries visit their website, **www.miami.edu/ touch-research** which will contain the answers to most if not all questions. If the website does not have the information you need, you can establish contact with the Institute at:

Touch Research Institute
Department of Pediatrics
P.O. Box 016820 (D-820)
1601 NW 12th Avenue
Miami, FL 33101
fax (305) 243-6488

Searchable Databases of Scientific Studies

For those wishing to do further research into published studies on massage and bodywork, the Internet has many resources that can help.

AMTA Foundation has created a searchable directory of published books and articles about the efficacy of massage at: **www.amtamassage.org/foundation/dbase.htm**

National Center for Complementary and Alternative Medicine maintains a page with several links to searchable databases. At **www.nccam.nih.gov/databases.html** you can find links to:

Complementary and Alternative Medicine on PubMed
www.nlm.nih.gov/nccam/camonpubmed.html

Combined Health Information Database: **www.chid.nih.gov**

Computer Retrieval of Information on Scientific Projects:
www.crisp.cit.nih.gov

The main website for the National Institutes of Health also has a searchable database at **www.search.nih.gov**

The growth of the Internet as a research tool is staggering; this list of websites gathered in 2002 may seem rudimentary to those seeking to do research later in the decade, but these sites can serve as a good starting point at present for those wishing to research the scientific literature about massage and bodywork.

21 Reimbursement For Your Service by Insurance Companies

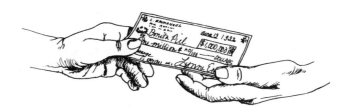

The Current Status of Insurance Reimbursement for Massage

The issue of insurance reimbursement is a source of confusion for many in the massage industry. The question "is your work covered by insurance" sounds like a simple question, but when you try to answer it, it can become quite complicated.

Consider, for example:

- Some health insurance policies cover massage, some do not.

- Some cover massage only if it is performed in a doctor's office.

- Some states license massage, and being in a non-licensed state may affect reimbursement.

- Automobile accident victims are under auto insurance, which has a different set of rules than health insurance.

- Within the automobile insurance industry, there are different rules in different states.

The variations in insurance policies, in types of insurance cases, and in state laws, combine to make the subject of insurance reimbursement for massage a difficult one to explain. However, it is not so difficult that it cannot be understood, and this chapter will give you the basics for understanding the insurance reimbursement system as it applies to massage therapy.

How big a part of the profession are we talking about?

In 1990, the AMTA surveyed its members about insurance reimbursement. Of those who answered the survey, 27% never participate in insurance billing. 9% have tried without success for insurance reimbursement. 34% report that they sometimes receive insurance reimbursement, and 20% receive reimbursement whenever they submit a claim. These results are from AMTA members, who are probably more oriented toward medical massage than the average massage therapist. The national averages for the entire massage community would undoubtedly show a smaller percentage of the total pursuing insurance reimbursement than is reflected by that study.

Some massage therapists do exclusively medical massage, and have mastered the skills required for insurance billing. These therapists routinely receive compensation for their services from insurance companies. Others, who may not do much insurance billing, and may not understand the correct procedures, become frustrated by what they perceive as roadblocks or red tape in the insurance billing field. They tend to shy away from insurance reimbursement clients. Still other therapists decline to undertake the extra work involved in obtaining pre-approval, charting each client's progress, reporting to insurance companies, tracking billings and payments, and following up on unpaid cases. These therapists choose not to participate at all in insurance billing.

Some of the political issues discussed in Chapter 3 have their effect in the insurance billing field. The issues of credentialing, certification, and standardization of educational requirements all have relevance in this field. However, even with the national picture unsettled at this time, you as a practitioner can still learn what is necessary to successfully do insurance billing and make this a part of your practice if you choose to do so.

Before exploring "how to" do insurance billing, we will consider the advantages and disadvantages of this type of practice.

Advantages and disadvantages

Insurance reimbursement for massage is a two-edged sword. On one side, people who could not otherwise afford massage, or who otherwise would not choose to pay for massage, become clients, and often repeat clients over a period of time. On the other side, your control over what you do as a massage therapist can be compromised, and each massage session you bill to insurance companies brings added paperwork for you.

These are the days of managed care. Doctors complain that managed care has ruined the practice of medicine. Insurance companies, eager to keep costs to a minimum, have become aggressive in telling doctors, psychotherapists and chiropractors what treatments will be paid for, at what rate, and under what conditions. Professionals who rely on insurance reimbursement are losing much of their freedom to practice as they see fit because they must conform to insurance company guidelines.

Another consideration is that you should expect at least some resistance by insurance companies to which you submit your claims for reimbursement. Insurance companies, like any other companies, make a profit by paying out less money than they take in. Most companies will pay legitimate claims, but they may require substantial paperwork to demonstrate that the claims are legitimate. Some companies resist even legitimate claims, requiring duplicative or excessive paperwork from the therapist.

Another hurdle some therapists have noticed in recent years is "bundling"— meaning that the insurance company that receives multiple claims on one client —for example chiropractic adjustment, massage therapy, and hot packs—

may "bundle" them all under the chiropractic adjustment code and pay only for that service. This can cause the massage therapist to be denied compensation. One solution is to have the patient receive massage and adjustment on different days. In that situation, the treatments cannot be "bundled".

The big advantages of working for insurance compensation are higher compensation and a stable client base. The billable hourly rate for clinical massage is usually between $60 and $130. (It is often closer to the high end in licensed states and closer to the low end in non-licensed states). The possibility of insurance compensation will also bring you clients who otherwise could not afford to use your services. These can be substantial advantages to an individual who is committed to the full-time practice of massage therapy.

It is up to you to decide whether the advantages to you outweigh the disadvantages, and you may not really know until you try it.

Your Role in the Health Care System

Massage therapists are not primary providers of health-care like physicians are. Massage therapists are "adjunct" therapists who work by prescription from a primary provider. Therefore, the doctor must provide a diagnosis and a prescription in order to initiate the process. Your therapy becomes part of the treatment plan of the referring doctor. He or she prescribes your services much the same as prescribing physical therapy or psychiatric care.

Some massage therapists have the knowledge and confidence to independently decide what a client needs and to make the insurance system work to reimburse them for what they do. Others work in a practice that can cast them more in the role of a technician, being told to work certain muscles only, or warm up an area for chiropractic adjustment. The kind of therapy you specialize in and your level of professional experience can make a large difference in this regard.

Relaxation Massage

Occasionally, a doctor will prescribe massage solely for its benefits in relaxing the client. Relaxation massage may or may not be reimbursable, depending on the patient's diagnosis and treatment plan.

Some chiropractors prescribe massage for patients who are too rigid to adjust, in hopes that the massage therapist will be able to help the patient release muscle tension, thus facilitating chiropractic care. A few medical doctors also prescribe massage for patients who are overly tense, as relaxation can help with a variety of medical problems that result from anxiety.

Medical Massage

Most prescriptions, however, are of a different sort, and involve what is commonly called "medical massage" or "clinical massage." This includes understanding of certain pathologies and knowledge of specific techniques that will be helpful in recovery from specific conditions and injuries. Some massage schools specialize in medical massage, and others offer some training in medical massage as part of their curriculum.

The newly-created Association of Manual Medicine Association, or AMMA (see page 134) is attempting to establish a standardized credential for medical massage, but at the current time there is no generally accepted industry standard for training in medical massage.

No *legal* requirement exists that you take a training in medical massage before working from a doctor's prescription. However, to attempt to do medical massage without proper training would be ill-advised, and would lead to frustration for you and for the doctor. Unless you have substantial training, you will not be able to understand the doctor's orders, and you will not know what to do to carry them out. Most doctors do not understand what massage therapists know and don't know, and therefore the responsibility to keep communication clear rests with you. Unless you are familiar with the terminology and procedures to be used in medical massage, problems will arise.

The AMMA (see page 134) is attempting to establish a standardized credential for medical massage, but at present there is still no widely accepted standard for medical massage training. Courses in pathology, medical terminology, neuromuscular therapy, trigger point therapy, cranio-sacral therapy, myofascial release, postural evaluation and deep tissue massage are useful. Also consider programs that include rehabilitative exercises and treatments for specific injuries and conditions. The medical massage component of your education could easily take 500 classroom hours, plus clinical practice.

Professional arrangements

A variety of professional arrangements are available to a massage therapist or bodyworker who wants to work with clients for insurance reimbursement.

1. The client pays the therapist at the time of service, and the client then submits the therapist's bill to the insurance company for reimbursement.

2. The therapist works by prescription of a physician, and the therapist deals directly with the insurance company for reimbursement.

3. The therapist works closely with the prescribing physician (or physical therapist) and the physician's office handles insurance reimbursement. The physician or physical therapist pays the therapist by the hour or by sub-contract. This arrangement is most common in non-licensed states, and is especially common when massage therapists work in chiropractors' offices.

No matter which of these arrangements you participate in, you should have a good understanding of insurance guidelines and the billing process. Even if the doctor's office does your billing, you should be able to supervise and assist the process, since the doctor's office person may not understand how to classify and bill for your services.

Procedures for Insurance Reimbursement

Assuming you have made the choice to work for insurance reimbursement, what follows is a nuts-and-bolts approach to the procedures you should follow. Note that there are entire manuals devoted to this topic, and the brief discussion in this chapter is meant to get you started, but cannot answer every question or cover every issue.

Step One — Preapproval

When a new client comes to you for insurance reimbursed work, your first task is to make sure they have a doctor's referral or prescription. It is possible to receive insurance reimbursement without a referral letter in some locations, but it is a safer practice to always have a referral letter.

A sample Physician's Prescription Letter of Referral is on Page 189. You should create your own Letter of Referral on your own letterhead. In the space titled "Treatment to include" create a list of the treatments you are able to do so the physician can check them off. Use accepted orthopedic language in this section so the physician will be comfortable with it.

Try to obtain a completed Letter of Referral for each client you will be working with. It establishes medical necessity, and it also lets the physician know what you do.

At your initial meeting with a client, in addition to reviewing the letter of referral, obtain the following information:
   Patient's name
   Date of birth
   Social Security Number
   Address and Phone Numbers
   Date of Injury
   Patient's Employer
   Insurance Company's Name, Address, Telephone Number
   Policy Number and Name of Insured Party

From the physician's referral or prescription note the following information:
   Diagnosis codes
   Frequency of Treatments
   Total Number of Treatments
   Name and UPIN# (Doctor's ID#) of Referring Physician
   Statement That Massage Therapy is Medically Necessary

Once you have the above information, contact the client's insurance company and ask for preapproval. State that you are a massage therapist, and that the treatment has been declared "medically necessary" by a physician. You may want to seek preapproval for "soft tissue mobilization" or "myofascial release" rather than "massage". Find out how many visits will be paid for, how much the company will pay per visit, what CPT code procedures are acceptable, and whether there are any restrictions on who performs the service or where it is performed.

Write down the name of the person you spoke with and the date. Make note of the answers to all of the above questions, and make sure you have the correct phone number and extension in case you need to reach this person again to follow up. Place the note in the client's file for future reference.

Step Two — Documentation

The first session should be documented in a separate report titled "Report of First Massage Therapy". Detail your objective findings, the client's symptoms, and any postural or range of motion measurements you made. This report will serve as a baseline from which you can measure future progress.

Each session should be individually documented. The customary format is the SOAP format. This stands for Subjective, Objective, Assessment, Plan/Prognosis.

> *Subjective* refers to the complaints and symptoms as the client expresses them. What pain is she having, and how often?

> *Objective* refers to postural distortions, gait pattern, and range of motion evaluation, and all measurable limitations.

> *Assessment* refers to the improvement resulting from this session. Did pain levels drop? Are there structural improvements? What aspects of the treatment plan are working ?

> *Plan/Prognosis* refers to the future treatment plans. Note goals for this client, including which muscles or regions of the body need treatment and what techniques are to be used.

Some therapists have modified the SOAP format to SOTAP format. The added "T" is for *Treatment,* and in this category they list the therapeutic procedures used in the session, such as massage (Mass), neuromuscular therapy (NMT), myofascial release (MFR), therapeutic exercise (Ther-X) for example. These prefixes are matched with insurance CPT codes for use on the HCFA insurance form.

After several visits, a "Progress Report" may be required to show the status of the client's treatment. This report compares all the objective client information to date with the measurements made at the initial visit, and reports on the change (if any) in the client's conditions and any circumstances that may be interfering with the client's progress.

Step Three — Billing the Company

Submit your bill for insurance reimbursement on HCFA Form 1500. This form must include the CPT codes used by practitioners of physical medicine, and should be filled out in the language used by health care providers nationally. The CPT code book is updated annually and is available from the American Medical Association.

The following codes listed in the 2001 CPT code book are the ones most commonly used by massage therapists and bodyworkers:

97124 Massage
97140 Manual Therapy
97112 Neuromuscular re-education (may require advanced training)

The following codes are less commonly used by massage therapists and bodyworkers, but may be appropriate for your work.

97010 Application of hot or cold packs

97039 Unlisted Modality

97139 Unlisted Therapeutic Procedure

97110 Therapeutic Exercises (may require advanced training)

97530 Therapeutic Activities (may require advanced training)

Note also that different codes will result in different rates of reimbursement. For example, 97112 usually is compensated substantially higher than 97124. If your work qualifies for this code, you will receive greater compensation by using this code instead of the one labeled "massage".

Consult the current edition of the *CPT Manual* to determine which codes are currently in use, and to find out the exact definitions of each code so you can assure you are using a code that correctly describes your work.

Most insurance companies base their allowable fees on a national or regional average, and will furnish you with their schedule of fees upon request.

Note that if you are providing services under a Worker's Compensation claim, lower fees are paid, different CPT codes are used, and different rules apply to insurance billing. An explanation of how to do Worker's compensation billing is beyond the scope of this chapter.

Step Four — Follow-up

If you do not receive payment within 45 days after you submit your bill, contact the representative at the insurance company (see the note you made when you called for preapproval). Make sure the bill has been received, and find out if there is any reason it has not been paid, or when you can expect payment. If forms have been incorrectly completed, your claim could be substantially delayed. Finding out about the error can help you clear it up.

Other times, simply drawing attention to your claim can help the wheels of bureaucracy turn a little faster; sometimes the "squeaky wheel" gets the oil. Send a written follow up or "tracer" stating "Tracer: please send payment or reason for non-payment".

If the company asks you to reduce your fee, you can send a "rebuttal" explaining in detail why your fees are appropriate. If your claim goes unpaid after you have sent two tracers, you have the option of filing a complaint with the state insurance commission. If the company is contacted by the state insurance commission, you can expect your claim to receive significant attention. Take this step only if diligent and reasonable collection efforts have failed.

Avoid Billing Pitfalls

Some common reasons that claims are rejected or delayed and how to avoid them:

Untimely billing. Send out bills every two to four weeks.

Incorrect dates. Carefully verify all dates on your billing forms.

Incomplete or unusual diagnosis. Doctor's diagnosis must be clear and follow coding books.

Diagnosis and treatment codes mismatched. Make sure your treatment codes are compatible with the Doctor's diagnosis codes and are appropriate for that condition.

Blank spaces on billing form. Fill in all spaces, indicating "N/A" or "none" when necessary.

Multiple same-day visits. Avoid submitting bills for different services of the same date. Schedule doctor visits and massage sessions on different days.

Unclear or excessive charges. Your fees must be itemized, and you must provide a total of your fees for each claim. Know the prevailing fees in your area for your kind of work.

Medical necessity. Send prescription or doctor's referral letter with your claim form.

Use standard forms. While the HCFA 1500 "superbill" is not required, and technically any form can be used to submit a claim for reimbursement, use the HCFA 1500 to avoid missing any required items and to avoid having your claim singled out for "special" attention.

Describe your work correctly. When speaking with insurance representatives, use the terms "soft tissue mobilization" or "neuromuscular re-education," since "massage" is often interpreted as relaxation massage and excluded from coverage.

Kinds of Insurance

One complicating aspect of this field is that there are different kinds of insurance carriers you may be submitting to. What follows is a brief discussion of the kinds of insurance you may encounter in this field, and how they differ.

Workers' Compensation. Generally a reliable payer; stay strictly within the authorized number of treatments, and work only on the regions of the body that are diagnosed and approved by the adjuster.

Automobile Insurance. Each policy will have a PIP (Personal Injury Protection) limit. This is the total amount available to pay all health care claims. Inquire at the time of preapproval as to the amount of PIP coverage, and whether the remaining balance is sufficient to pay for your treatment. Generally a reliable payer; when benefits expire, client will be responsible for balance if Financial Responsibility Form has been signed (see below). It is also possible to file a lien against the client's recovery for the cost of your services.

Liability Insurance. In rare cases, liability insurance will be responsible for payment for massage, such as a slip-and-fall in a grocery store. When preapproved, these carriers are usually reliable in paying for treatment. Sometimes payment is withheld until the end of treatment.

Group Health Insurance/Indemnity Policies. These policies usually have an annual deductible that must be met before benefits are paid to the insured, as well as a client co-pay amount, such as 20% of your fee. You would then bill 80% of your fee to the insurance company, and if the deductible is not yet satisfied, your fee would go toward the deductible. Billing this type of insurance carrier involves more details and restrictions than the types described above. These carriers are usually reliable payers after proper preapproval.

Financial Responsibility Form

Except as to Workers' Compensation, all clients may be made responsible to pay fees that insurance will not reimburse. This form should be signed at the first office visit. Many clients have never considered that they might be responsible for fees insurance will not pay, and some therapists choose not to use a Financial Responsibility Form, choosing instead to waive their fee if insurance will not pay.

If you choose to have a Financial Responsibility Form, either consult an attorney to have a form drawn up, or if you are comfortable with your ability to write clearly, create your own form by which your clients acknowledge that they are financially responsible to pay for your services if insurance reimbursement is denied for any reason.

States With Licensure vs. States Without Licensure

Practitioners in Washington State benefit from a 1996 law that requires insurance companies to cover expenses for health care by *any* licensed health professionals, including massage therapists. Therefore, all health insurance policies in Washington State must reimburse for massage therapy.

In the other states, the right to reimbursement for massage is not as well established. However, when all the proper procedures are followed, insurance reimbursement for massage should be received in states with massage licensure (see State Licensing Chart on page 154) and may also be available in states that do not have statewide massage licensing.

Litigation and the "Letter of Protection"

In a personal injury case, you may be asked to wait until the conclusion of the lawsuit to be paid for your work. Your client's attorney may offer you a Letter of Protection that guarantees you will be paid out of the settlement or judgment.

Be aware, however, that there is not always enough money available to pay everyone. Claims may be paid in the order they are received, and if the funds are exhausted before yours is paid, you can lose out. Some litigation cases guarantee 100% payment, but usually you must wait until massage therapy treatment is completed.

Most of these claims are paid eventually, and if you can do without the money at present, it can be a welcome surprise to finally receive a large check for work long since completed.

Fees and rate structures — legal and practical issues

Legally, you are *not* permitted to charge different rates for cash clients and for insurance reimbursement clients. Doing so constitutes insurance fraud.

This creates the unfair situation that the record-keeping, progress notes, billing and follow-up needed for insurance reimbursement work all go unpaid. As a result, working for insurance reimbursement can result in a substantially lower hourly rate when all of the additional tasks are figured in.

There are a couple of things you can legitimately do about this. First, while it is fraudulent to bill different charges to cash and insurance clients for the *same* service, it is not fraudulent to bill different charges for *different* services. Therefore, if you offer "relaxation massage" to cash clients for $60.00 per hour and "injury treatment" to insurance clients for $105.00 per hour, there is no fraud involved, assuming the two kinds of sessions you offer really are different.

Another possible solution is to establish a co-pay policy for insurance clients. Choose an amount that reasonably compensates you for the extra work involved in insurance billing, and establish that amount as a co-pay from your client at the time of service. You will then secure your customary fee for all the time you spend. The client may actually benefit from having a personal investment in the outcome of the therapy, becoming more involved in the healing process as a result.

A Word About Electronic Filing

If you submit your claims to insurance companies on paper, the following does not apply to you. However, if you choose to submit your claims on line or via e-mail, be aware that as of February, 2003, new federal regulations went into effect governing the formats and requirements for electronic filing of claims for health care reimbursement. For a summary of the requirements, you can visit: http://www.aspe.hhs.gov/admnsimp/faqtx.htm

This chapter has provided you with "the basics."

You may feel comfortable taking this information and beginning to bill insurance companies, or you may feel that you need additional information and guidance. See the resources on pages 208, 209 and 212 and consider also people in your community who have expertise in insurance billing who could give you some help or instruction as you get started.

Myofascial Associates

Specializing in Neuromuscular & CranioSacral Therapy Injury Rehabilitation

123 Maple Street · Suite ABC · Local Medical Park · Smallville, New York, 12345
t. (555) 296-7566 · f. (555) 296-1657

PRESCRIPTION/LETTER OF REFERRAL

Patient's Name	Address		
	City	State	Zip

Date of Birth	Date of Accident	Sex: Male ☐ Female ☐	S.S. #

ICD-9-CM Principal Diagnosis	Date

Treatment to include:

Treatment for the following area(s)/Diagnosis Codes

_____784.0 Headaches _____847.0 Cervical Strain/Sprain _____840.0 Shoulder Strain/Sprain _____840.9 Unspecified Upper Extremities: R_____
L_____ B_____ 842.0 Wrist Strain/Sprain: R_____ L_____ B_____ 847.1 Thoracic Strain/Sprain _____847.2 Lumbar Strain/Sprain
_____846.0 Lumbosacral Strain/Sprain _____724.3 Sciatica (pain in leg, no back pain) _____844.9 Unspecified site of knee and leg (strain/sprain): R_____
L_____ _____848.5 Pelvic Strain/Sprain _____723.4 Cervical Radiculitis _____354.0 Carpal Tunnel Syndrome
_____Other:_____
Safety Measures:_____
_____

Orders of Discipline and Treatment Plan

Duration: _____8 weeks _____6 weeks _____4 weeks _____Other_____
Frequency: _____Daily _____3x/weekly _____2x/weekly _____Weekly _____Biweekly _____Monthly

Medically Necessary: _____Yes _____No
Start of Care:_____

Physician's Name, Address, and Telepohne

Physician's Signature	Date

Physician's U.P.I.N.

22 Keeping Client and Financial Records

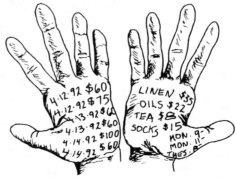

There are three basic kinds of records to keep; records you need to file your taxes, records about the operation of your practice, and records about each individual client.

Tax records

These are your records of all the money you earn and all the money you spend on deductible items. If you should be called on one day to demonstrate to the IRS the truth of all the entries in your tax return, you will need to produce accurate records of your income and deductions. These records should be kept four years after your return is filed in case the IRS chooses to audit your return at a later date.

Business records

These are the records you keep to give you a better understanding of your own practice. Different practices have different slow and busy times. Your practice may slow down for three weeks every August, which would make that a perfect time for your vacation in the Colorado Rockies. If you don't keep accurate records, you might not see that pattern, and might wind up staying in town during your slow season and leaving when clients will miss you more.

Client records

Client records allow you to better know and serve each client. Your records will let you know basic personal and medical information about each client, and will show you their history of receiving treatments from you. When appropriate, your records will give you an at-a-glance view of how your treatments affected specific problems or situations in your clients' lives.

This chapter discusses how to keep each of these three kinds of records, and suggests some ways to design your own record-keeping system that will make the whole process easier and more efficient. Sample forms appear at the end of the chapter. You may copy and use these forms, modify them to suit you, or create your own.

Record-keeping For Tax-Time

The records you need to keep are those proving your *income* and your *deductions*. Chapter 19 explains income and deductions.

The main things you should do to support proper tax record-keeping are 1) write down every payment you receive for your work in some type of ledger, 2) keep track of your automobile business mileage in a ledger, and 3) keep bills, receipts and canceled checks in one container until the end of the year, when you can sort them into categories and tally them up.

SHOE by Jeff MacNelly

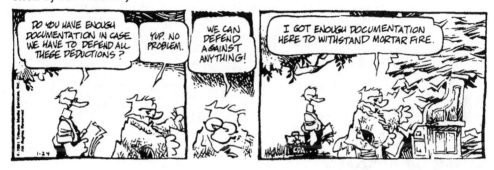

Recording income and business mileage

There is no required form for these records. The only requirement is that they be *accurate* and *complete*. If your car has a trip odometer, you can easily compute miles for each business trip by resetting the trip odometer to zero when you begin, and reading the trip odometer when you finish. Keep your log in the car, and record the mileage when you finish each business trip.

No matter what system you decide to use, take the time *each day* to record all of the day's business activity. Record the day's business mileage, and all income you receive each day. Get in the habit of recording each day's business activity before you go to sleep.

Records of Business Activity

Your records should show you your business activity for each day, each week, each month, and each year. It takes a minimum amount of effort to translate your business records into a useful chart, and the rewards can be substantial.

If you do not have a convenient source of graph paper, do an internet search for "printable graph paper" at **www.google.com** and you will locate several sites offering free printable graph paper you can use.

Charting your business activity gives you information about when you can expect seasonal ups and downs, it tells you whether your overall business activity is going up, going down, or staying about the same, and it can give you feedback about whether particular promotions produced results, and to what extent.

During some slow weeks, I could have become depressed or pessimistic about the progress of my practice. Instead, I glanced at my business activity chart, and I saw that last month I had a slow week and it was in-between two better weeks.

Instead of thinking my practice was going sour, I realized I was experiencing a normal fluctuation and nothing was going wrong. That insight did a lot for my emotional health.

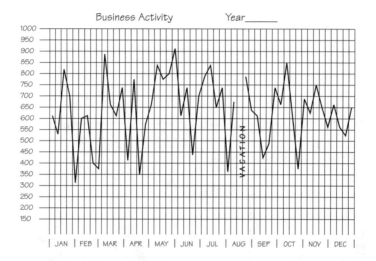

Keeping Client Records

If you or your clients are going to bill insurance companies for your services, you need to keep detailed records for each treatment you perform. See Chapter 21 dealing with billing insurance companies, and see pages 208–209 for resources to help with record-keeping for insurance clients.

Even if you are not dealing with insurance billing, you should keep client records. For each client, you should have a completed intake form that includes the following basic information:

- Date of first treatment

- Client's name, address, phone numbers and e-mail address

- Medical history (as much as you feel is necessary)

- Previous experience with massage or bodywork

- Current symptoms or problems

- Reason for seeking treatment

Date of first treatment will be useful to you later as you review your records on a particular client.

The address is necessary if you ever want to mail something to the client (such as a Christmas card, promotional flyer, or bill) or do a house call.

The phone number is necessary in the event of cancellation or change of plans on short notice.

Medical history gives you a better sense of how your treatment can fit into this person's whole picture, and can be useful in discovering contraindications for part or all of the treatment you will give.

Whether the person has previously had bodywork helps you to know how to approach this session.

Current symptoms or problems, and reason for seeking treatment give you information about what this client wants from you. Failure to get this information can result in doing a session that does not satisfy a client. They will not usually spontaneously tell you what they expect from your work.

The sample intake form on the next page is one you can modify to suit your own needs. If you do remedial work, you may want substantially more medical information. Keep in mind that the intake form has two basic purposes. First, it provides you with contact information and essential data about your clients. Second, it serves to open a dialogue between you and your client, and thereby begin the therapeutic relationship. It is a tool for communication.

If the client's care does not involve insurance billing, you may not need to keep further records for this client, except those necessary for business activity and tax purposes. If you do need to keep further records, you can use the back of the client's intake form, or create a separate file for records about continuing care clients.

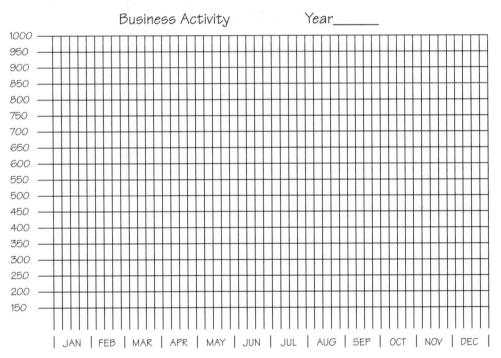

Client_____ Date of birth _____

Address_____

_____Phone (_____) _____

Date of first treatment_____

Occupation_____

Medical History:
Previous major Illnesses:

Previous broken bones or other
injuries:

Are you currently under a physician's
care?

    Physician _____

    For what condition? _____

    Are you taking any medications? _____

Current Condition:
Areas of pain or discomfort:

Reasons for seeking massage:

Have you previously had massage or
other bodywork? What type?

What do you do to manage your stress?

What is your routine of exercise?

Weekly Business Log

Week of _____

Date	Client	fee	miles

23 Managing Your Money
Some Ideas On Financial Planning

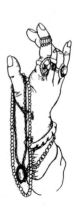

In the early years of your massage career, you will not have much money to manage. Spare dollars will go to necessities, and to improvements in your professional equipment.

In time, however, success will bring with it prosperity, and when it does, you will need to give at least a little thought to how to manage your money.

Savings

One of the hardest things for a self-employed person to do is to put money into a savings account. However, it is a very important habit to get into. Consider the following expenses you will have:

1. Quarterly estimated tax payments

2. Health insurance, auto insurance

3. Professional association dues

These expenses come quarterly, semi-annually, or annually. They can put a strain on your budget if you are living from month to month. Having a reserve in your savings (or checking) account makes life easier when these expenses come due.

Open a savings account at your bank. Start it with at least $100, and add whatever amounts you can. Avoid making withdrawals unless absolutely necessary. The fact that you have a few hundred dollars, or a couple of thousand dollars, can be very comforting when the mechanic tells you that you need a transmission overhaul.

Beyond this issue of emergency reserves to meet unforeseen expenses, you will also want to consider the larger financial reserves you will need to meet the major expenses you can expect sooner or later:

4. Buying a new car

5. Buying a home

6. Rearing children

7. Retirement

These are the expenses that require you to make, and save, substantial sums of money, and to manage that money in a way that gives you the most advantage out of it.

Long-range planning

As a rule of thumb, there are two critical points in the careers of many would-be massage therapists—two years into a career and five years into a career.

Many practitioners give up somewhere near the two-year mark. Either they failed to pursue any organized marketing approach, or they gave up before getting the benefit of the approach they were using.

Those who survive the two-year mark usually find some degree of success in the field. Another critical point often comes at the five-year mark, when the physical nature of the work may begin to take its toll, or the practitioner may decide to branch off into another kind of work.

Practitioners who stay with the work longer than five years can usually keep doing the work practically indefinitely. Some keep working into their seventies. If you are staying in the field longer than five years, you will do well to take up the study of estate planning and investment.

You can't live on Social Security

Consider what you will have to live on when you retire.

Social security may be enough to keep a roof over your head, and bread on the table, but it is not enough money to *live* on. Before you reach retirement age, you should have put aside enough to create your own retirement plan. The earlier you start, the easier it will be.

Kinds of Savings Plans

Savings plans can take many forms.

1. You can stockpile cash, but if you do so you earn no interest, and can lose everything in a theft or fire.

2. You can keep your money in a savings account, certificate of deposit, or money market account. These will earn interest, and your money will be basically safe.

3. You can choose a "tax shelter" keyed to retirement. While you must still pay self-employment tax on the money you put into your retirement plan, you do not pay federal income tax on this money. You pay income tax on the retirement money only when you receive it, at retirement. Tax breaks available to retired persons may help you pay lower taxes on your money at retirement time than you would now.

Tax Shelter Retirement Plans

One major advantage of tax shelter retirement plans is that they force you to keep your money invested until you retire. Because of high penalties for withdrawing money prior to age 59½, you are forced to keep your "nest egg" safe for your future.

You lose the flexibility to deal with your money on a whim; you have fewer options now, but more security later.

The government makes this appealing by giving you a slightly better tax treatment if you put your money into a retirement plan. Consider the following example:

It is April 14th, and you are preparing your tax return for the previous year. You do all your computations, find out you owe $2,104 in income tax (we are ignoring social security tax in this example, because retirement plans do not change your social security tax).

If you use some money you have saved to make a contribution of $2,000 to a qualified retirement plan, your income tax bill will be reduced to $1,804 (assuming you pay 15% income tax). You therefore reduce your tax by $300 by placing $2,000 in a retirement plan. As long as you make this contribution by April 15, it counts as a deduction for the preceding year's taxes.

Save now, save later

To take the example a step further, consider the long-term effects of this decision. If you *do not* make the contribution to your retirement plan, you must spend $300 of the $2,000 on taxes. This leaves you with $1,700.

Assume that you keep this $1,700 invested at "average" interest rates for thirty years. Interest rates are always changing, but as a rule of thumb, you can figure that money well-invested will double itself every ten years. Therefore, in 30 years, an investment should grow to eight times the original amount. (After 10 years, the original investment will double; after 20 years it will double again, or be four times the original amount; after 30 years it will double a third time, and be eight times the original amount).

This rule of thumb tells us that $1,700 today will be $13,600 in 30 years.

Now consider the alternative where you put $2,000 in a retirement account. The same rule of thumb tells us that the $2,000 today will turn into $16,000 in 30 years. However, this $16,000 will be subject to income tax when you receive it at retirement. Current rates of income tax, 15%, would reduce that $16,000 to $13,600 — exactly the same amount as if you had paid your $300 tax in the first place and left the $1,700 invested.

However, unless you are a person of incredible will power, you *will not* leave that $1,700 alone for 30 years to gain interest. What you will wind up with will be somewhat less than the $13,600 you know you can count on if you sock the money away in a retirement plan where you cannot reach it without substantial penalties.

In addition, tax breaks available to retired persons may make it possible for you to pay less than 15% tax on the money when you receive it at retirement. Any such breaks you get make it definitely advantageous to have your money in a retirement account.

Kinds of Retirement Plans

There are three kinds of retirement plans available to you as a self-employed person: The IRA (Individual Retirement Account), the SEP (Simplified Employee Pension Plan, a form of IRA); and the Keogh.

IRA and ROTH IRA

Easy to set up and widely available, an IRA or Roth IRA allows you to shelter up to a maximum of $3,000 per year. IRA's are designed for people without large incomes.

SEP

Also easy to set up and widely available, the SEP allows you to shelter up to 15% of your earnings (to a maximum contribution of $30,000 in any one year)

Keogh

Two types of plans exist, one which requires a set contribution each year, and one which does not. The maximum contributions are 20% of income or a maximum of $40,000 per year. Keogh's are more complicated to set up, and can be more expensive to create and maintain than IRA's or SEP's.

IRA's and SEP's can be set up any time before April 15, and will still be valid for the previous year's taxes. Keogh's must be *set up* by December 31 in order to be valid for that tax year, although contributions can still be made until April 15 of the next year.

You also have the option of setting up a 401(k) as a self-employed individual. This allows almost unlimited contributions to your retirement account, but it is costly to set up and maintain. If you have very high income, consult with a financial professional about whether this might be the best option for you.

If you are interested in establishing a retirement account, start with your local bank, savings and loan, or insurance advisor. Chances are, they can advise you and set up an account for you, often at no charge. Also check with your accountant or financial advisor. Once established, these accounts cannot be modified, so be very careful that you understand how your account will fit into your future plans.

V

Equipment
and Other
Professional
Resources

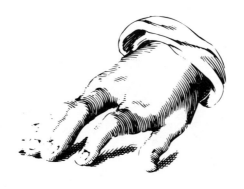

Massage Tables and Chairs

All of the following companies ship their products nationwide. They will all send you brochures or information packets about their massage tables and other products at your request.

Massage Table / Chair Manufacturers

Astra Lite Tables
120 Manfree Rd.
Watsonville, CA 95076
(800) 368-5483 or (831) 763-0397
www.astra-lite.com

Extremely lightweight, portable table; stationary table; fixed or push-button adjustable height, with recessed legs and cables and built-in face cradles; bolsters, carrying cases

Blue Ridge Tables
2679 S. Harper Rd.
South Industrial Park
Corinth, MS 38834
(800) 447-2723 or (662) 286-7007
www.blueridgetables.com

Full line of massage equipment; portable, tables and chairs.

Colorado Healing Arts
P.O. Box 2247
Boulder, CO 80306
(800) 728-2426 or (303) 449-2425
www.coloradohealingartsproducts.com

Portable and non-portable tables, oils, linens, bolsters, massage tools, charts, professional office forms and other items. Free brochure includes "How to select a massage table."

Creative Touch
1713 G Street #1
Sacramento, CA 95814
(800) 441-6759 or (916) 441-6759
www.massageresources.com

Lightweight, adjustable height, oval massage tables and accessories

Custom Craftworks
P.O. Box 24621
Eugene, OR 97402
(541) 345-2712
(800) 627-2387
www.customcraftworks.com

A selection of stationary and adjustable height portable tables; on-site chair, electric lift table, desktop portable support, bolsters, carrying cases, — and accessories. Lifetime warranty on all wood tables

Earthlite
3210 Executive Ridge Dr.
Vista, CA 92083
(800) 872-0560
www.earthlite.com

Full line of portable, stationary and electric lift massage tables; bolsters fleece pads, table skate, carry case, stools, headrest covers, flannel sheets

Galaxy Enterprises, Inc.
5411 Sheila St.
Los Angeles, CA 90040
(323) 728-3980 or (800) 876-4599
www.galaxymfg.com

Lightweight, portable, adjustable height massage table

Golden Ratio Woodworks
P.O Box 297
Emigrant, MT 59027
(800) 345-1129
www.goldenratio.com

Full line of stationary and portable tables, spa tables, on-site chair, 14-pound on-site chair, covers, oils, bolsters, charts, books and other accessories.

Living Earth Crafts
5800 Redwood Dr.
Rohnert Park, CA 94928
(800) 358-8292 or (707) 584-4443
www.livingearthcrafts.com

Complete line of stationary and portable tables, including very inexpensive portable, on-site chair, desk-top face cradle, oils, linens, books, charts, music, videos, and more.

New Generation Products
c/o The Unexerciser
(800) 326-2724

Basic and deluxe lightweight adjustable height massage tables; carry case, fitted face cradle covers, oil pouch belt (lifetime guarantee except for vinyl)

Northern Touch, Inc
(877) 948-6824 or (780) 921-2299
www.northerntouch.net

Massage tables with lifetime warranty on structure and foam

Oakworks, Inc.
P.O. Box 238
Shrewsbury, PA 17361
(717) 235-6807 or (800) 558-8850
www.oakworks.net

Complete line of stationary and portable tables, on-site chair, carrying cases, bolsters and sheets

Pisces Productions
380 Morris St., Suite A
Sebastopol, CA 95472
(800) 822-5333 or (707) 829-1496
www.piscespro.com

Vertical to horizontal, adjusting on-site chair, portable tables ultra-light tables, and accessories

Robert Hunter Bodywork Tables
910 SE Stark St.
Portland, OR 97214
(800) 284-3988
www.RobertHunter.com

Stationary and portable adjustable height tables, sheets, massage oil, carrying cases, customization available

Stronglite Massage Table Kits
255 Davidson St.
Cottage Grove, OR 97424
(541) 942-0130
(800) BUY-KITS (800-289-5487)
www.stronglite.com

Portable, lightweight adjustable height, inexpensive tables, on-site partially assembled tables and kits at substantially lower cost. Stronglite also makes the ComforTable line of massage tables.

Tatum Table
305 S.W. 250th St.
Newberry, FL 32669
(800) 382-8530
www.tatumtable.com

Portable, adjustable height massage table, on-site chair, accessories.

Touch America
P.O. Box 1304
Hillsborough, NC 27278
(919) 732-6968
(800) 678-6824
www.touchamerica.com

Complete line of stationary and portable tables, spa products, acoustic music table, on-site chair, stool, sheets, miscellaneous items workshop series, spa therapies, hydrokinetic vichy.

Powered Height Adjustment Tables

Care-Tech Research Corp.
4337 River Road W.
Delta, BC., V4K 1R9, Canada
(604) 946-1574

Comfort Craft Bodywork Tables
P.O. Box 520638
Longwood, FL 32752
(407) 830-7332 or (800) 858-2838
www.comfortcraft.com

Custom Craftworks
P.O. Box 24621
Eugene, OR 97402
(541) 345-2712 or (800) 627-2387
www.customcraftworks.com

Earthlite
3210 Executive Ridge Dr.
Vista, CA 92083
(800) 872-0560
www.earthlite.com

Integrated Medical, Inc.
8100 S. Akron, Ste. 320
Englewood, CO 80112
(800) 333-7617

Very Light Portable Tables (25 lbs. or less)

Astra Lite Tables
120 Manfree Rd.
Watsonville, CA 95076
(800) 368-5483 or (831) 763-0397
www.astra-lite.com

Golden Ratio Woodworks
P.O Box 297
Emigrant, MT 59027
(800) 345-1129
www.goldenratio.com

Pisces Productions
380 Morris St., Ste. A
Sebastopol, CA 95472
(800) 822-5333 or (707) 829-1496
www.piscespro.com

Stronglite Massage Table Kits
255 Davidson St.
Cottage Grove, OR 97424
(541) 942-0130 or (800) 289-5487
www.stronglite.com

Ultra-Light Inc.
4975 Crescent Technical Court
St. Augustine, FL 32086
(904) 749-7979 or (800) 999-1971
www.ultralightcorp.com

Specialty Tables

Somatron Corp.
8503 N. 29th St.
Tampa, FL 33604
(800) 544-4294
www.somatron.com

Vibro-acoustic massage table that directs vibrations through the client's body during the massage

Massage Supply Stores and Catalogue Services

Alternative Essentials
P.O. Box 54
Coopers Mills, ME 04341
(207) 623-4551

Massage and physical therapy supplies, books, charts music, gift certificates, accessories, massage tables and chairs, aromatherapy supplies

Banner Therapy Products
524 Hendersonville Rd.
Asheville, NC 28803
(888) 277-1188 or (828) 277-1188
www.BannerTherapy.com

Aromatherapy, massage tools, oils, gels, lotions, vibrators, hot and cold packs, hydrocollators, pack chillers, paraffin baths, charts, supports, pillows, desktop portal, 30-day money back guarantee.

Best of Nature
176 Broadway
Long Branch, NJ 07740
(800) 228-6457 or (732) 728-0004
www.bestofnature.com

Massage tables and chairs, oils, creams, lotions, liniments, essential oils, linens, self-massage tools, incense, books, videos, music, bottles and pillows

BML (Basic Massage Lines)
501 W. Kingshighway
Paragould, AR 72450
(800) 643-4751
www.bmlbasic.com

Oils, lotions, hydrocollators, vibrators, paraffin baths, hot and cold packs, massage tables and chairs, linens, bolsters, pillows, stools, other accessories

The Body Shop
2051 Hilltop Dr., suite A-5
Redding, CA 96002
(530) 221-1031 or (800) 736-6897

Massage Holster, aqua-relief pad, sunfresh soap, stronglite tables, aromatherapy supplies, oils, lotions, charts, face rest covers (fitted and flat).

Buymassage.com
Core Institute (FL)
www.buymassage.com

Supplies, equipment, accessories, books, workshops, large variety of products

Gotyourback
4442 Main St.
Philadelphia, PA 19127
(800) 677-9830 or (215) 483-9802
www.gotyourback.com

Massage tables and on-site chairs, accessories, oils & lotions. Large inventory, same-day shipping.

Bodywork Central
5519 College Avenue
Oakland, CA 94618
(510) 547-4313
orders: (888) 226-8500
www.bodyworkcentral.com

Variety of massage tables and on-site chairs, bolsters, Biotone oil & lotions, carrycase, table skate, table carrier, spa supplies, body support cushion, table selection assistance, yoga products.

Bodywork Emporium   www.bodyworkemporium.com   1-800-TABLE-4-U

338 North Coast Highway	1011451 Morena Blvd.	414 Broadway
Leucadia, CA 92024	San Diego, CA 92110	Santa Monica, CA 90401
(760) 942-9565	(619) 276-2608	(310) 394-4475
1804C Newport Blvd.	4529 Sepulveda Blvd.	1329 State Street
Costa Mesa, CA 92627	Sherman Oaks, CA 91403	Santa Barbara, CA 93101
(949) 548-0220	(818) 990-6155	(805) 965-5546

Large selection of massage tables and on-site chairs, massage oils and lotions, videos, books, charts, music and other supplies, on-site massage therapy.

Edcat Enterprises
P.O. Box 168
Daytona Beach, FL 32115
(386) 253-2385 or (800) 274-3566

Large selection of anatomical and other charts, self-massage tools, oils, lotions, tables, chairs, anatomy models, hydrocollators, hot & cold packs.

Educating Hands School of Massage Bookstore Catalogue
120 Southwest 8th Street
Miami, FL 33130
(800) 999-6991

Books, massage tables, massage oils charts, audio cassettes, videos, hot and cold application equipment, self-massage tools, linen and hand cleaners, misc. items.

HANDSON BOOKSTORE™
QWL Services
POB 20795
NY, NY 10025
(212) 222-4240

Located at www.qwl.com/mtwc/handson, this is a virtual bookstore specializing in books for the massage and bodywork professional. Large selection, On-line ordering.

Hands on Health Care Catalog
Acupressure Institute
1533 Shattuck Ave.
Berkeley, CA 94709
(800) 422-2232 or (510) 845-1059
www.acupressure.com

Books, reference charts, flash cards, videos, audio tapes, massage and self-massage tools, magnet devices, acupressure model, music

Hands-on-supply
Connecticut Center for MT Bookstore
(800) 842-9874
www.hands-on-supply.com

Oils, brochures, linens, pillows, videos, charts, books, music.

The Health Touch
261 Main St.
Royersford, PA 19468
(800) 890-6195

Oils, lotions, creams, aromatherapy supplies, massage products, massage tools, massage tables. Free catalogue.

Here's The Rub
66 Evergreen Ave.
Warminster, PA 18974
(877) 484-3782
www.herestherub.net

Massage equipment, linens and pads, charts, oils, books, music, videos, aromatherapy, spa, hot and cold therapy

Massage Central
12235 Santa Monica Blvd.
Los Angeles, CA 90025
(310) 826-2209
www.mcla.com

Large display of massage tables and on-site chairs, and other supplies, spa and salon equipment.

Massage King
(800) 290-3932
www.massageking.com

Tables, chairs, other supplies and specials

MassageTableWarehouse
(800) 224-5555
www.mtswarehouse.com

Massage tables and chairs from numerous makers, same-day shipping from Texas warehouse

MassageWarehouse.com
5965 Peachtree Corners E., Bldg #C-3
Norcross, GA 30071
(770) 582-9191
www.massagewarehouse.com

Large selection of tables, chairs, oils, books, and supplies for massage practitioners

New England Massage Tables and Chairs
20 Bridge St.
Manchester, NH 03101
(800) 545-8497
www.massagestore.com

Massage tables, massage chairs, oils, lotions, gels, essential oils, charts, books, self-massage tools, bolsters, hot and cold applications products, flash cards, other accessories

Rosenthal Clinic Massage Tables & Chairs
141 N. Meramec
St. Louis, MO 63105
(800) 833-3603

Distributor of most brands of massage tables and chairs; table selection service

Sunset Park Massage Supply
2302 S. Hubert Ave.
Tampa, FL 33629
(800) 344-7677 or (813) 251-0320
www.massagesupplies.com

Massage tables and chairs from 12 companies, accessories, charts, books, aromatherapy supplies, videos, hydrocollators, paraffin baths, lotions, oils, body & pregnancy cushions, CEU home study, etc.

West Coast Massage Tables and Chairs
209 Pacific Ave.
Rodeo, CA 94572
(510) 799-4704 or (888) 670-9720

Tables and chairs at 5% discount below retail. Oils, linens, fountains, fleece table covers, stools, white noise devices, etc.

Miscellaneous Massage Items

Table covers, sheets and related items:

Innerpeace
P.O. Box 940
Walpole, NH 03608
1-800-949-7650
www.innerpeace.com

100% cotton flannel sheets, face cradle
covers, bolster slip covers and more

Daffodil's Associates
12 Shelby Rd.
East Northport, L.I., NY 11731
(631) 368-1197

Disposable 40" x 90" massage sheets in car-
tons of 50; AcuPlus electro-stimulator for pain
relief sold only to LMT's

Printed items such as brochures about massage and gift certificates:

Information for people
P.O. Box 1038
Olympia, WA 98507
(800) 754-9790 or (360) 754-9799
www.info4people.com

(Marketing materials, including brochures, selection of books and compassionate touch
videos, display cases, gift certificates, greeting cards, post cards, sculptures)

Touch, Ink. MicroPublishing
847 S. Liman
Oak Park, IL 60304
(800) 296-3968
www.touchink.com

(Touch, Ink. is a promotional newsletter aimed at massage clients. It is personalized with
the name of the massage therapist on the front page, and contains informative articles
about massage and related topics) Gift certificates, templates emphasizing topics such as
stretching, carpal tunnel, stress & self care, breast massage.

Practice Management Software:

Customer Pro-File—Keeps track of clients, notes, scheduling, business records.
Inexpensive program to computerize your practice.

Land Software
5163 Fulton St. NW
Washington, D.C. 20016
(202) 237-2733   www.landsw.com

Easy Billing—Produces SOAP notes and HCFA 1500 forms for insurance billing, prints letters and reports

Marla Productions
524 Don Gaspar
Santa Fe, NM 87501
(800) 618-6136   www.nets.com/easybilling

Elite Software—Keeps track of clients, sales, inventory, appointments, payroll,
marketing.

Elite Software
(800) 662-ELITE
www.elite-usa.com

MassageSOFT 5.1—Daily appointment book, mailing lists, billing and follow-up, SOAP notes and HSCF forms.

Get Physical! Software, Inc.
(800) 622-0025
15 E. Putnam Ave., Ste. 376
Greenwich, CT
www.massageSOFT.com

Massage Office 2.2—Keeps track of clients, scheduling and records; will print SOAP notes onto anatomical chart and will print HCFA 1500 forms for insurance billing

Island Software
(877) 384-0295 or (972) 241-0705
www.islandsoftwareco.com

MediSoft—The Medical Massage Office Billing System— Keeps track of clients, scheduling and records, produces documentation and will print HCFA 1500 forms for insurance billing

Compmed Billing
(888) 322-5520 or (561) 697-8414

Assorted products and services:

My Receptionist—The service provides you with a toll-free number, and you arrange call forwarding to have your appointment line ring in their offices. A professional receptionist answers your line with your business name, and can answer basic questions about your services, schedule your appointments, make reminder calls, take credit cards, and sell gift certificates. The service costs $29.95 per month plus a charge of seventy cents per minute for usage.

My Receptionist
P.O. Box 0161 / 408 Riverside Ave.
Eau Claire, WI 54702
(800) 686-0162
www.myreceptionist.com

Khepra Foot Balm—A preparation for use in massaging the feet, that creates a skin texture with a subtle resistance for better massage, eliminates foot odor, and conditions and refreshes the feet:

Khepra Skin Care, Inc.
500 E. 36th St.
Minneapolis, MN 55408
(800) 367-9799
www.khepracare.com

BodyCushion™—a contoured system of support that positions the body comfortably, prone, supine or laterally; useful for pregnancy, geriatric, disabled, on-site and seated massage:

Body Support Systems, Inc.
P.O. Box 337
Ashland, OR 97520
(800) 448-2400
www.bodysupport.com

Magazines, Journals, Newsletters and Books

Magazines

Massage Magazine covers a broad range of news and features of general interest to massage practitioners. Each issue also contains up-to-date nationwide licensing information. Published six times a year. Subscriptions (800) 533-4263

AMTA's *Massage Therapy Journal*, available by subscription to non-members, contains articles of interest to the general massage community, and items of special interest to AMTA members. Published four times a year. Subscriptions (847) 864-0123

ABMP's *Massage & Bodywork* Magazine, available by subscription to non-members, contains articles of interest to the general massage community, and items of special interest to ABMP members. Published four times a year. Subscriptions (303) 674-8478

Journals

The Journal of Soft Tissue Manipulation This is an international, multidisciplinary journal highlighting research, clinical change, aspects of the client/practitioner relationship, precautions and contraindications, and philosophical issues concerning massage and related disciplines. It is a publication of the Ontario (Canada) Massage Therapist Association. Subscriptions (416) 968-6487

Touch Research Abstracts—Touchpoints This is the quarterly publication of the Touch Research Institute, Tiffany M. Field, Ph.D., director. The publication reports on the work of the Touch Research Institute in scientifically documenting the health benefits of touch, and also provides information on programs sponsored by the Institute. Subscriptions are $10.00 per year. Touchpoints/Touch Research Institute, Department of Pediatrics (D820), University of Miami School of Medicine, P.O. Box 016820, Miami, FL 33101, (305) 243-6781. **www.miami.edu/touch-research**.

On-line employment directory

www.portablepractitioner.com is an on-line service listing employment opportunities worldwide

Books for Bodyworkers

The library of books for massage and bodywork seems to grow by the day. The books in the following list were selected because they can assist you with the career of massage.

Self-Care Books

Save Your Hands! by Lauriann Greene. This book covers reasons for injury, common injuries, how to use your body, techniques to use or avoid, exercises, stretching and treatment. It retails for $17.95. Published by Guilded Age Press, 1-877-261-1500 or (970) 493-3793 **www.saveyourhands.com.**

National Certification Review Books:

Complete Review Guide for National & State Certification Examinations, by Dr. Patrick Barron, $21.95. Publisher: Futurmed, available from **www.buymassage.com**

Massage Board Review Book, by Don Newton, M.A., D.C., instruction on exam topics and sample questions, $19.95, available from **www.simran.com**

Massage Therapy Exam Questions, by Daphna Moore, Hugnes Henshaw Publications, $38.00, available at **www.hugheshenshaw.com**

Questions & Answers, by Daphna Moore, Hugnes Henshaw Publications, $39.95, available at **www.hugheshenshaw.com**

Questions and Answers for Passing State and National Therapeutic Massage Examinations and *More Questions and Answers for Passing State and National Therapeutic Massage Examination*, by Massage Review Publications, (954) 578-5055, **www.massagereview.com.** Spiral bound, each book $49.95 or both for $79.95.

Therapeutic Massage & Bodywork (Exam Review for the NCETMB), by Jane Garofano, Ph.D., Appleton & Lange $28.00, includes a computer diskette.

Pathology for Massage and Bodywork

Clinical Pathology for the Professional Bodyworker, 2nd edition, by Don Newton, M.A., D.C., Simran Publications, $24.95. Each condition is discussed separately, along with suggestions for massage techniques and movements to assist with that malady. Available from **www.simran.com**

Massage Therapist's Guide to Pathology, by Ruth Werner, includes practice suggestions for each malady, $41.95, Lippincott Williams & Wilkins, availabe at **www.lww.com**

Pathology A to Z, a Handbook for Massage Therapists, 2nd edition, by Kalyani Premkumar, M.D. This book is arranged alphabetically. For each pathology, it discusses the cause, signs & symptoms, risk factors, cautions & recommendations, and notes. Optional CD-ROM. Published by VanPub Books, 1640 16th Ave., suite 205 N.W., Calgary, AB, T2M0L6, Canada, 1-877-VANPUB-1, **www.meducational.com/vanpub**

Pocket Book of Pathology—a quick reference, by Kalyani Premkumar, M.D., a brief version of *Pathology A to Z*, also available with a companion CD-ROM, Published by VanPub Books, 1640 16th Ave., suite 205 N.W., Calgary, AB, T2M0L6, Canada, 1-877-VANPUB-1, **www.meducational.com/vanpub**

Recognizing Health and Illness, Pathology for Massage Therapists and Bodyworkers, by Sharon Burch. This oversize textbook is well-organized, with each chapter covering a physiological system. It contains illustrations, study questions, references and chapter reviews. It is available from Health Positive! Publishing, P.O. Box 3818 Road, Lawrence, KS 66046, fax (888) 797-5594. $50.00 **www.healthpositive.com/ schools.htm**

Medical Massage / Clinical Massage

The Insurance Reimbursement Manual by Christine Rosche, M.P.H. The author is also available for telephone consultations at (800) 888-1516; to order phone (800) 297-5943

The Medical Massage Office Manual, 2nd edition, by Margery M. Callahan and David W. Luther, $59.95; to order (888) 322-5520, complete guidelines for insurance billing and reimbursement procedures, including sample forms and letters. Includes a diskette with printable forms. Also available is "MediSoft" software (see Practice Management Software, above).

Hands Heal: Documentation for Massage Therapy: A Guide to SOAP Charting by Diana L. Thompson, LMP. $23.95 postpaid from Diana L. Thompson, All You Knead 1518 Broadway Seattle, WA 98122 (206) 328-3412 (Forms pack and teacher's manual also available)

Basic Clinical Massage: Integrating Anatomy and Treatment by James H. Clay and David M. Pounds, $42.95 from Lippincott Williams & Wilkins, ISBN: 0683306537, published August, 2002

Scientific Studies on the Effectiveness of Massage

Touch Therapy, by Tiffany Field, PhD, 2000, hardcover $32.95. Publisher: Churchill Livingstone, Inc. Summarizes and analyzes the scientific evidence of benefits of massage to health, wellness and healing. Written by the leader in touch research.

Massage Therapy: The Evidence for Practice, by Grant Jewell Rich, $34.95 from Mosby. Information about both books at **www.harcourt-international.com**

Ethical issues for Massage and Bodywork

The Educated Heart, by Nina McIntosh, MSW, Decatur Bainbridge Press 1999, $22.95. Nina McIntosh, a certified Rolfer, has written a comprehensive volume on ethics for bodyworkers, emphasizing the need for strong boundaries and strict avoidance of dual relationships. Much of the advice in the book is most useful for bodyworkers who engage the client psychologically as well as physically, as this type of work requires stricter adherence to proper boundaries. However, all bodyworkers will benefit from reading this treatise on ethics for the profession. **www.educatedheart.com**

Massage for Cancer Patients

Medicine Hands, by Gayle MacDonald, M.S., LMT, Findhorn Press, 1999, $23.95. Massage schools typically teach that cancer is a "contraindication" for massage, because mechanical pressure on the tumor might cause it to dislodge partially and further metastasize. MacDonald reviews the medical literature and presents a different view, giving both a scientific and humanistic discussion of the benefits of using massage with cancer patients. If your work does or may include hospital massage, medical massage, hospice work or simply a general practice in which you may massage cancer patients, this volume is an invaluable resource to add to your bookshelf. **www.findhornpress.com**

Networking, Marketing and Promotional Services

The Quiet Touch International Massage Network
(800) 946-2772 or (561) 379-3224
P.O. Box 7613
West Palm Beach, FL 33405
www.massageinc.com

Accepts: Licensed Massage Therapists with current membership in AMTA, ABMP, IMA or you can get corporate discounts through The Quiet Touch from ABMP.

Service Provided: The company markets massage and makes agreements to provide massage services to clients in hotels, offices, health spas, the company's own massage offices and clients' homes. The company started in New York, spread quickly to New Jersey, Connecticut and Florida, and now has clients in all 50 states, and in foreign countries.
  Clients schedule appointments through the company's 800 number and participating massage therapists are told where and when to report to fill these appointments. The therapist receives up to 70% of the fee paid by the client. Therapists need not have their own office to participate. Therapists are charged a $250.00 annual fee to participate.

ASSOCIATED MTssm
Bruria Ginton, LicMT
212-222-4240
www.qwl.com/mtwc/amts

Membership Categories: Active, Student and Supportive.

Service Provided: This is a co-operative promotional, mentoring and advocacy network, created in NYC, 1992, to enhance the reputation, professional status and economic opportunities for licensed massage therapists. The organization maintains a website and places advertisements in national publications. Active members are included in the online global directory, MTs NEAR YOUtm. They can use the company logo and other promotional materials. In addition, members may also participate in online and offline co-operative promotions in which several massage therapists share the cost of a specific promotional effort.

Active Membership dues: $120.00 first year, $65.00 per year renewal

Student Membership: $25 per year, upgrade to Active Membership at renewal rate.

VI

Bodywork Organizations and Trainings

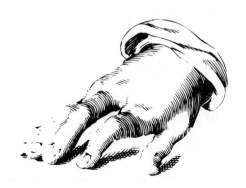

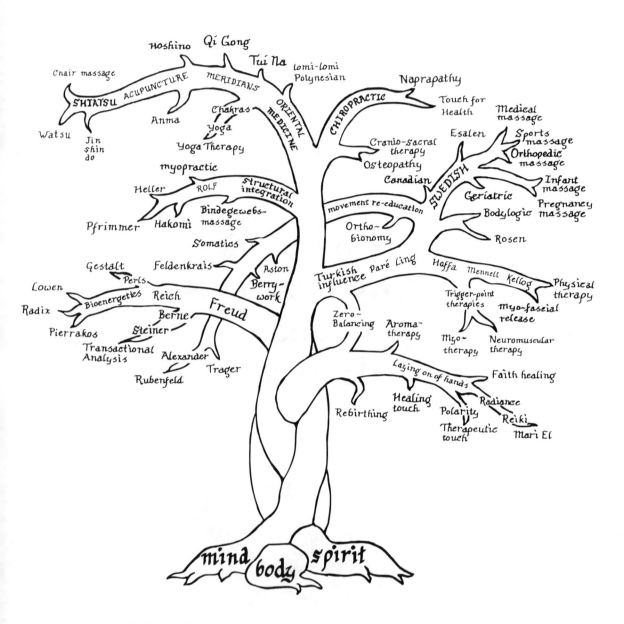

The Bodywork Tree © 1999

Based on a concept by David Linton

Bodywork Systems, Organizations and Trainings

For purposes of this Directory, "bodywork" refers to a body-centered therapy that is different from Swedish massage.

Some of the forms listed below are very similar to Swedish massage—for example, sports massage, Esalen, pregnancy massage. Some are entirely different from Swedish massage—for example, Alexander Technique, Reiki, Somatics Psychology.

For each form of bodywork, the listing includes a brief explanation of the nature of the work, the name and address of an official organization representing the form, if available, and in some cases, contact information for trainings and supplies.

New forms of bodywork are continually created as imaginative and dedicated bodyworkers explore their own unique gifts and systematize their work. Factors that go into the decision to include a form in this directory include how long the form has been in existence, how widely it is practiced, and whether it is taught in mainstream massage schools. Appearing for the first time in this edition is "Hot Stone Massage."

For a listing with even more modalities than I have included in this book, you can visit **www.thebodyworker.com**.

Acupressure

See Shiatsu

Alexander Technique

The Alexander technique is an educational method for improving coordination, and for developing awareness of unnecessary tensions in the body.

F. M. Alexander was an actor who had a problem with losing his voice. By studying his habitual movements in a mirror, he discovered ways he was using his body that created his vocal problem and was able to resolve the difficulty. He went on to create a system for enhancing balance, posture and the use of the body, which is called the Alexander technique. Practitioners refer to themselves as teachers of the Alexander method and refer to sessions as lessons.

Three websites that provide good resources concerning the Alexander technique are:

> www.alexandercenter.com
> www.alexandertech.com
> www.ATI-net.com

AMMA® Therapy (or ANMA)

AMMA therapy is a method of restoring the flow of life energy in the body, and is used to treat a wide range of medical conditions. It combines Oriental medical principles with a Western approach to organ dysfunction. AMMA therapy may include dietary plans, detoxification, herbs and vitamins, and therapeutic exercises.

Applied Kinesiology (see also Touch for Health)

Applied Kinesiology is a technique used mainly by chiropractors to gain diagnostic information through muscle testing and to strengthen muscles to aid in structural correction. Muscles are related to specific organs or systems through the acupuncture meridian network. The site **www.kinesiology.net** has many links to related methods of muscle testing.

Aquatic Bodywork

See Watsu

Aromatherapy

Aromatherapy involves working with aroma as a healing modality by using pure essential oils, each distilled from a single botanical source. Aromatherapy is often done in conjunction with massage, but not always. The major professional organizations for aromatherapy are:

National Association for Holistic Aromatherapy (NAHA)
4509 Interlake Ave., N., Ste. 233
Seattle, WA 98103
(888) ASK-NAHA or (206) 547-2164
www.naha.org

Internataional Aromatherapy and Herb Association
3541 W. Acapulco Lane
Phoenix, AZ 85053
(602) 938-4439

Suppliers of essential oils

There are many suppliers of essential oils. The companies listed below have been recommended by practitioners as having a good reputation in the industry and supplying good quality oils:

Amrita Aromatherapy Inc.
1900 W. Stone
Fairfield, IA 52556
(641) 472-9136
www.amrita.net

Fragrant Earth
2000 Second Ave., Ste. 206
Seattle, WA 98121
(800) 260-7401
www.fragrantearth.com

Nature's Gifts Custom Aromatherapy
1040 Cheyenne Blvd.
Madison, TN 37115
(615) 612-4270
www.naturesgift.com

Samara Botane
1811 Queen Anne Ave. N., Ste. 104
Seattle, WA 98109
(800) 782-4532
www.wingedseed.com

Time Laboratories
P.O. Box 3243
South Pasadena, CA 91031
(877)-TIMELABS (877-846-3522)
www.timelabs.com

Elizabeth Van Buren, Inc.
P.O. Box 7542
Santa Cruz, CA 95061
(800) 710-7759 or (831) 425-8218
www.evb-aromatherapy.com

Leydet Aromatics
P.O. Box 2345
Fair Oaks, CA 95628
(916) 965-7546
http://leydet.com

Prima Fleur
1525 E. Francisco Blvd., Ste. 16
San Rafael, CA 94901
(415) 455-0957
www.primafleur.com

Snow Lotus Inc.
875 Alpine Avenue, Suite 5
Boulder, CO 80304
(303) 443-9289 or (800) 628-8827
www.snowlotus.org

Warren Botanicals
73-4689 Kahualani Rd.
Kailua-Kona, HI 96740
(888) 848-0642 or (808) 334-1112
www.warrenbotanicals.com

Selected Aromatherapy trainings

Some massage schools teach aromatherapy as part of their curriculum. In addition, the following schools offer specialized instruction in aromatherapy:

CA: **Pacific Institute of Aromatherapy**
P.O. Box 6723, San Rafael, CA 94903, (415) 479-9120

FL: **Atlantic Institute of Aromatherapy**
16018 Saddlestring Dr., Tampa, FL 33618, (813) 265-2222

The National Coalition of Certified Aromatherapist and Aromatologist Practitioners
(NCCAAP), P.O. Box 835025, Miami, FL 33283, (305) 595-4776

NJ: **Institute of Aromatherapy**
3108 Route 10 West, Denville, NJ 07834, (201) 989-1999   **www.aromatherapy4u.com**

OR: **Australian College of Herbal Studies**
P.O. Box 57, Lake Oswego, OR 97034, 1-800-48-STUDY (1-800-487-8839)   **www.herbed.com**

WA: **Institute of Dynamic Aromatherapy**
4925 6th Ave. NW, Marysville, WA 98271, (360) 651-9809   **www.theida.com.**

Asian Bodywork

A number of forms of Asian bodywork are described under separate headings, such as Jin Shin Do, Jin Shin Jyutsu, Qi Gong, Shiatsu, Thai Massage and Tui Na. The major organizations for practitioners of these modalities are:

**American Association of
Oriental Medicine**
433 Front St.
Catasauqua, PA 18032
(610) 266-1433 **www.aaom.org**

**American Orgnaization for Bodywork
Therapies of Asia**
1010 Haddonfield-Berlin Rd., Ste. 408
Voorhees, NJ 08043
(856) 782-1616 **www.aobta.org**

Aston-Patterning® www.astonenterprises.com

Aston-Patterning aims to increase the body's grace, resiliency and ease of movement by releasing layers of tension throughout the body. It uses movement education, bodywork, environmental design and fitness training. For information about trainings and certification, contact:

Aston-Patterning
P.O. Box 3568
Incline Village, NV 89450
(775) 831-8228

Bindegewebsmassage

Bindegewebsmassage is a type of connective tissue massage originated in Germany. It is an adjunctive therapy in the treatment of organic and musculo-skeletal disorders.

Bioenergetics www.bioenergetic-therapy.com

Bioenergetics was created by Alexander Lowen, M.D., an outgrowth of his work with Wilhelm Reich, M.D. Bioenergetics is a way of understanding personality in terms of the body and its energetic processes. Bioenergetics therapy works with the mind and the body to release chronic stresses and chronic muscular tensions.

Dr. Lowen has written 14 books. An excellent introduction to bioenergetics is *Bioenergetics*, available at most bookstores and libraries.

For a brochure listing centers, workshops and books on bioenergetics, contact:

> **International Institute for Bioenergetic Analysis**
> 155 Main St., Ste. 304
> Brewster, NY 10509
> (845) 279-8474

Biokinetics/Hanna Somatics www.somatics.com

Biokinetics uses a composite of techniques for rehabilitation through neuromuscular retraining. It is designed to release chronic muscular contraction and restore voluntary control of the muscular system. For further information about Biokinetics and training, contact:

> **Association for Hanna Somatics**   **Novato Instiutute**
> 925 Golden Gate Dr.   1516 Grant Ave., Ste. 212
> Napa, CA 94558   Novato, CA 94945
> (707) 255-2473   (415) 897-0336
>
> **Workshops: Lawrence Gold**
> 8236 Old Waterloo Rd.
> Warrenton, VA 20186
> (540) 351-0874

Body Logic^SM

Body Logic is a system of bodywork and body understanding developed by Yamuna Zake. It uses the principle of "space making" whereby space is created around joints and locked areas to allow the body to unfold and finds its own balance, enhancing freedom of movement, posture, strength and energy. For information on Body Logic, trainings and practitioners, contact:

> **Body Logic**
> 295 West 11th Street, apt. 1F
> New York, NY 10014
> (212) 633-2143 or (888) 226-9616
> www.bodylogic.com

Body-Mind (also see "Somatics")

"Body-mind" is a term used to acknowledge the intimate connection between the state of the mind and the state of the body. This is an awareness that is present in most forms of massage and bodywork, and many massage schools teach massage from a "body-mind" perspective. However, some forms make it the focus of the work. The programs listed below are designed as advanced programs for massage therapists, and focus on the body-mind connection.

> **Body Synergy Institute, Inc.**
> Bala Cynwyd, PA
> (610) 667-3070
> www.bodysynergyinstitute.com

Curriculum includes deep tissue bodywork, body reading, using a floor-length mirror as an educational tool, working with postural history and attitudes, and using your body with awareness and ease.

School for Body-Mind Centering
189 Pond View Dr.
Amherst, MA 01002
(413) 256-8615
www.bodymindcentering.com

The school, founded by Bonnie Bainbridge Cohen, offers introductory and certification training programs in many locations. The course includes study of the body systems and how they support and initiate movement, as well as movement re-education to correct problems at their root level.

Bowen Technique

This technique was developed in Australia by Thomas Bowen. It combines energy work with gentle soft tissue manipulation. **www.bowtech.com** is the home page of the founders of the Bowen Therapy Academy of Australia.

Breema www.breema.com

Breema takes its name from the Kurdish mountain village of Breemava where it originated and was passed down from generation to generation. It is a comprehensive system of bodywork, done on the floor, with a variety of techniques ranging from simple holding points on the body to techniques requiring flexibility and dexterity. This work is taught at:

The Breema Center
6076 Claremont Ave.
Oakland, CA 94618
(510) 428-0937

Canadian Deep Muscle Massage

This work was created by Will Green, founder of the International Massage Association (IMA Group) and owner of Georgetown Bodyworks in Washington, DC. It is derived from a system of cross-fiber massage that began in northern Canada in the 1940s. Will added insights gained from the works of Therese Pfrimmer, Joseph Pliates, Ida Rolf, Dr. Samuel West, and Debra Smith.

For more information on Canadian Massage, visit **www.learnmassage.com**.

Chair Massage (or on-site or seated massage)

This refers to a brief bodywork session, usually a shiatsu-based routine, done in a special chair in which the client sits facing toward the cushions, exposing the scalp, shoulders, neck, back and hips. Sessions may last between five and thirty minutes.

Originally pioneered as "on-site massage", a modality for the workplace, it has expanded into many other environments. Chair massage is now offered in storefronts, health food stores, airports, airplanes, health fairs, grand openings, sporting events, and other locations. It has therefore come to be called "chair massage" or "seated massage" instead of "on-site."

Because of the relatively low cost of a brief session, it is more affordable than the usual full-body massage. Because it is done fully clothed, it attracts some clients who would be too uncomfortable for table massage. Because it is done in locations where the client is already present, it is more convenient than table massage. For all these reasons, the practice of chair massage has grown so fast that many of the massage table companies report they are selling more on-site chairs than massage tables. The large number of massage schools including chair massage in their curriculum is another indication of the popularity and wide-spread acceptance of this branch of the profession.

Two U.S. companies conduct workshops on chair massage technique and marketing. These are:

TouchPro Chair Massage Seminars
1-800-999-5026   www.touchpro.org
Instructors certified and supervised by David Palmer

Seated Massage Experience®
1-800-868-2448   1-800-TOUCH-4-U
Workshops are taught by Raymond Blaylock

A Canadian company offers 2-week residential trainings in Ontario:

Relax to the Max
251 Davenport Road
Toronto, Ontario M5R 1J9, CANADA
(416) 962-7441 or (877) 222-5782   www.chairmassagetraining.com

Chi Kung/Chi Gong

See Qi gong

Colon Hydrotherapy (also called colonics or high colonics or colonic irrigation)

A cleansing procedure for the colon, using purified water at controlled temperature and controlled pressure, providing a gentle, deep cleansing of the colon. Practitioners often use massage, reflexology or visceral manipulation skills during a session. Of the 50 states, only Florida licenses colon hydrotherapy. Certification is available through:

International Association of Colon HydroTherapy
P.O. Box 461285
San Antonio, TX 78246
(210) 366-2888   www.i-act.org

Cranio-Sacral Therapy (also called cranial-sacral)

A technique for finding and correcting cerebral and spinal imbalances or blockages that may cause sensory, motor or intellectual dysfunction. Practitioners work with the subtle articulations of skull sutures, and the flow of cerebro-spinal fluid.

In addition, Cranio-sacral techniques are taught by the following institutions:

Colorado Cranial Institute
1080 Hawthorne Ave.
Boulder, CO 80304
(303) 449-0322

The Craniosacral Institute
800 Polhemus Rd., Ste. 22
San Mateo, CA 94402
(650) 573-0527 or (888) 627-2642
www.cranial.org

National Institute of Craniosacral Studies, Inc.
7827 N. Armenia Ave.
Tampa, FL 33604-3806
(888) 824-7025 or (813) 933-6335

Shea Educational Group
13878 Oleander Avenue
Juno Beach, FL 33408
(561) 863-3350   **www.sheacranial.com**

The Upledger Institute
11211 Prosperity Farms Road
Palm Beach Gardens, FL 33410
(561) 622-4334   **www.upledger.com**

The American CranioSacral Therapy Association can be reached at (877) 942-2782, and at **www.acsta.com**

Equine Sports Massage

Massage or other bodywork can adapted to horses for the purpose of enhancing performance and preventing injuries. This field has recently been developed and shows signs of gaining rapidly in popularity, as breeders are interested in any techniques that can give them a competitive edge. The Rolf Institute (see Rolfing, below) also refers rolfers who practice on horses.

According to Jack Meagher, author of *Beating Muscle Injuries for Horses* (available for $16.45 postpaid from Lynnwoodpublishing—P.O. Box 8296, Lynn, MA 01904; by credit card at 1-877-SHOWTAC; on line at **www.MyHorseStable.com**), an equine sports massage practitioner applies techniques of human massage, especially sports massage, to horses. A pioneer in the fields of sports massage and equine sports massage, Jack Meagher turned to working with horses as a way of proving the value of sports massage techniques for athletes. By using the techniques on horses and achieving demonstrable results, he was able to rebut the contention that results with humans were due to psychological factors.

International Association of Equine Sports Massage Therapists
P.O. Box 447
Round Hill, VA 20141
(800) 843-0224   **www.iaesmt.com**

Equine sports massage is taught at the following locations:

Don Doran's Equine Sports Massage Program
9791 NW 160th St.
Reddick, FL 32686
(352) 591-4735
www.equinesportsmassage.com

Equinology
P.O. Box 1248
Grover Beach, CA 93483
(805) 474-9044
www.equinology.com

Equissage School
15715 Southern Cross Lane, P.O. Box 447
Round Hill, VA 20141
(800) 843-0224 or (540) 338-1917
www.equissage.com

EquiTouch Systems
Loveland, CO
(800) 483-0577
www.equitouch.net

Hands On Horses School of Equine Massage
Mississippi Gulf Coast
(888) 452-8828

Integrated Touch Therapy
Circleville, OH
(800) 251-0007
www.integratedtouchtherapy.com

TT.E.A.M.ˢᵐ Training International
(Tellington-Touch Equine Awareness Method)
P.O. Box 3793
Santa Fe., NM 87501
(505) 455-2945 or (800) 854-8326
www.lindatellintonjones.com

Esalen® massage www.esalen.org

Esalen is a variant of Swedish massage pioneered at Esalen Institute in Big Sur, California. Esalen is the place where many therapies were tested or launched in the '60s and '70s, including gestalt therapy and rolfing. The unique brand of massage practiced there typically involves total nudity and long flowing stokes. Esalen is known for its original, honest, nurturing and probing atmosphere. Esalen massage tends to be nurturing, trance-like and meditative, allowing the greatest possible unfoldment to take place in the client. For information contact:

Esalen Institute
Hwy. 1
Big Sur, CA 93920
(408) 667-3000

Facial Rejuvenation

This bodywork was developed by Linda Burnham, N.D. It involves sculpting the face and affecting the twelve major nerve centers on the head. On another level, it involves shedding beliefs and thoughts that aren't ours and the emotions that no longer serve us.

For information about professional certification, contact:

Burnham Systems Facial Rejuvenationˢᵐ
University of Natural Medicine
(505) 424-7800   **www.UniversityNaturalMedicine.org/BSFR.html**

Feldenkrais® www.feldenkrais.com

Moshe Feldendrais was an Israeli physicist who began developing this system in mid-life. Feldenkrais work emphasizes having a coherent body image and thinking a movement through. It also uses micro-movements for neuromuscular re-education. The system is most effective for pain relief, and also promotes grace and ease of movement. For further information contact:

The Feldenkrais Guild of North America
3611 SW Hood Ave., Ste. 100
Portland, OR 97201
(800) 775-2118

Geriatric Massage

Working with the elderly and the ill, often in a long-term care setting. A therapist doing geriatric massage should understand the physical and psychological characteristics of aging, and should also be familiar with the diseases that commonly afflict the elderly.

Some resources in the field of geriatric massage are:

Daybreak Geriatric Massage Project
(954) 578-5055   www.daybreak-massage.com

Foundation for Long Term Care
150 State Street, Albany NY 12207
(518) 449-7873
Carol Hegemen, Director.

Compassionate Touch
20 Swan Ct., Walnut Creek, CA 94596
(925) 935-3906

A massage therapist with extensive experience in nursing home and long term facility care was recruited by Elder Health HMO to establish an insurance-based program of massage for nursing home residents who are on Medicare or Medicaid. Her company, SeniorTouchllc, has been successful in setting up massage at a string of nursing homes in the Baltimore, MD area.

Hakomi bodywork www.hakomi.com

Hakomi bodywork regards body, mind and spirit as one, and blends bodywork and psychotherapy into a simultaneous process. The work serves to lead a person to an awareness of limitations in his physical and psychological patterns, bringing the possibility of new openness and freedom.

P.O. Box 1873
Boulder, CO 80306
(888) 421-6699

Healing Touch www.healingtouch.net

Healing touch is an energy-based, hands-on technique done to balance and align the human energy field. The technique is approved by the American Holistic Nurses Association. Information about the technique, trainings, and organization membership can be obtained from:

Healing Touch International, Inc.
12477 W. Cedar Drive, Suite #202
Lakewood, Colorado 80228
(303) 989-7982

Hellerwork® www.hellerwork.com

Hellerwork is an outgrowth of Rolfing (see below), created by Joseph Heller. It integrates movement and verbal communication with connective tissue work. Information about Hellerwork can be obtained from:

Hellerwork, Inc.
3435 M Street, Eureka, CA 95503
(800) 392-3900 or (707) 441-4949

Horse Massage

See Equine Sports Massage

Hot Stone Massage

Heated Stones are placed on the body to achieve relaxation. This modality has recently become very popular in spas and salons. Workshops are taught in many massage schools, and some stand-alone trainings and videos are also available. Below is a listing of resources for stones and educational videos:

Carol Gilmore
2095 Mesquite Ave., Ste. 25
Lake Havasu City, AZ 86403
(928) 854-8101
www.islandstonetherapy.com

European Stone Massage, LLC
P.O. Box 817
Augusta, ME 04332
(207) 240-4671
www.europeanstonemassage.com

LaStone Therapy
PMB #287, 7850 N. Silverbell, #114
Tucson, AZ 85743
(520) 572-9537
www.lastonetherapy.com

Hot Stone Massage
Professional Development and Supplies
Institute for Therapeutic Massage (NJ)
(973) 839-6131
www.hotstonevideo.com

Hawaiian Hot Stones
(808) 573-3103
www.hawaiianhotstones.com

Real Bodywork
(888) 505-5511 or (805) 564-7073
www.deeptissue.com/stone/stone.htm

RiverStones
(877) 384-0295 or (972) 241-0705
www.islandsoftwareco.com/stones.htm

Therapeutic Stones
(561) 361-3966 or (866) 680-5149
www.thstone.com

Spa Equip, Inc.
2436 Foothill Blvd., Ste. G
Calistoga, CA 94515
(877) 778-1686 or (707) 942-1223
www.spaequip.com

Hydrotherapy

See Spa Treatments

Infant Massage

Infant massage instructors teach parents the art of infant massage. Trainings are offered to certify people as infant massage instructors. For information, contact:

**International Association of
Infant Massage**
1891 Goodyear Ave., Ste. 622
Ventura, CA 93003
(800) 248-5432 or (415) 752-4920
www.iaim-us.com

**International Loving Touch
Foundation, Inc.**
P.O. Box 16374
Portland, OR 97292
(503) 253-8482
www.lovingtouch.com

Also offering information and contacts are:

www.infantmassage.com
www.lastingi.com

Jin Shin Do®

Jin Shin Do is a synthesis of acupressure theory, psychology, Taoist philosophy, and breathing methods, which helps release physical and emotional tensions and armoring. The Jin Shin Do Foundation has information about trainings and practitioners, as well as books, charts, videos and audiotapes.

> **Jin Shin Do Foundation for Bodymind Acupressure**
> P.O. Box 416, Idyllwild, CA 92549
> www.jinshindo.org
> (for Canadian trainings visit **www.jinshindo.com**)

Jin Shin Jyutsu® www.jinshinjyutsu.com

This is an ancient art promoting harmony of life energy and the body. It was revived and systematized in the early 1900s by Master Jiro Murai. It was brought to the US in the 1950s by Mary Burmeister. It is an energy technique done with a light touch, and is often used as a self-treatment. For further information contact:

> **Jin Shin Jyutsu, Inc.**
> 8719 E. San Alberto
> Scottsdale, AZ 85258
> (602) 998-9331

Lomilomi

The traditional massage of Hawaii, it is taught at massage schools in Hawaii and some schools on the mainland. The Hawaiian Lomilomi Association maintains a directory of practitioners and teachers and links to informational websites about lomilomi.

> Hawaiian Lomilomi Association
> 15-156 Puni Kahakai Loop
> Pahoa, HI 96778
> (808) 965-8917   **www.lomilomi.org**

Lymphatic drainage (manual lymphatic drainage℠ or MLD®)

The lymphatic system is a vital part of the immune system in the body. Lymphatic drainage massage assists the operation of the lymphatic system. The system was devised in the 1930s by a Danish massage therapist, Dr. Emil Vodder, and is popular and well established as a health modality in Germany and Austria. Two organizations certify practitioners and teachers of manual lymphatic drainage:

> **North American Vodder Association of Lymphatic Therapy™ (NAVALT®)**
> (888) 4-NAVALT (1-888-462-8258)   **www.navalt.com**
> recent trainings held in CA, GA, ID, MA, MD, NJ, NY, OH, TX, VA, VT, WA

> **Kessler Lerner Lymphedema Academy**
> Attention: Terry McKeon, PT
> 304 Chestnut Street
> Nedham, MA 02492
> (800) 232-5542 or (781) 444-1108
> **www.lymphedemaservices.com   www.kessler-rehab.com**
> recent trainings held in NJ and FL

Medical Massage (clinical massage)

Working with injuries, pathologies and rehabilitation; working by physician's prescription. A program of instruction in medical massage is very desirable for a therapist interested in working in the health care system and obtaining insurance reimbursement for massage services. See chapter 21 for further information.

Also offering certification in Medical Dysfunction is:

> **Kurashova Institute for Studies in Physical Medicine**
> P.O. Box 6246
> Rock Island, IL 61201
> (309) 786-4888 or (800) 791-9248   **www.kurashova.com**

Founded in 1999, the Amercian Manual Medicine Association is designed for the advancement of medical massage as a specialization within the practice of massage.

> **American Manual Medicine Association**
> 2040 Raybrook, SE, Ste. 104
> Grand Rapids, MI 49546
> (888) 375-7245
> **www.americanmedicalmassage.com**

Myofascial Release

Myofascial release (MFR) is a technique for working with fascia as a means of achieving pain relief, restoring function and reducing stress. The system is taught in a series of seminars in various locations. It is designed to be used by massage therapists and physical therapists. For information about trainings contact:

> **John F. Barnes' MFR Seminars**
> www.myofascialrelease.com

Myopractic® www.myopractic.com

This is a system of posture balancing and deep relaxation developed and taught by Robert Petteway. The three basic techniques are 1. releasing tension and holding patterns; 2. clearing scar tissue, trigger points and other obstructions in soft tissue; and 3. separating to release myofascial adhesions and balance muscles. The practitioner does deep muscle therapy while keeping her own body and hands relaxed, and the system relieves chronic pain and postural imbalances. Trainings are offered through:

> **The Myopractic Institute**
> 5644 Westheimer, Suite 217
> Houston, TX 77056
> (713) 869-5151 or (888) 696-9898

Myotherapy℠

See Trigger Point Therapies

Neuromuscular Therapy

See Trigger Point Therapies

On-Site Massage

See Chair Massage

Ortho-Bionomy™

This system seeks to remind the body of its ability to find balance. The work involves positioning the client, working with points of tension in the body, and using movement. Results can include relieving pain, promoting emotional release, and improving structural alignment. For information, contact:

Society of Ortho-Bionomy International
P.O. Box 257899
Chicago, IL 60625
(800) 743-4890 or (773) 506-6540
www.ortho-bionomy.org

Creative Healing Institute
2848 W. Gregory St.
Chicago, IL 60625
(877) 650-3160
www.healingcreatively.com

Wellness & Massage Training Institute
1051 Internationale Parkway
Woodridge, IL 60517
(630) 739-WMTI or (630) 739-9684
www.wmti.com

New Mexico Academy of Healing Arts
(888) 808-5188
www.nmhealingarts.org

AKS Massage School (Virginia)
(877) 306-342 or (703) 464-0333
www.aksmassageschool.com

Maui Center for Ortho-Bionomy
(808) 242-9162
www.maui.net /~zoee

Orthopedic Massage   www.omeri.com

This term is used by Whitney W. Lowe and Benny Vaughn to describe their work. Ten modalities are combined to create a comprehensive approach to the treatment of soft-tissue pain and injury conditions. The work shares some elements of sports massage and some elements of medical massage. The Institute offers a 100-hour certification program several times each year at various locations, and also publishes a newsletter "Orthopedic & Sports Massage Reviews". For further information, contact:

Orthopedic Massage Education & Research Institute
P.O. Box 1468
Bend, OR 97709
(541) 317-9855 or (888) 340-1614

Pfrimmer Deep Muscle Therapy® www.pfrimmer.com

Pfrimmer Deep Muscle Therapy is a system of corrective treatment to aid in the restoration of damaged muscles and soft tissue. It is intended to be used as one aspect of treatment for a wide range of muscular and soft-tissue conditions.

It is currently taught at Alexandria School in Indiana and Pennsylvania School of Muscle Therapy in Oaks, Pennsylvania. Further information can be obtained from these schools or the website.

Polarity www.PolarityTherapy.org

Developed by Dr. Randolph Stone, polarity focuses on the energy currents that exist in all life. The polarity therapist uses her hands as conductors of energy. The intention is to balance the electromagnetic energy in the body, toward the ultimate goal of uniting the body, emotions, mind and soul.

Polarity is commonly taught in massage schools, but programs also exist to teach polarity that have no connection to massage schools. Although many massage schools offer an introduction to polarity as part of their training, few offer a substantial amount of training.

The American Polarity Therapy Association (APTA) is a non-profit organization that distributes educational material, registers practitioners, hosts educational conferences and publishes a regular newsletter. The APTA also certifies schools as meeting their educational standards, and will supply a list of approved schools upon request. For further information contact:

> **American Polarity Therapy Association**
> P.O. Box 19858
> Boulder, CO 80308
> (303) 545-2080

Postural Integration

See Structural Integration

Pregnancy Massage (or prenatal massage)

This is an adaptation of Swedish massage for the needs of pregnant women. It is sometimes called prenatal or perinatal massage, or massage for the child-bearing year.

> **National Association of Pregnancy Massage Therapy**
> 1007 Mopoc Circle
> Austin, TX 78758
> (888) 451-4945

Qi Gong (or Chi Kung)

This may be the most commonly practiced modality in the world. It is routinely used in Chinese hospitals as a healing modality. It involves a system of exercises designed to induce a state of mindfulness that can be used to generate Qi (or chi)—life energy. The name literally means "skill with life energy" and it evolved over two thousand years ago in Tibet and China.

Qi gong is related to Tui Na (below).

For further information, you can explore the following websites:

> **www.nqa.org** (National Qi gong association)
> **www.qi.org**
> **www.chilel-qigong.com**
> **www.qigonginstitute.org**

Radiance Technique www.authenticreiki.org

The Radiance Technique was formerly called The Official Reiki Program. For further information, contact:

The Radiance Technique International Assn.
P.O. Box 40570
St. Petersburg Fl 33743
(727) 347-2106   www.trtia.org

Reflexology www.reflexology.org   www.reflexolgy-usa.org

Reflexology is a system of massaging the feet, or feet and hands, with the intention of affecting other parts of the body. The feet and hands are regarded much like maps of the body, with points on the feet and hands corresponding to organs and tissues in the body. It is thought that sensitivity or tenderness in the feet or hands indicates imbalances in the corresponding body part, and by working with the point on the foot or hand, beneficial results can be achieved in the corresponding body part.

While many reflexologists spend an entire therapy session working only on the hands and feet (and sometimes ears), some spend approximately half of their time on the feet, and half on Swedish massage. Reflexology is taught at more US massage schools than any other form of bodywork.

Independent certification in reflexology is offered by:

American Reflexology Certification Board (ARCB)
P.O. Box 740879
Arvada, CO 80006
(303) 933-6921   www.ARCB.net

Reiki www.reiki.org

Reiki is an energy process for restoring and balancing life energy and promoting healing and personal transformation. The approach is thousands of years old, and was systematized in the 1800s by Dr. Mikao Usui. The practitioner attunes to and transmits reiki energy. Further information can be obtained from:

**International Association of
Reiki Professionals**
P.O. Box 481, Winchester, MA 01890
(781) 729-3530   www.IARP.org

The Reiki Alliance
P.O. Box 41, Cataldo, ID 83810
(208) 783-3535

Reiki Council
420 Stone Road, Suite A1
Villa Park, IL 60181
(630) 926-5891   www.reikicouncil.com

American Reiki Masters Association
P.O. Box 130, Lake City, FL 32056
(904) 755-9638

Rolfing® www.rolf.org

Ida Rolf was the first to create, practice and teach a system of bodywork aimed toward working with the connective tissue of the body to achieve structural changes in the client. She originally called her system Structural Integration, but it came to be called Rolfing and is taught by:

The Rolf Institute
205 Canyon Blvd.
Boulder, CO 80302
(800) 530-8875 or (303) 449-5903

Rosen Method Bodywork® www.rosenmethod.org   www.rosenmethod.com

Developed by Marion Rosen, this work emphasizes simplicity. The practitioner contacts contracted muscles and matches the muscle tension. The practitioner follows changes in the client's breathing as a means of guiding the client's inner process. The work can bring up buried feelings and memories, and can be a tool for pain relief and personal growth.

Below are the current contacts for Rosen Method Bodywork. They can give you information about trainings and practitioners in their areas:

California:	**The Berkeley Center** (510) 845-6606
Connecticut:	**Rosen Center East, LLC.** (860) 859-0574
Florida:	**Rosen Center Florida** (941) 541-0558
New Mexico:	**Rosen Method Center Southwest** (505) 982-7149
North Carolina:	**Rosen Method Bodywork Carolina Center** (919) 967-0870

Rubenfeld Synergy™ www.rubenfeldsynergy.com

This method integrates elements of Alexander, Feldenkrais, gestalt and hypnotherapy into a body-mind therapy that helps clients contact and release energy blocks, tensions and imbalances. Rather than treating illnesses, the practitioner treats the psychophysical problems people carry with them. By dealing with the emotional body, the practitioner can often abate physical symptoms. For information, contact:

National Association of Rubenfeld Synergists
7 Kendall Road, Kendall Park, NJ 08824
(877) RSM-2468 code 8516

Seated Massage

See Chair Massage

Shiatsu or acupressure

Shiatsu is a Japanese bodywork which uses pressure to points on acupuncture meridians. Practice of shiatsu is usually accompanied by study of Chinese five-element theory and meridians, and it involves a way of looking at the body that is completely different from the "muscles, bones and blood" view of Western science, focusing instead on the flow of life energy through meridians.

The name "Acupressure" is sometimes used to mean shiatsu, and is sometimes used to describe a finger-pressure technique similar to shiatsu but not identical.

Somatics (also called Somatics Psychology or Somatic Therapy)

"Somatic" literally means "of or pertaining to the body." In the context of Somatics Psychology, it refers to the mind-body connection and makes use of techniques to bring awareness of the mind and the body to each other. It is therefore related to the form "Body-Mind" which is described above. For further information, you may wish to obtain "Somatics Magazine":

Somatics Magazine
1516 Grant Ave., Ste. 212
Novato, CA 94945
(415) 892-0617   www.somaticsed.com

United States Association for Body Psychotherapy (USABP)
7831 Woodmont Ave., Ste. 294
Bethesda, Maryland 20814
(202) 466-1619   www.usabp.org

Spa Treatments

Spa, or Health Spa, refers to an establishment that provides rejuvenating treatments in a residential setting (or non-residential at a day spa). Often at a resort and often luxurious in setting, spas aim for relaxation, therapeutic treatments, and beautification treatments. Modalities such as herbal wraps, seaweed wraps, mud baths, loofa scrubs and salt glows are designed to detoxify and refresh the system.

Related to spa treatments is Hydrotherapy, meaning "water therapy." It includes treatments like contrast baths (alternating hot and cold water), and wet sheet wraps. Hydrotherapy is a required course for massage licensure in Texas and Florida.

Sports Massage

Sports massage is an adaptation of Swedish massage. Its purpose is to prepare athletes for sporting activity and help them recover from the exertion of sporting activity.

Sports massage trainings vary widely in length, and there is no standard training length, although the American Massage Therapy Association and the United States Sports Massage Federation both have standards for approving trainings.

U.S. Sports Massage Federation
2156 Newport Blvd.
Costa Mesa, CA 92627
(949) 642-0735

Structural Integration (or Postural Integration)

This is a generic term for therapies that are related to Rolfing, in that they aim to improve the structure or posture of the client. See also Hellerwork.

The Guild For Structural Integration can be contacted at:

3107 28th St., Boulder, CO 80301
(303) 447-0122 or (800) 447-0150   www.rolfguild.org

Thai Massage

The traditional massage of Thailand includes passive stretching as well as stroking.

International Thai Therapists Association, Inc.
C/O Luma Center, 3600 S. 60th Ave. Shelby, MI 49455
(231) 861-0481   www.thaimassage.com

Following is a sampling of trainings in Thai Massage:

Florida and New Jersey, **The Institute of Thai Massage**   www.thai-massage.org
Northern California, **Spirit Winds School of Thai Massage**   www.spiritwinds.net
Mill Valley, CA, **School of Thai Traditional Medical Massage**   www.thai-massage.com
San Rafael, CA, **The Center for Thai Massage**   www.thaimassagecenter.com
Hawaii, Valerie Passion Flower   www.thaimassagetherapy.com
New York and New Jersey, **The Lotus Heart**   www.thelotusheart.com
Kathmandu, **The Healing Hands Center**   www.ancientmassage.com
Various locations, **The Thai Massage Center**   www.thai-massage.net

Therapeutic Touch (TT)

TT is a means of attuning to and directing the universal life energy. The goal is to release congestion and balance areas where the flow of life energy has become disordered. Removal of these blockages facilitates the person's intrinsic healing powers.

TT is most commonly taught to, and used by nurses. However, some massage therapists study TT and incorporate it into their work.

Several books are available on TT, including *Therapeutic Touch: A Practical Guide* by J. Macrae, Knopf, 1988; *The Therapeutic Touch* by D. Krieger, Prentice-Hall 1979; *Therapeutic Touch* by Borelli and Heidt, Springer Co., 1981.

The Nurse-Healers Association maintains a website that has useful information about TT, at:

www.therapeutic-touch.org

Touch For Health (see also Applied Kinesiology)

This is a system for using applied kinesiology to aid the bodyworker. Applied kinesiology makes use of the fact that certain conditions result in weakening of specific muscles. Through muscle testing, the bodyworker gains information about the specifics of the client's condition. Further information is available from:

Touch For Health® Kinesiology Association
PO Box 392
New Carlisle, Oh 45344-0392
(800) 466-8342 or (937) 845-3404   **www.tfhka.org**

Trager®

Dr. Milton Trager, M.D., had a gift for bodywork from a young age, and developed his own system of bodywork which emphasizes gentle rocking of the client, and rolling body parts to encourage release and loosening and softening.

Some massage schools offer brief introductory trainings in Trager bodywork, giving the massage therapist a glimpse into the system. Massage therapists with introductory training often integrate a bit of the Trager awareness into their massage work. However, Trager practitioners practice only Trager, at least during a Trager session. Information about becoming a Trager practitioner can be obtained from:

Trager Association
3800 Park East Dr., Suite 100, Room 1
Beachwood, OH 44122
(216) 896-9383   www.trager.com

Trigger Point Therapies (Myotherapy℠ or neuromuscular therapy)

This refers to any of several systems of working with trigger points. Trigger points are tender congested spots in muscle tissue, which may radiate pain to other areas. Significant relief results when the trigger point is treated.

The techniques used in trigger point therapies are similar to those used in Shiatsu or acupressure, but trigger point therapies are based on western anatomy and physiology. Many schools listed in the State-by-State directory offer training in trigger-point therapies. Several institutions have refined the art of trigger point therapy into a self-contained modality, and teach their therapy in a non-massage context. These schools are:

Bonnie Prudden™ School of Physical Fitness and Myotherapy
P.O. Box 65240
Tucson, AZ 85728
(520) 529-3979 or (800) 221-4634
www.bonnieprudden.com

The Academy For Myofascial Trigger Point Therapy
1312 East Carson St.
Pittsburgh, PA 15203
(412) 481-2553

International Academy of NeuroMuscular Therapies
C/O NMT Center
900 14th Ave N.
St. Petersburg, FL 33705
(727) 821-7167
www.nmtcenter.com

St. John Neuromuscular Therapy Seminars
10710 Seminole Blvd., Suite #1
Largo, FL 33778
1-888-NMT-HEAL(668-4325)
www.stjohnnmtseminars.com

Tui Na

Tui Na is an Oriental bodywork related to Qi Gong. It is sometimes called Chinese medical massage.

Vibrational Healing Massage Therapy®

This modality was developed by Patricia Cramer, founder of the World School of Massage in San Francisco. It is based on the Fluid Body Model, and brings liquid consciousness to movement and breathing. Focusing on fluidity frees up tensions and stresses which have been held in the body. Thinking, speaking, listening and bodywork are all part of the system.

Watsu™ (aquatic shiatsu)

Watsu (from "water" and "shiatsu") began when Harold Dull started floating people, applying the moves and stretches of the zen shiatsu he had studied in Japan. Physical and emotional blocks are removed by the work, which can be done even by small individuals since the client's body in water is buoyant. It is done in chest-high, 94-degree water.

Certification can be obtained by taking three week-long workshops at:

School of Shiatsu and Massage
P.O. Box 889
Middletown, CA 95461
(707) 987-3801   **www.waba.edu**

Yoga therapy

In this method, yoga asanas are used to facilitate healing.

Zero-Balancing

Developed by Fritz Smith, MD, osteopath, Rolfer and acupuncturist, zero balancing works with the relationship between a person's physical structure and their energy. The practitioner works with fulcrums, points where structure and energy can be accessed together, to bring about change.

For fuller information about zero-balancing, trainings or practitioners, contact:

The Zero Balancing Association
801 West Main St., Ste. 202,
Charlottesville, VA 22903
(434) 244-2458   **www.zerobalancing.com**

VII

State-by-State
Directory

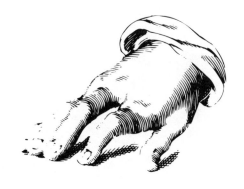

About the State-by-State Directory

The specific information about each school in the directory was provided by the school itself. The information was accurate as of June, 2002. Each school received the questionnaire below, and the answers provided by the schools comprise the school's listing. If no questionnaire was returned, then the only information listed is name, address, phone and Internet address, if any.

1. School Name _____

2. Address _____

3. Telephone _____ Internet address _____

4. Classroom hours of instruction (includes supervised practice) _____

   Total program hours (if different) _____

   Degree granted (if any) _____

5. Cost of program _____ Cost includes books, supplies, etc.?

   Specify _____

6. School offers: day program (yes/no)   night program (yes/no)

   weekend program (yes/no) other (specify) _____

7. Scholarships (yes/no)   grants (yes/no)   no-interest loans (yes/no)

   payment plans (yes/no)

8. Program emphasis (can circle more than one):

   relaxation massage (yes/no)   sports massage (yes/no)

   medical massage (yes/no)   deep tissue (yes/no)

   energy work (yes/no)   Eastern or Asian systems (yes/no)

   other (specify) _____

9. School statement or description (optional)—up to 25 words to say what-

   ever you wish about your school: _____

   _____

   _____

   _____

   _____

   _____

Degree-Granting Schools

Forty-one schools offer Associates degrees in massage. They are:

Arizona
Apollo College

California
Monterey Peninsula College
Weimar College
Western Institute of Science and Health

Colorado
Boulder College of Massage Therapy
Colorado School of Healing Arts
Community College of Denver
Heritage College

Florida
Florida College of Natural Health

Illinois
Illinois Central College
Wellness & Massage Training Institute

Indiana
Ivy Tech State College
Vibrant Life Resources School of Massage

Maryland
Allegany College of Maryland
Community College of Baltimore County

Massachusetts
Springfield Technical Community College

Michigan
Kirtland Community College
Oakland Community College

Minnesota
Minnesota School of Business – Brooklyn Ctr
Minnesota School of Business – Richfield

New Jersey
Lourdes Institute of Wholistic Studies

New Mexico
The Medicine Wheel

New York
Finger Lakes Community College
Orange County Community College
Rockland Community College
Swedish Institute
Trocaire College

North Carolina
Carteret Community College
Lenoir Community College
Sand Hills Community College

North Dakota
Williston State College

Ohio
Cuyahoga Community College
Ohio College of Massotherapy
Stark State College of Technology

Oregon
Central Oregon Community College

Pennsylvania
Academy of Medical Arts and Business
Allied Medical & Technical Careers
Pennsylvania School of Muscle Therapy

South Dakota
National American University

Utah
Provo College

Vermont
Community College of Vermont

About Accreditations and Financial Aid

Currently, five accrediting bodies actively accredit massage schools in the United States. Three of them are independent agencies recognized by the U.S. Department of Education, and two are agencies affiliated with massage professional associations.

Accreditations that can affect financial aid

The agencies recognized by the U.S. Department of Education are Accrediting Bureau of Health Education Schools or "ABHES" (**www.abhes.org**); Accrediting Commission of Career Schools and Colleges of Technology "ACCSCT" (**www.accsct.org**); and Accrediting Council for Continuing Education and Training "ACCET" (**http://accet.org**). Accreditation by one of these agencies makes schools eligible to offer federal financial aid to students. COMTA (see below) has also applied to the U.S. Department of Education for official recognition, but as of deadline for this Edition, that application had not been finally acted upon.

Federal (U.S.) financial aid comes in several forms, such as Pell Grants, Stafford loans, and PLUS loans. A student can receive federal financial aid only when attending a school which is qualified under the U.S. government's guidelines. That is why accreditation by ABHES, ACCSCT or ACCET is required for federal financial aid.

Other forms of financial aid are available, both through governmental and private funding. Some examples are Veterans rehabilitation benefits, private foundation grants and loans, and direct financial aid from massage schools.

As to all forms of financial aid, questions should be directed first to the massage school you plan to attend. They can tell you what types of financial aid are available. You may also want to explore private foundations or social groups that may have money available for tuition assistance. Check with local sources such as business leaders and charities to find out if any organizations in your area have such funds available.

Accreditations by massage professional associations

The two other accrediting bodies are Commission on Massage Therapy Accreditation "COMTA" (**www.amtamassage.org**); and Integrative Massage and Somatic Therapies Accreditation Council "IMSTAC" (**www.abmp.com**). Some state laws (Connecticut, North Dakota, Rhode Island and Utah) specify attendance at a COMTA-accredited school.

At the beginning of each state's listing in this Directory, there is a chart listing the accredited schools in that state, if any, and indicating which agencies accredit which schools.

ALABAMA

Accredited Schools	COMTA	IMSTAC	ABHES	ACCET	ACCSCT
Capps College			•		

Advanced Academy of Therapeutic Massage
1209 Mulberry St.
Montgomery, AL 36106
(334) 834-2278

Birmingham School of Massage
1776 Independence Court, Ste. 202
Birmingham, AL 35216
(205) 414-1477

Blue Cliff School of Therapeutic Massage
3737 Government Blvd., Ste. 517
Mobile, AL 36693
(251) 665-9900

CLASSROOM HOURS: 670

COST: $5,600.00 including books, massage table (payment plan)—day/night

EMPHASIS: relaxation, sports, medical, deep tissue, energy, Eastern/Asian, lomi lomi

SCHOOL STATEMENT: Blue Cliff School of Therapeutic Massage has been offering high-quality professional training for massage therapists since 1987.

Capps College
3590 Pleasant Valley Rd.
Mobile, AL 36609
(massage school at 1365 Government St.)
(251) 344-1203 (main) or (251) 438-2690 (massage)
www.poweroftouch.net

Massage Therapy Institute
1403 Beltline Rd. S.W., Ste. 1
Decatur, AL 35601
(256) 306-0444 or (800) 713-4162

Mobile Institute of Soft Tissue Therapy
1365 Government St., Ste. 1
Mobile, AL 36604
(334) 438-2600   www.mistt.com

Montgomery School of Massage Therapy
512 George Todd Dr.
Montgomery, AL 36117
(334) 396-1600   www.msmtmass.com

CLASSROOM HOURS: 1005

COST: $10,250.00 including books and supplies (no-int. loans, payment plan)—day/night

EMPHASIS: relaxation, sports, medical, deep tissue, energy

SCHOOL STATEMENT: MSMT provides quality education in a professional environment. Our curriculum certifies students in Medical, Swedish, and Esalen Massage. Introductories: Reiki, Sports, Pregnancy and Chair Massage.

North Alabama Wellness School of Massage
190 Ana Dr.
Florence, AL 35630
(256) 767-1890

Red Mountain Institute
1900 20th Ave. S., Ste. 220
Birmingham, AL 35209
(205) 933-0702

ALASKA

Accredited Schools	COMTA	IMSTAC	ABHES	ACCET	ACCSCT
University of Alaska	•				

Alaska Learning Institute
Day's Inn, 321 E. 5th Ave.
Anchorage, AK 99501
(800) 264-9835   www.healinghands.net

GateKey School of Mind-Body Integration Studies
4041 B St., Ste. 302
Anchorage, AK 99503
(907) 561-7327

CLASSROOM HOURS: 1200–1800

COST: $8,300 + (payment plans)—day program, some night and weekend classes

EMPHASIS: relaxation, sports, medical, deep tissue, energy, Eastern/Asian

SCHOOL STATEMENT: GateKey school has pioneered the healing arts and complementary medicine in Alaska since 1982. We provide a well proven, successful foundation for these professions.

Ida's Massage Therapy School
4141 B Street Ste. 302
Anchorage, AK 99503
(907) 561-7327

University of Alaska
3211 Providence Dr.
Anchorage, AK 99508
Office: (907) 786-1800
Massage: (907) 786-6542   www.uaa.alaska.edu

Accredited Schools	COMTA	IMSTAC	ABHES	ACCET	ACCSCT
Apollo College			•		
Arizona School of Massage Therapy	•		•		
The Bryman School					•
Desert Institute of the Healing Arts	•				•
Phoenix Therapeutic Massage College				•	
Rainstar University		•			•
Southwest Institute of Healing Arts					•

Schools Offering Associate's Degree

Apollo College

Apollo College
2701 West Bethany Home Rd.
Phoenix, AZ 85017
(602) 433-1333   www.apollocollege.com

CLASSROOM HOURS: 720 (Associate's degree, Tucson campus)—day/night/afternoon

EMPHASIS: relaxation, sports, medical, deep tissue, energy, Eastern/Asian

SCHOOL STATEMENT: The massage therapist diploma and degree program combine a complete and comprehensive study of Swedish massage with other manual and energetic therapies and supporting courses.

Massage also offered at:
Mesa campus (480) 831-6585
Tucson campus (520) 888-5885

Arizona School of Acupuncture & Oriental Medicine
4646 E. Ft. Lowell
Tucson, AZ 85712
(520) 795-0787   www.azschacu.edu

Arizona School of Integrative Studies
701 S. Broadway
Clarkdale, AZ 86324
(520) 639-3455

Arizona School of Massage Therapy
1409 West Southern Ave., Ste. 6
Tempe, AZ 85282
(877) 969-BODY or (480) 983-2222   www.arizonasmt.com

Bio-Link Massage Institute
627 S. 48th St., Ste. 110
Tempe, AZ 85281
(480) 966-2120   www.biolinktherapy.com

The Bryman School (High Tech Institute)
2250 W. Peoria Ave.
Phoenix, AZ 85029
(800) 987-0110   www.hightechschools.com

Charles of Italy School of Massage
1987 McCulloch Blvd.
Lake Havasu City, AZ 86403
(928) 453-6666   www.charlesofitaly.com

Desert Institute of the Healing Arts
140 E. 4th St.
Tucson, AZ 85705
(800) 733-8098   www.desertinstitute.org

CLASSROOM HOURS: 650 (zen shiatsu)/1000 (massage)

COST: $9,756.00 (grants, payment plan)—day (full-time)/night (part-time)

EMPHASIS: relaxation, sports, medical, deep tissue, energy, Eastern/Asian

SCHOOL STATEMENT: Dedicated to providing quality personal instruction in the art and science of massage therapy and shiatsu, thereby providing the public with highly skilled professionals.

Institute for Natural Therapeutics, Inc.
217 W. University
Mesa, AZ 85201
(602) 844-2255

Northern Arizona Muscle Therapy Institute
215 Coffee Pot Dr., Ste. A
Sedona, AZ
(928) 526-0832   www.namti.com

Phoenix College Therapeutic Massage Program
1202 W. Thomas Rd.
Phoenix, AZ 85013
(602) 285-7611   www.maricopa.edu

Phoenix Therapeutic Massage College
www.ptmcaz.com

609 N. Scottsdale Rd.
Scottsdale, AZ 85257
(480) 945-9461

9201 N. 29th Ave.
Phoenix, AZ 85051
(602) 395-9494

1000 N. Humphreys, Ste. 204
Flagstaff, AZ 86001
(502) 213-0010   www.ptmcflagstaff.com

Providence Institute
1126 N. Jones Blvd.
Tucson, AZ 85716
(520) 323-0203 or (866) 280-5713
www.providenceinstitute.com

Rainstar University
4110-4130 N. Goldwater Blvd.
Scottsdale, AZ 85251
(480) 423-0375   www.rainstaruniversity.com

Southwest Institute of Healing Arts
1402 N. Miller Rd. Ste. D
Scottsdale, AZ 85257
(480) 994-9244   www.swiha.org

West-Wind Academy of Massage Therapy
6511 N. 7th St.
Phoenix, AZ 85014
(602) 265-4466   www.westwindmassageacademy.com

West Valley Massage College
518 N. 35th Ave.
Phoenix, AZ 85009
(602) 269-1741

ARKANSAS

American Academy of Healing Arts
8201 Cantrell Rd., Ste. 300
Little Rock, AR 72227
(501) 666-9100 or (888) 669-9101

CLASSROOM HOURS: 500

COST: $4,100.00 including textbooks (no-int. loans, payment plan)—day/weekend

EMPHASIS: relaxation, sports, medical, deep tissue, energy, hydrotherapy, hygiene, business & marketing

SCHOOL STATEMENT: AAHA provides comprehensive high quality training in massage therapy. AAHA is a state-approved institution of higher learning with high educational standards and ethics.

Body Wellness Therapeutic Massage Academy
11323 Arcade Dr., Ste. D
Little Rock, AR 72212
(800) 280-6138

Fort Smith School of Massage
6108 S. 31st St.
Fort Smith, AR 72908
(501) 648-1107

Jean's School of Therapy Technology, Inc.
655 Park Ave.
Hot Springs, AR 71901
(501) 623-9686

CLASSROOM HOURS: 500—day program

EMPHASIS: relaxation, sports, deep tissue, Eastern/Asian, zen shiatsu

SCHOOL STATEMENT: The school has an organized comprehensive curriculum dealing with body systems and functions. Techniques taught with creativity based on long-standing knowledge of varied massage therapies.

Medicine Mountain Massage
4810 Central-Sunbay Resort
Hot Springs, AR 71913
(501) 525-8209

**Northwest Arkansas School
of Massage Therapy**
28 S. College, Ste. 8
Fayetteville, AR 72701
(501) 582-4341   www.nwasm.com

**Touching America—Hot Springs School
of Massage & Bodywork**
3000 Kavanaugh, Ste. A
Little Rock, AR 72205
(800) 844-0667 or (501) 663-3353
www.touchingamerica.com

A Touch for Health
502 East 24th St
Texarkana, AR 71854
(870) 774-1000   www.atouchforhealth.com

**Touch of Health School of
Massage and Bodywork**
P.O. Box 1420
Camden, AR 71711
(870) 836-0980

Valley of Vapors School of Massage
3909 Central Ave. Unit 7
Hot Springs, AR 71913
(501) 525-6883

White River School of Massage
48 Colt Square Dr.
Fayetteville, AR 72703
(501) 521-2550   www.wrsm.com

CLASSROOM HOURS: 500+

COST: $3,500.00 (scholarships, grants, no-int. loans, payment plan)—day/weekend/summer intensive

EMPHASIS: relaxation, sports, medical, deep tissue, Eastern/Asian, other modalities

SCHOOL STATEMENT: State-licensed professional training program offers outstanding value in education. Highly qualified faculty, balanced curriculum, comfortable modern facility, supportive learning environment. AMTA member. FREE CATALOG.

CALIFORNIA					

Accredited Schools	COMTA	IMSTAC	ABHES	ACCET	ACCSCT
Academy of Professional Careers				•	
Bryman College					•
California Healing Arts College					•
Career Networks Institute			•		
Concorde Career Institute					•
Glendale Career College				•	
Golden State				•	
Heartwood Institute				•	
Mueller College	•				
National Holistic Institute				•	
National Institute of Technology					•
Silicon Valley College					•
Western Institute of Sci & Health *Rohnert Park*			•		
Western Institute of Sci & Health *San Francisco*			•		

Schools Offering Associate's Degree
Monterey Peninsula College
Weimar College
Western Institute of Science and Health

Abrams College
Admissions: 101 College Ave., Ste. 4
Classroom: 961 N. Emerald, Ste. C
Modesto, CA 95350
(800) 953-6277   www.abramscollege.com

Academy of Professional Careers
(619) 461-5100   www.academyofhealthcareers.com

340 Rancheros Drive, Ste. 260
San Marcos, CA 92069

6784 El Cajon Blvd.
San Diego, CA 92115

8376 Hercules St.
La Mesa, CA 91942

CLASSROOM HOURS: contact school; day/night

EMPHASIS: relaxation, sports, deep tissue, energy, reflexology, shiatsu

SCHOOL STATEMENT: APC offers a year-round 730-hour massage therapy program and a 1000-hour holistic health practitioner program. Financial aid is available to those who qualify.

Acupressure Institute
1533 Shattuck Ave.
Berkeley, CA 94709
(800) 442-2232   www.acupressure.com

CLASSROOM HOURS: 150 (basic)/200 (specialized)/850 (acupressure)

COST: $1,450.00/$1,950.00/$5,950.00 (payment plan)—day/night/weekend/intensives

EMPHASIS: energy, Eastern/Asian, emotional balancing, Women's Health Issues, sports acupressure

SCHOOL STATEMENT: Internationally acclaimed Asian Bodywork trainings. Learn both Eastern and Western massage, over 80 bilateral points and ten bodywork styles. Call our school counselors.

A Diamond Holistic Massage Institute
140 Mayhew Way, Ste. 202
Pleasant Hill, CA 94523
(925) 609-8888   www.adiamondmassage.com

Advanced School of Massage Therapy
1414 E. Thousand Oaks Blvd., Ste. 213
Thousand Oaks, CA 91362
(805) 495-1353   www.asmt.net

Aesclepion Massage Institute
1314 Lincoln Ave., Ste. B
San Rafael, CA 94901
(415) 453-6196   www.aesclepion.org/massage.html

Agape School of Massage
3899 Stockdale Hwy., Ste. A
Bakersfield, CA 93309
(661) 832-8190

Ahern's Massage Therapy School
Offices: 4615 Indian Peak Rd.
Classroom: 5009 5th St.
Mariposa, CA 95338
(800) 578-2822   http://ahernsmassagetherapyschool.com

Alive & Well! Institute of Conscious Bodywork
100 Shaw Dr.
San Anselmo, CA 94960
(888) 259-5961   www.alivewell.com

All About Massage
74-121 Highway 111
Palm Desert, CA 92260
(760) 346-7949   www.allaboutmassage.com

(Spa Massage classes only)

Alternative Healthcare and School of Massage
197 East Ave
Chico, CA 95926
(530) 894-5457

American Institute of Massage Therapy Inc.
2156 Newport Blvd.
Costa Mesa, CA 92627
(949) 642-0735

American University of Complementary Medicine
11543 Olympic Blvd.
Los Angeles, CA 90064
(310) 914-4116   www.aucm.org

Auburn School of Health & Wellness
11960 Heritage Oak Place, Ste. 21
Auburn, CA 95603
(530) 823-6905 or (877) 611-5521   www.yogassage.net

Banning Massage School
66705 East Sixth St.
Desert Hot Springs, CA 92240
(760) 329-5066   www.tagnet.org/dstc

CLASSROOM HOURS: 100/150/250 (500 total hours)—day program

EMPHASIS: relaxation, sports, medical, deep tissue, energy

SCHOOL STATEMENT: We are happy to announce that our students have well-grounded knowledge of anatomy, physiology, pathology and hydrotherapy, and a well-balanced study on therapeutic massage.

Birdywhaw's Bodyworks Massage School
37748 Rio Vista Rd.
Springville, CA 93265
(559) 539-2053

CLASSROOM HOURS: 2 levels, each 24 classroom hours (each 100 total hours)

COST: $800.00 per level (payment plan)—day/night/weekend—arranged to fit students' needs

EMPHASIS: relaxation, sports, medical, deep tissue, energy

SCHOOL STATEMENT: Owned and operated by Teresa Glover, C.M.T., who offers basic and advanced classes from a holistic, medically based approach with small classes for individualized training.

BOD-E-WORK
3500 El Camino Real
Atascadero, CA 93422
(805) 461-4808   www.bod-e-work.com

Body Electric School of Massage and Rebirthing
6527A Telegraph Ave.
Oakland, CA 94609
(510) 653-1594   www.bodyelectric.org

Body Institute School of Massage Therapy
8331 Sierra College, Ste. 210
Granite Bay, CA 95746
(916) 791-1951

Body Mind College
5440 Morehouse Dr., Ste. 2700
San Diego, CA 92121
(858) 453-3295   www.BodyMindCollege.com

CLASSROOM HOURS: contact school; day/night

EMPHASIS: relaxation, sports, deep tissue, energy, Eastern/Asian

SCHOOL STATEMENT: Our classes are designed to provide profound experiences—both in your own personal healing and in learning to facilitate others, a truly holistic approach.

Body Therapy Center
368 California Ave.
Palo Alto, CA 94306
(650) 328-9400   www.bodymindspirit.net

Body Tune Up School of Therapeutic Massage
1955 Lucille St., Ste. D
Stockton, CA 95209
(209) 473-4993

Bryman College
www.bryman-college.com
Central Office: (888) 741-4271

Locations offering massage programs:

3000 S. Robertson Blvd., Ste. 300, Los Angeles, CA 90034
(310) 840-5777

511 N. Brookhurst St., Ste. 300, Anaheim, CA 92801
(714) 953-6500

12449 Putnam St., Whittier, CA 90602
(562) 945-9191

520 N. Euclid Ave., Ontario, CA 91762
(909) 984-5027

22336 Main St., Hayward, CA 94541
(510) 582-9500

Calaveras College of Therapeutic Massage
P.O. Box 274 (classroom 96 Court St.)
San Andreas, CA 95249
(209) 754-4876

California College of Physical Arts
18582 Beach Blvd., Ste.11
Huntington Beach, CA 92648
(714) 964-7744 or (800) 884-7744   www.calcopa.com

California Healing Arts College
12217 Santa Monica Blvd., Ste. 206
West Los Angeles, CA 90025
(310) 826-7622   www.chacmassage.com

California Massage Schools

The following index is arranged roughly from north to south, and grouped by area code for easy reference

North of Greater San Francisco

(530)
Alternative Healthcare and School of Massage
Auburn School of Health & Wellness
Chico Therapy: Wellness Ctr. Inst. of Healing Arts
Foothills Massage School
Lake Tahoe Massage School
Makoto Kai Healing Arts
Massage Therapy Institute
Mount Shasta Institute of Holistic Therapies
New Life Institute of Massage Therapy
Phillips School of Massage
School of Alternative Health Care
Weimar College

(707)
California Institute of Massage & Spa Services
Calistoga Massage Therapy School
Heartwood Institute
Lifestream Massage School
Loving Hands Institute of Healing Arts
Mendocino School of Holistic Massage
Napa Valley School of Massage
Pacific School of Massage
School of Shiatsu & Massage
Sebastopol Massage Center
Trinity College
Wellness Holistic School of Massage
Western Institute of Science and Health

Greater San Francisco Area

(408)
Central Coast Massage Institute
DeAnza College
Just For Your Health College of Massage
Milpitas College of Massage Therapy and
Electrolysis
Pacific College of Alternative Therapies
The Royal Touch Massage Therapy School
Silicon Valley College
Trinity College

(415)
Aesclepion Massage Institute
Alive & Well! Institute of Conscious Bodywork
Care Through Touch Institute
Diamond Light School of Massage & Healing Arts
San Francisco School of Massage
School for Self-Healing
School of Thai Traditional Medical Massage
Western Institute of Science and Health
World School of Massage and Advanced Healing
Arts

(510)
Acupressure Institute
Body Electric School of Massage and Rebirthing
Bryman College
Chi Nei Tsang Institute
Institute of Orthopedic Massage
McKinnon Institute
National Holistic Institute
reSource
School of Healing Touch
Silicon Valley College

(650)
Body Therapy Center

(925)
A Diamond Holistic Massage Institute
Silicon Valley College

Sacramento/Stockton Area

(209)
Abrams College
Ahern's Massage Therapy School
Body Tune Up School of Therapeutic Massage
Calaveras College of Therapeutic Massage
Massage School of Healing Arts
Oakendell School of Massage & Healing Arts
Touching for Health Center School of Prof. Bodywork

(916)
Body Institute School of Massage Therapy
California Institute of the Healing Arts and Sciences
Clinical Touch School of Massage Therapy
Fair Oaks Massage Institute
Healing Arts Institute
Western Career College

Between Greater SF and Greater LA

(559)
Birdywhaw's Bodyworks Massage School
Golden State Business College
Heavenly Touch Massage Therapy & Learning Center
Quality College of Vocational Careers
Therapeutic Learning Center

(805)
Advanced School of Massage Therapy
BOD-E-WORK
Hirudaya Holistic Life Center
Kali Institute for Massage & Somatic Therapies
Lu Ross Academy
Ojai School of Massage
Thousand Oaks Healing Arts Center

(831)
Cypress Health Institute
Esalen Institute
Lupin Massage Institute
Monterey Institute of Touch
Monterey Peninsula College
Twin Lakes College of the Healing Arts

Southeastern California

(760)
All About Massage
Banning Massage School
Desert Resorts School of Somatherapy
Healing Hands School of Holistic Health
Natural Healing Institute of Naturopathy
West Coast College

Greater Los Angeles Area

(213)
J.H.J. Education College
Los Angeles Vocational Institute

(310)
American University of Complementary Medicine
Brynam College
California Healing Arts College
Emperor's College of Traditional Oriental Medicine
Harbor Medical College
Institute of Professional Practical Therapy
Institute of Psycho-Structural Balancing
Massage School of Santa Monica

South Bay Massage College
Southern California College of Holistic Health

(323)
Hahm Therapeutic Massage Institute
Meridian Institute of Massage
National Polytechnic College

(562)
Bryman College
Cerritos College Community Education
National Institute of Technology

(626)
East-West Institute of Hand Therapy
Oriental Medicine Institute in America
United Beauty College
USA Pain Care College

(661)
Agape School of Massage
Career Care Institute
Massage Training Institute

(714)
Bryman College
California College of Physical Arts
Career Networks Institute
College of Physical Arts & Cosmetology
Golden Acupressure and Therapeutic Massage Coll.
Golden West Coll., Community Ed. Div
Lincoln Institute
Mesa Institute
West Pacific Institute

(805)
Halcyon Center
Santa Barbara Body Therapy Institute
Santa Barbara School of Massage

(818)
Glendale Career College
Hands on Healing Institute
Integrative Healing Arts Academy
The Touch Therapy Institute

(909)
Bryman College
Concorde Career Institute Inc.
Southern California School of Massage, Inc.

(949)
American Institute of Massage Therapy Inc.
The Western Institute of Neuromuscular Therapy

South of Los Angeles

(619)
Academy of Professional Careers
Mueller College of Holistic Studies
Pacific College of Oriental Medicine

(858)
Body Mind College
California Naturopathic College
International Professional School of Bodywork
School of Healing Arts
Vitality Training Center

California Institute of Massage & Spa Services
P.O. Box 673/730 Broadway
Sonoma, CA 95476
(707) 939-9431   www.calmassage.com

CLASSROOM HOURS: 165 (basic); 100 (spa); 100 (shiatsu); 100; 135 (advanced)

COST: $1,349.00; $1,139.00; $1,084.00; $1,104.00; $1,975.00 (approx.) including books and supplies (payment plan)—day/night/weekend

EMPHASIS: relaxation, sports, medical, deep tissue, energy, Eastern/Asian, spa services, pregnancy massage, body mechanics

SCHOOL STATEMENT: Loving touch lightens every heart. Let it lighten yours. CIMSS provides an inspirational environment in which students excel and enjoy the healing power of touch.

California Institute of the Healing Arts and Sciences
3550 Watt Avenue, Ste. 140
Sacramento, CA 95821
(916) 484-1700   http://californiainstitute.net

California Naturopathic College
1228 Camino Del Mar
Del Mar, CA 92014
(858) 259-1222 or (800) 354-8166

CLASSROOM HOURS: 100/200/500/1000/1500

COST: $1,000.00 to $25,000.00 (scholarships, payment plan)—day/night/weekend

EMPHASIS: relaxation, medical, deep tissue, energy, Eastern/Asian

SCHOOL STATEMENT: Unique Naturopathic training programs in Nutrition, Herbology, Homeopathy, Energetic Healing and Bodywork; small classes and personalized attention; enthusiastic teachers; oceanview location; loans available; state-approved.

Calistoga Massage Therapy School
5959 Commerce Blvd., No. 13
Rohnert Park, CA 94928
(707) 586-1953   www.calistogamts.com

CLASSROOM HOURS: 100

COST: $900.00 (payment plan)—day/night

EMPHASIS: therapeutic spa massage

SCHOOL STATEMENT: Basic 100-course teaching massage utilized in spas

Career Care Institute
43770 15th St. West, Ste. 230
Lancaster, CA 93534
(661) 942-6204

Career Networks Institute
986 Town and Country Rd.
Orange, CA 92868
(714) 568-1566 or (800) 455-4700   www.cniworks.com

Care Through Touch Institute
P.O. Box 420427
San Francisco, CA 94142
(415) 345-9265

Central Coast Massage Institute
1263 South Padre Dr.
Salinas, CA 93901
(408) 422-8240   www.taxwright.com/CCMI

Cerritos College Community Education
11110 E. Alondra Blvd.
Norwalk, CA 90650
(562) 860-2451 ext. 2521   www.cerritos.edu

Chico Therapy: Wellness Ctr. Inst. of Healing Arts
1215 Mangrove Ave., Ste. B
Chico, CA 95926
(530) 891-4301

Chi Nei Tsang Institute
2218 Woolsey St.
Berkeley, CA 94705
(800) 495-7797 or (510) 848-9558   www.chineitsang.com

Clinical Touch School of Massage Therapy
6815 Five Star Blvd., Ste. 105
Rocklin, CA 95677
(916) 630-1215

CLASSROOM HOURS: 130

COST: $999.00 (payment plan)—night program

EMPHASIS: sports, medical, deep tissue

SCHOOL STATEMENT: Located 15 miles northeast of Sacramento, Clinical Touch emphasizes proper technique, body mechanics, and "hands-on" supervised practice. Class size is limited to 14.

College of Physical Arts & Cosmetology
14600 Goldenwest St., Ste. 114
Westminster, CA 92683
(714) 799-9161

Concorde Career Institute Inc.
570 W. 4th St., Ste. 107
San Bernardino, CA 92401
(909) 884-8891   www.concordecareercolleges.com

Cypress Health Institute
P.O. Box 2941
Santa Cruz, CA 95063
(831) 476-2115   www.cyprushealthinstitute.com

CLASSROOM HOURS: 170/200

COST: $1,250.00 including books and supplies (payment plan)—night/weekend

EMPHASIS: relaxation, sports, medical, deep tissue, energy, Eastern/Asian, polarity

SCHOOL STATEMENT: Cypress provides opportunities to acquire professional training in therapeutic skills useful in facilitating a high level of physical, mental and emotional well-being in themselves and others.

DeAnza College
21250 Sevens Creek Blvd.
Cupertino, CA 95014
(408) 864-5678   www.deanza.fhda.edu

Desert Resorts School of Somatherapy
13100 Palm Dr.
Desert Hot Springs, CA 92246
(760) 329-1175   www.somatherapy.com

CLASSROOM HOURS: 300-1000

COST: $1,815.00 per 300 hours (payment plan)—day/night/weekend

EMPHASIS: relaxation, sports, deep tissue, energy, Eastern/Asian, lymphatic

SCHOOL STATEMENT: Our school offers courses of 300 to 1000 hours, including more than a dozen modalities as well as anatomy, physiology, business, ethics, holistic theory.

Diamond Light School of Massage & Healing Arts
P.O. Box 5443
Mill Valley, CA 94942
(415) 454-6651   www.diamondlight.net

CLASSROOM HOURS: 150-500

COST: $1,275.00-$5,500.00 (no-int. loans, payment plan)—day/night/weekend

EMPHASIS: relaxation, deep tissue, energy, Eastern/Asian

SCHOOL STATEMENT: We offer a heart centered, meditative approach to bodywork and healing, integrating the physical, emotional, spiritual and creative aspects of massage.

East-West Institute of Hand Therapy
7728 E Garvey Ave., Ste. 6
Rosemead, CA 91770
(626) 288-6797

Emperor's College of Traditional Oriental Medicine
1807-B Wilshire Blvd.
Santa Monica, CA 90403
(310) 453-8300   www.emperors.edu

Esalen Institute
Coast Rt. 1
Big Sur, CA 93920
(831) 667-3000   www.esalen.org

CLASSROOM HOURS: 26/150/250/500

COST: 150 hours $3,900.00 including books and supplies (scholarships)—Residential programs of 5 days, 28 days, etc.

EMPHASIS: relaxation, sports, deep tissue, energy, Eastern/Asian

SCHOOL STATEMENT: Esalen offers the original mind-body-spirit concept of massage.

Fair Oaks Massage Institute
4136 Pennsylvania Ave.
Fair Oaks, CA 95628
(916) 965-4063   www.fairoaksmassageinstitute.com

CLASSROOM HOURS: 126 basic/124 advanced (250 total)

COST: $1,150.00 basic/$1,150.00 advanced (payment plan)—day/night/night + weekend

EMPHASIS: relaxation, sports, medical, deep tissue, energy, Eastern/Asian

SCHOOL STATEMENT: Providing an avenue for helping others

Foothills Massage School
12794 Tyler Foote Xing Rd.
Nevada City, CA 95959
(530) 292-3123

Glendale Career College
1015 Grandview Ave.
Glendale, CA 91201
(818) 243-1131 or (800) 498-1818   www.success.edu

Golden Acupressure and Therapeutic Massage College
2525 N. Grand Ave., Ste. J & K
Santa Ana, CA 92750
(714) 771-4400

Golden State Business College
(559) 733-4040   www.goldenstatecollege.com

1320 E. Shaw Ave., Ste. 18
Fresno, CA 93726

3356 S. Fairway
Visalia, CA 93277

CLASSROOM HOURS: contact school; day/night

EMPHASIS: relaxation, sports, deep tissue, energy, reflexology, shiatsu

SCHOOL STATEMENT: GSBC offers a year round 730-hour massage therapy program. Financial aid is available to those who qualify.

Golden West College, Community Ed. Div.
15744 Goldenwest St.
Huntington Beach, CA 92647
(714) 892-7711   www.gwc.cccd.edu

Hahm Therapeutic Massage Institute
8474 W. 3rd St., Ste. 204
Los Angeles, CA 90048
(323) 966-4141

Halcyon Center
1129 State St. Ste. 5
Santa Barbara, CA 93101
(805) 962-3581

Hands on Healing Institute
2817 Montrose Ave.
La Crescenta, CA 91214
(818) 248-6979

Harbor Medical College
1231 Cabrillo Ave., Ste. 201
Torrance, CA 90501
(310) 320-3200   www.petersons.com/cci/155.html

Healing Arts Institute
112 Douglas Blvd.
Roseville, CA 95678
(916) 782-1275 or (800) 718-6824
www.healingartsinstitute.com

CLASSROOM HOURS: 126

COST: $1,270.00 including books (payment plan)—day/night

EMPHASIS: integrative massage

Healing Hands School of Holistic Health
(800) 355-6463 or (760) 746-9364
www.healinghandsschool.com

Office:
11064 Pala Loma
Valley Center, CA 92082

Classrooms:

125 W. Mission Ave. Ste. 212
Escondido, CA 92025

23022 La Cadena, Ste. 204
Laguna Hills, CA 92653

Heartwood Institute
220 Harmony Lane
Garberville, CA 95542
(707) 923-5000 or (877) 936-9663
www.heartwoodinstitute.com

Heavenly Touch Massage Therapy & Learning Center
709 N. Irwin St.
Hanford, CA 93230
(559) 584-9234

Hirudaya Holistic Life Center
11555 Los Osos Valley Rd., No. 201
San Luis Obispo, CA 93405
(805) 549-0951

CLASSROOM HOURS: 200/550/1000

COST: $875.00/$3,400.00/$6,750.00 (payment plan)

CLASSROOM HOURS: contact school; day (summer only)/night (year-round)/weekend (year-round)

EMPHASIS: relaxation, sports, deep tissue, Eastern/Asian

SCHOOL STATEMENT: Hirudaya School of Healing Arts provides thorough training in massage and holistic health practices, offering a balance of Eastern and Western techniques and theories.

Institute of Orthopedic Massage
406 Berkeley Park Blvd.
Kensington, CA 94706
(510) 524-3107   www.orthopedicmassage.com

Institute of Professional Practical Therapy
1835 South La Cienega Blvd., Ste. 260
Los Angeles, CA 90035
(310) 836-8811   www.ippt.com

Institute of Psycho-Structural Balancing
5817 Uplander Way
Culver City, CA 90230
(310) 342-7130   www.ipsb.com

CLASSROOM HOURS: 150/500/advanced classes

COST: $1,275.00/$5,068.00—day/night/weekend

EMPHASIS: relaxation, deep tissue, energy

SCHOOL STATEMENT: School's holistic approach allows students to learn eclectic hands-on techniques, body psychology and movement awareness in an environment of self-exploration.

Integrative Healing Arts Academy
7620 Lindley Ave.
Reseda, CA 91335
(818) 344-7184   www.a2zhealth.com

CLASSROOM HOURS: 300

COST: $1,500.00 (payment plan)—day/night/weekend/advanced courses

EMPHASIS: relaxation, sports, deep tissue, Swedish techniques

International Professional School of Bodywork
1366 Hornblend St.
San Diego, CA 92109
(858) 272-4142 or (800) 748-6497   www.ipsb.edu

J.H.J. Education College
2551 Beverly Blvd.
Los Angeles, CA 90057
(213) 384-0414

Just For Your Health College of Massage
2075 Lincoln Ave., Ste. E
San Jose, CA 95125
(408) 723-2570 or 723-2131
http://members.tripod.com/just4yourhealth

Kali Institute for Massage & Somatic Therapies
746 E. Main St.
Ventura, CA 93001
(805) 648-6204

CLASSROOM HOURS: 200/650

COST: $1,600.00 (no-int. loans, payment plan)—day/night

EMPHASIS: relaxation, sports, medical, deep tissue, energy, Eastern/Asian, Neuro Structural

SCHOOL STATEMENT: "Be the best, attend the best"

Lake Tahoe Massage School
PO Box 9927/1113 Emerald Bay Rd.
South Lake Tahoe, CA 96158
(530) 544-1227   www.laketahoemassageschool.com

Lifestream Massage School
2744 Jefferson Street
Napa, CA 94558
(707) 226-2090   www.lstreammassageschool.com

Lincoln Institute
202 W. Lincoln Ave., Ste. G
Orange, CA 92865
(714) 998-4943   www.lincolnmassage.com

CLASSROOM HOURS: 400+

COST: $600.00 to $800.00 per 100-hour course (payment plan)—day/night/weekend

EMPHASIS: relaxation, sports, deep tissue, energy, Eastern/Asian

SCHOOL STATEMENT: State Approved, EZ payment plan. Day, Evening, Weekend classes. First 100-hour basic circulatory massage course is self-paced with flexible schedule. Students love our classes!

Los Angeles Vocational Institute
3540 Wilshire Blvd., Ste. 410
Los Angeles, CA 90010
(213) 480-4882   www.lavocational.com

CLASSROOM HOURS: 300/500—day/night/weekend

EMPHASIS: relaxation, sports, deep tissue, energy, Eastern/Asian, trigger point, chair

SCHOOL STATEMENT: Our flexible schedules, affordable payments and diverse staff provide students with the best possible training in massage therapy, for a successful, rewarding career.

Loving Hands Institute of Healing Arts
639 11th St.
Fortuna, CA 95540-2346
(707) 725-9627   www.lovinghandsinstitute.com

CLASSROOM HOURS: 150 to 940

COST: $600.00 to $1,900.00 including books—nights and Saturdays

EMPHASIS: relaxation, sports, medical, deep tissue, energy, Eastern/Asian, Esalen, acupressure, trigger point, lymph drainage

SCHOOL STATEMENT: To teach natural healing techniques that enhance the quality of life. To educate for knowledge and mastery of massage therapy and holistic health education.

Lupin Massage Institute
P.O. Box 1274
Los Gatos, CA 95031
(831) 234-5791   www.lupin.com/lmi.html

CLASSROOM HOURS: 115 (125 total hours)—day/night/weekend/ modular and intensive programs

EMPHASIS: relaxation, sports, medical, deep tissue, energy, Eastern/Asian

SCHOOL STATEMENT: Located on relaxing 110-acre Santa Cruz Mountain Naturist Resort, LMI offers weekend and longer courses in many massage styles, healing arts and medical Qigong.

Lu Ross Academy
470 E. Thompson Blvd.
Ventura, CA 93001
(805) 643-2401   www.lurossacademy.com

Makoto Kai Healing Arts
443 First St.
Woodland, CA 95695
(530) 662-5662

CLASSROOM HOURS: 150 hours, each Module (300 total hours)

COST: $900.00 (payment plan)—weekend program

EMPHASIS: Eastern/Asian

SCHOOL STATEMENT: 150 hour basic course in Okazaki Restorative Massage (module 1). Additional 150 hours training in treatments (module 2). An American Judo and Jujitsu Federation school.

Massage School of Healing Arts
330 S. Fairmont, Ste. 2
Lodi, CA 95240
(209) 365-0679

Massage School of Santa Monica
1452 Third St. Promenade, Ste. 340
Santa Monica, CA 90401
(310) 393-7461   www.MassageSchoolSantaMonica.com

CLASSROOM HOURS: 500—day/night/weekend

EMPHASIS: relaxation, sports, deep tissue, energy, Eastern/Asian

SCHOOL STATEMENT: The Massage School of Santa Monica believes that learning the art of massage is first and foremost a journey of exploration into your own self.

Massage Therapy Institute
424 F. St., Ste. B
Davis, CA 95616
(530) 753-4428

Massage Training Institute
2427 G. St
Bakersfield, CA 93301
(661) 631-1966

McKinnon Institute
2940 Webster St.
Oakland, CA 94609
(510) 465-3488   www.mckinnonmassage.com

CLASSROOM HOURS: 100 (Swedish)/142 (Asian)/142 (sports)/ 134 (subtle touch)

COST: $1,075/$1,430.00/$1,350.00/$1,340.00 (scholarships, payment plan)—day/night/weekend/intensives

EMPHASIS: sports, deep tissue, Easter/Asian/touch for diverse populations

SCHOOL STATEMENT: We offer four certification courses and advanced trainings, introductory courses and general interest classes for the community. We offer 105 hours of anatomy and physiology.

Mendocino School of Holistic Massage
2680 Road B
Redwood Valley, CA 95470
(707) 485-8197

Meridian Institute of Massage
922 N. Vine St., Ste. 107
Los Angeles, CA 90038
(323) 467-3671

CLASSROOM HOURS: 350

COST: $2,485.00 including books and supplies (no-int payment plan)—day/night

EMPHASIS: relaxation, sports, medical, deep tissue, Eastern/Asian

SCHOOL STATEMENT: Small classes allow for personal attention to each individual. Scheduling can be flexible. 99% placement rate.

Mesa Institute
150 N. Feldner
Orange, CA 92868
(714) 937-4161

Milpitas College of Massage Therapy and Electrolysis
500 E. Calaveras Blvd., Ste. 333
Milpitas, CA 95035
(408) 946-9522   www.milpitascollege.net

Monterey Institute of Touch
27820 Dorris Dr.
Carmel, CA 93923
(831) 624-1006   www.montereyinstituteoftouch.com

Monterey Peninsula College
980 Fremont St.
Monterey, CA 93940
(831) 646-4231   www.mpc.edu

CLASSROOM HOURS: 160/800 (28 units)/800 (60 units; associates degree)

COST: CA residents: $100.00/$300.00/$700.00; non-residents $850.00/$4,000.00/$8,500.00 (scholarships, grants)—day/night/summer intensive

EMPHASIS: relaxation, sports, medical, deep tissue

SCHOOL STATEMENT: Monterey Peninsula College Massage Therapy Program offers professional training, exceptional affordability, and is located in one of the most beautiful areas on the planet.

Mount Shasta Institute of Holistic Therapies
212 E. Lake
Mount Shasta, CA 96067
(530) 926-4055

Mueller College of Holistic Studies
4607 Park Blvd.
San Diego, CA 92116
(619) 291-9811 or (800) 245-1976
www.muellercollege.com

Napa Valley School of Massage
1131 Trancas St.
Napa, CA 94558
(888) 282-1212 or (707) 253-0627
www.napamassageschool.com

National Holistic Institute
5900 Hollis St., Ste. J
Emeryville, CA 94608
(510) 547-6442 or (800) 315-3552   www.nhimassage.com

National Institute of Technology
236 E. Third St.
Long Beach, CA 90802
(562) 437-0501

National Polytechnic College
2465 W. Whittier Blvd., Ste. 201
Montebello, CA 90640
(323) 728-9636   www.npcollege.com

Natural Healing Institute of Naturopathy
1470 Encinitas Blvd.
Encinitas, CA 92024
(760) 943-8485

CLASSROOM HOURS: 100–1000 (H.H.P.)

COST: $745.00–$9.000.00 (payment plan)—day/night/weekend

EMPHASIS: relaxation, sports, medical, deep tissue, energy, Eastern/Asian, cranial-sacral, somatics

SCHOOL STATEMENT: State approved school of natural healing offering license and certification programs in massage therapy, nutrition, herbology, aromatherapy, holistic health, oriental therapies, sports and shamanic healing.

New Life Institute of Massage Therapy
1159 Hilltop Dr.
Redding, CA 96003
(530) 222-1467   www.newlifeinstitute.com

CLASSROOM HOURS: 170 (basic)/348 (additional) (605 total hours)

COST: $4,770.00 for total program (payment plan)—day/night/weekend

EMPHASIS: relaxation, sports, medical, deep tissue, energy, myofascial, cranio-sacral, neuromuscular, lymphatic, reflexology

SCHOOL STATEMENT: We focus on the how and why each massage technique works. From understanding comes the most successful therapy. Please visit us in our scenic location.

Oakendell School of Massage & Healing Arts
3585 Hawver Rd./Box 1144
San Andreas, CA 95249
(209) 754-0244

Ojai School of Massage
619 West El Roblar Dr.
Ojai, CA 93023
(805) 640-9798   www.ojaischoolofmassage.com

CLASSROOM HOURS: 250/500

COST: $1,500.00 per 250 hours (payment plan)—night/weekend

EMPHASIS: relaxation, sports, deep tissue, energy, Eastern/Asian, animal massage, equine massage, aromatherapy

SCHOOL STATEMENT: Our goal is to provide professional, high quality training in massage therapy and aromatherapy while enhancing the spiritual, mental and physical well-being of each student.

Oriental Medicine Institute in America
701 W. Valley Blvd., No. 222
Alhambra, CA 91803
(626) 281-8640

CLASSROOM HOURS: 150/400 (500 total hours)

COST: $1,000.00 including books (payment plan)—day/weekend

EMPHASIS: relaxation, sports, medical, deep tissue, Eastern/Asian

SCHOOL STATEMENT: Have a sincere commitment to provide the highest quality of massage and bodywork educational services.

Pacific College of Alternative Therapies
19997 Stevens Creek Blvd, Ste. 2
Cupertino, CA 95014
(408) 777-0102

Pacific College of Oriental Medicine
7445 Mission Valley Rd., Ste. 105
San Diego, CA 92108
(619) 574-6909 or (800) 729-0941   www.ormed.edu

Pacific School of Massage
44800 Fish Rock Rd.
Gualala, CA 95445
(707) 884-3138

CLASSROOM HOURS: 110

COST: $2,000.00 including books and supplies (payment plan)—2 residential weeks with one month in-between, residential cost $600 to $1,200 for both weeks)

EMPHASIS: relaxation, deep tissue, energy, Eastern/Asian, transformational bodywork

SCHOOL STATEMENT: Maximum class size is 12 students with a unique holistic approach addressing body, mind and spirit.

Phillips School of Massage
101 Broad St., Ste. B/P.O. Box 1999
Nevada City, CA 95959
(530) 265-4645   www.handsinharmony.com

CLASSROOM HOURS: 230 (level I)/230 (level II)/140 (level III) (600 total hours)—day/night/weekend

EMPHASIS: relaxation, sports, medical, deep tissue, energy, Eastern/Asian

SCHOOL STATEMENT: A healing, learning retreat offering technical and intuitive development, quality instruction in various bodywork modalities, and extensive massage experience with students and the public.

Quality College of Vocational Careers
1570 N. Wishon Ave.
Fresno, CA 92728
(559) 497-5050 or (800) 542-2225
www.qualityschool.com

reSource
Box 5398
Berkeley, CA 94705
(510) 433-7917

CLASSROOM HOURS: 200–1000

COST: $500.00–$1,000.00 (payment plan)—weekend program

EMPHASIS: holistic massage

SCHOOL STATEMENT: Since 1982, providing training and continuing education in bodywork and massage. Licensed to provide CA certification (200 hours) plus 500-hour and 1000-hour diplomas.

The Royal Touch Massage Therapy School
254 E. Main St., Ste. A
Los Gasos, CA 95031
(408) 354-7779   www.theroyaltouch.com

San Francisco School of Massage
1327 Chestnut St., Ste.s A & B
San Francisco, CA 94123
(415) 474-4600   www.sfsm.net

Santa Barbara Body Therapy Institute
516 N. Quarantina St.
Santa Barbara, CA 93103
(805) 966-5802   www.sbbti.com

CLASSROOM HOURS: 200/650/1000

COST: $1,200.00/$5,200.00/$7,700.00 (payment plan)—day/night/weekend

EMPHASIS: relaxation, deep tissue, energy, Eastern/Asian

SCHOOL STATEMENT: Holistic, experiential education blending awareness, compassion and anatomical understanding with skillful technique and dynamic body mechanics.

Santa Barbara School of Massage
1018 Garden St. Ste. 104
Santa Barbara, CA 93101
(805) 962-4748

School for Self-Healing
2218 48th Ave.
San Francisco, CA 94116
(415) 665-9574   www.self-healing.org

CLASSROOM HOURS: 760—day program

EMPHASIS: Meir Schneider Self-Healing method of massage, movement therapy and eye exercises

SCHOOL STATEMENT: Self-healing is body-mind work. It offers powerful combinations of massage, movement therapy, visualization, breathing exercises, and for those who need it, vision improvement techniques.

School of Alternative Health Care
197 East Ave
Chico, CA 95926
(530) 894-5457

School of Healing Arts
1001 Garnet Ave., Ste. 200
San Diego, CA 92109
(858) 581-9429   www.schoolofhealingarts.com

School of Healing Touch
2881 Castro Valley Blvd., Ste. 1
Castro Valley, CA 94546
(510) 886-0893   www.schoolofhealing.com

CLASSROOM HOURS: 100 to 500

COST: $10.00 per hour including books (payment plan)—day/night/weekend

EMPHASIS: relaxation, deep tissue, energy, Eastern/Asian, spa, pre-natal

SCHOOL STATEMENT: One of the few schools which offers spa and massage therapy, enables students to combine Eastern and Western knowledge for the well being of all.

School of Shiatsu & Massage
P.O. Box 570
Middletown, CA 95461
(707) 987-3801   www.schoolofshiatsuandmassage.com

CLASSROOM HOURS: 100/300/500/1000

COST: $750.00 per 50 hours (no-int. loans, payment plan)—Cost includes lodging at Harbin Hot Springs

EMPHASIS: relaxation, sports, deep tissue, energy, Eastern/Asian, Watsu(r)

SCHOOL STATEMENT: Our classes are based on a holistic and innovative approach to bodywork. We support our students to creatively develop their techniques and styles.

School of Thai Traditional Medical Massage
9 Homestead Blvd.
Mill Valley, CA 94941
(415) 383-4492   www.thai-massage.com

(Thai Medical Massage only)

Sebastopol Massage Center
108 N. Main St., Ste. 5
Sebastopol, CA 95472
(707) 823-3550

Silicon Valley College
www.siliconvalley.edu

Locations offering massage education:

1400 65th St. Ste. 200, Emeryville, CA 94608
(510) 601-0133

41350 Christy Street, Fremont, CA 94538
(510) 623-9966

6201 San Ignacio Ave., San Jose, CA 95119
(408) 360-0840

2800 Mitchell Dr., Walnut Creek, CA 94598
(925) 280-0235

South Bay Massage College
120 South Sepulveda, Ste. B
Manhattan Beach, CA 90266
(310) 546-8774

Southern California College of Holistic Health
730 So. Pacific Coast Hwy, Ste. 101
Redondo Beach, CA 90277
(310) 540-3355   www.SCCHH.org

CLASSROOM HOURS: 800 (1624 total hours)

COST: $9.50 per hour (payment plan)—day/night/weekend

EMPHASIS: relaxation, sports, medical, deep tissue, energy, Eastern/Asian

SCHOOL STATEMENT: We strive to teach our students to be true healers. We want them to truly want to help people feel better.

Southern California School of Massage, Inc.
12702 Magnolia Ave., Ste. 21
Riverside, CA 92503
(909) 340-3336

CLASSROOM HOURS: 100/250/500/1000/1150

COST: $795.00/$2,155.00/$4,220.00/$7,490.00/$8,490.00 (payment plan)—day/night/weekend/9-day intensives

EMPHASIS: relaxation, sports, medical, deep tissue, energy, Eastern/Asian

SCHOOL STATEMENT: SCSM individualizes student curriculums to meet the individual's scheduling needs. SCSM offers five programs, or individual classes may also be attended.

Therapeutic Learning Center
3636 N. First St., Ste. 154
Fresno, CA 93726
(559) 225-7772   www.tlcmassageschool.com

CLASSROOM HOURS: 250 hour program plus four 100-hr. classes

COST: 250 hours $3,150/100-hr class $1,250.00 (payment plan)—day/night/weekend

EMPHASIS: relaxation, deep tissue, energy, Eastern/Asian, reflexology

SCHOOL STATEMENT: Individuals are encouraged through love and high professional standards to improve their capacity for hands-on healing techniques and to open to greater self-realization.

Thousand Oaks Healing Arts Center
2955 Moorpark Rd.
Thousand Oaks, CA 91360
(805) 241-4194

Touching for Health Center School of Professional Bodywork
628 Lincoln Center
Stockton, CA 95207
(209) 474-9559

CLASSROOM HOURS: 105/500—night/Saturday

EMPHASIS: medical, deep tissue, energy, Eastern/Asian, structural integration, relaxation

SCHOOL STATEMENT: We are dedicated to the highest standards of teaching. Excellence is our goal as well as our standard of practice.

The Touch Therapy Institute
15720 Ventura Blvd., Ste. 101
Encino, CA 91436
(818) 788-0824   www.touchtherapyinstitute.com

CLASSROOM HOURS: 200/500/1000

COST: 200 hours $1,800.00 (no-int. loans, payment plan)—day/night/weekend

EMPHASIS: relaxation, sports, medical, deep tissue, energy, Eastern/Asian

SCHOOL STATEMENT: State Approved school. Registered with NCBTMB, member of ABMP, GI benefits, CEUs for nurses and acupuncturists, M-1 visa for foreign students.

Trinity College
www.trinitycollege.com

25 North 14th St., Ste. 60
San Jose, CA 95112
(408) 287-5100

804 W. Texas St.
Fairfield, CA 94533
(707) 425-2288

CLASSROOM HOURS: contact school; day/night

EMPHASIS: relaxation, sports, deep tissue, energy

SCHOOL STATEMENT: Trinity College offers a 730-hour massage therapy and a 1000-hour holistic health practitioner programs. Financial aid is available to those who qualify.

Twin Lakes College of the Healing Arts
1210 Brommer St.
Santa Cruz, CA 95062
(831) 476-2152

CLASSROOM HOURS: 200–750—day/night

EMPHASIS: relaxation, sports, clinical applications, deep tissue, energy, Eastern/Asian, prenatal/post-partum, geriatric

SCHOOL STATEMENT: Celebrating our 20th year—innovators of "Client-Centered Approach to Massage Therapy"™ promoting wellness orientation, client empowerment, and therapists who value and practice self-care.

United Beauty College
9324 Garvey Ave., Ste. H
South El Monte, CA 91733
(626) 433-1371

USA Pain Care College
19091 E. Colima Rd.
Rowland Heights, CA 91748
(626) 854-2898

Vitality Training Center
243 N. Hwy. 101 (Boardwalk Ctr)
Solana Beach, CA 92075
(858) 259-9491   www.vitalitytrainingcenter.com

Weimar College
www.weimar.org/college
20601 W. Paoli Ln./P.O. Box 486
Weimar, CA 95736
(530) 637-4111 or (800) 525-9192 ext. 7710
(Associate's Degree offered)

Wellness Holistic School of Massage
345 South E. St.
Santa Rosa, CA 95404
(707) 546-8115

CLASSROOM HOURS: 120

COST: $1,040.00 (no-int. loans)—night/weekend

EMPHASIS: energy

SCHOOL STATEMENT: Our program includes three levels: Certified Massage therapist; Certified Wellness Coach; Certified Master Wellness Coach, and four hands-on systems: Swedish, Polarity, Reflexology, Touch for Health.

West Coast College
14725 7th St., Ste. 1100
Victorville, CA 92392
(760) 241-7332

Western Career College
8909 Folsom Blvd.
Sacramento, CA 98109
(916) 361-1660 or (800) 321-2386
www.westerncollege.com

The Western Institute of Neuromuscular Therapy
22981 Mill Creek Dr., Ste. A
Laguna Hills, CA 92653
(949) 830-6151   www.wintherapy.com

CLASSROOM HOURS: 500/1000

COST: $5,000.00/$8,000.00 (scholarships, payment plan)—day/night

EMPHASIS: relaxation, sports, medical, deep tissue, Body Mechanics, Professional Development

SCHOOL STATEMENT: The mission of Western Institute of Neuromuscular Therapy is to provide a comprehensive, academic, and challenging program in the art and science of massage.

Western Institute of Science and Health
www.westerni.org/massage.htm

78 First St.
San Francisco, CA 94105
(415) 543-1883

130 Avram Ave
Rohnert Park, CA 94928
(707) 664-9267 or (800) 437-9474
(Associate's degree offered)

West Pacific Institute
243 S. Lakeview Ave.
Placentia, CA 92870
(714) 223-7122   www.TheBodycentre.com

CLASSROOM HOURS: 500

COST: $2,750.00 ($550.00 per 100 hours) (no-int. loans, payment plan)—day/weekend

EMPHASIS: relaxation, sports, deep tissue

SCHOOL STATEMENT: Private training only

World School of Massage and Advanced Healing Arts
401 32nd Ave.
San Francisco, CA 94121
(415) 221-2533   www.worldschoolmassage.com

CLASSROOM HOURS: 175–1041—day/night/weekend

EMPHASIS: relaxation, sports, medical, deep tissue, energy, Eastern/Asian

SCHOOL STATEMENT: We've taught a holistic approach to health for twenty years, offering massage therapy, advanced healing and master bodywork classes, 175-1000 hours of training.

COLORADO

Accredited Schools	COMTA	IMSTAC	ABHES	ACCET	ACCSCT
Boulder College of Massage Therapy					•
Cambrian College					•
Center of Advanced Therapeutics					•
Colorado School of Healing Arts	•				•
Denver Career College					•
Heritage College					•

Schools Offering Associate's Degree

Boulder College of Massage Therapy
Colorado School of Healing Arts
Community College of Denver
Heritage College

Academy of Advanced Healing
1004 Badger Rd., Box 637
Crestone, CO 81131
(719) 256-4667

Academy of Natural Therapy
123 Elm Ave.
Eaton, CO 80615
(970) 454-2628   www.natural-therapy.com

CLASSROOM HOURS: 1000

COST: $7,500.00 including books and supplies (scholarships, no-int. loans, payment plan)—afternoon program

EMPHASIS: relaxation, sports, medical, deep tissue, Eastern/Asian

SCHOOL STATEMENT: Our sole purpose is to help the industry through graduating the most qualified, caring people anywhere.

Boulder College of Massage Therapy
6755 Longrow Dr.
Boulder, CO 80301
(303) 530-2100

CLASSROOM HOURS: 1000 (CMT), 1200 (Associate's degree)

COST: $10,900.00 (grants, no-int. loans)—day/night/weekend

EMPHASIS: relaxation, sports, medical, deep tissue, energy, Eastern/Asian

Cambridge College
12500 East Iliff Ave.
Aurora, CO 80014
(303) 338-9700 or (800) 322-4132
www.hightechschools.com

Center of Advanced Therapeutics
1221 S. Clarkson St., Ste. Ste. 414
Denver, CO 80210
(303) 765-2201

Collinson School of Therapeutics and Massage
2596 Palmer Park Blvd.
Colorado Springs, CO 80909
(719) 473-0145

Colorado Institute of Massage Therapy
1490 W. Fillmore St.
Colorado Springs, CO 80909
(719) 634-7347   www.coimt.com

CLASSROOM HOURS: 590 (1150 total hours)

COST: $7,200.00 including books and supplies (no-int. loans, payment plan)—day/night

EMPHASIS: relaxation, sports, medical, deep tissue

SCHOOL STATEMENT: International Neuromuscular Therapy Certification (IANMT) included in the 1,150 hour program. Internships include clinical hospitals, and professional sports team settings. Continuing education and retail store.

Colorado School of Healing Arts
7655 W. Mississippi, Ste. 100
Lakewood, CO 80226
(303) 986-2320   www.csha.net

CLASSROOM HOURS: 700/1000/93+ credit hours (Associate's degree)

COST: $8,800.00 (700 hours) (grants, no-int. loans, payment plan)—day/night

EMPHASIS: relaxation, sports, medical, neuromuscular

SCHOOL STATEMENT: CSHA is exalted for its authenticity, sense of community, and delivery of a curriculum that is expansive and on the cutting edge of the industry.

Colorado Springs Academy of Therapeutic Massage
3612 Galley Rd., Ste. A
Colorado Springs, CO 80909
(719) 597-3414

Community College of Denver
1070 Yosemite St., Building 849
Denver, CO 80230
(303) 365-8376   http://ccd.rightchoice.org
(Associate's degree offered)

Connecting Point School of Massage
P.O. Box 2101/104 Society Dr.
Telluride, CO 81435
(970) 728-6424

Cottonwood School of Massage Therapy
11100 E. Mississippi Ave., Ste. B-100
Aurora, CO 80012
(800) 272-7484 or (303) 745-7725
www.cottonwoodschool.com

Crestone Healing Arts Center
P.O. Box 156
Crestone, CO 81131
(719) 256-4036

CLASSROOM HOURS: 630

COST: $6,850.00 including books and housing—12-week residential intensive

EMPHASIS: relaxation, energy, Eastern/Asian, acupressure, reflexology

SCHOOL STATEMENT: Our unique certification program includes 7 massage modalities and 8 support courses taught within a 12-week intensive format. Experience personal transformation and self-discovery. Call today.

Denver Career College
1401 19th St.
Denver, CO 80202
(303) 295-0550 or (800) 848-0550
www.denvercareercollege.com

CLASSROOM HOURS: 720 (55 credit hours)

COST: $7,950.00 including books and supplies (scholarships, grants, payment plan)—day/night

EMPHASIS: relaxation, sports, energy, hydrotherapy

SCHOOL STATEMENT: Our program is designed to prepare students for entry level massage therapist positions in a variety of settings. Emphasis is small class size, quality instruction.

Full Circle School of Alternative Therapies
P.O. Box 2005
Edwards, CO 81632
(970) 926-6210 or (877) 926-1341
www.fullcircleschool.com

(massage program also offered in Basalt, Steamboat Springs, and Frisco)

Golden Door School of Massage
136 Country Club Dr. P.O. Box 2702
Telluride, CO 81435
(970) 728-6800 X6704

Healing Arts Institute
4007 Automation Way
Fort Collins, CO 80525
(970) 223-9741 or (800) 444-8244   www.hai-colo.com

Healing Spirits Massage Training Program
33 S. Boulder Circle, Ste. 307
Boulder, CO 80303
(303) 525-5213 or (800) 974-9464

Heritage College
12 Lakeside Lane
Denver, CO 80212
(800) 887-8556   www.Heritage-Education.com

CLASSROOM HOURS: 840/1200 (Associate's degree)—day/night

EMPHASIS: relaxation, sports, medical, deep tissue, Eastern/Asian, neuro-muscular

SCHOOL STATEMENT: Heritage has the largest and most comprehensive Nationally Accredited and State Approved massage program in Colorado. Other Schools in Jacksonville, Fort Myers, Oklahoma City and Kansas City.

The Holistic Learning Center (Sequoia Spa)
2932 Evergreen Parkway, Ste. 102
Evergreen, CO 80439
(303) 674-6902   www.sequoiaspaholistic.com

CLASSROOM HOURS: 282

COST: $2,630.00 (payment plan)—day/night/weekend

EMPHASIS: relaxation, sports, holistic health

SCHOOL STATEMENT: The Holistic Learning Center offers an educational alternative for individuals to increase their knowledge of mind body spirit health through massage and energy field medicine.

Institute of Therapeutic Massage of Western Colorado
204 North 12th, Ste. 21-23
Grand Junction, CO 81501
(970) 255-8037

CLASSROOM HOURS: 500

COST: $5,000.00 (payment plan)—day/night/weekend (flexible scheduling)

EMPHASIS: relaxation, energy

SCHOOL STATEMENT: The Institute of Therapeutic Massage offers their students flexible hours that enhances their capability of learning a career during transitional times.

International Beauty Academy
1360 N. Academy Blvd.
Colorado Springs, CO 80909
(719) 597-1413

Massage Therapy Institute of Colorado
1441 York St., No. 301
Denver, CO 80206
(303) 329-6345   www.traditionalhealing.net

CLASSROOM HOURS: 1000

COST: $5,900.00—day/night

EMPHASIS: relaxation, deep tissue, Eastern/Asian, neuromuscular, myofascial, structural

SCHOOL STATEMENT: Our goal is to train a professional who is well-grounded in the fundamentals of massage with specialization in soft tissue and neuro-muscular remediation.

Morgan Community College
17800 Road 20
Ft. Morgan, CO 80701
(800) 622-0216 or (970) 542-3100   www.mcc.cccoes.edu

MountainHeart School of Bodywork and Transformational Therapy
P.O. Box 575, 719 Fifth St., Ste. 1 Upstairs
Crested Butte, CO 81224
(970) 349-0473 or (800) 673-0539
www.mountainheart.org

CLASSROOM HOURS: 748 (850 total hours)

COST: $6,600.00 (payment plan)—3 days + 2 evenings per week

EMPHASIS: relaxation, sports, medical, deep tissue, energy, Eastern/Asian, somatic/mind body, neuromuscular

SCHOOL STATEMENT: MountainHeart School offers one of the most current, comprehensive, and integrated Massage Therapy programs available. This program integrates the leading trends in massage therapy today!

Rocky Mountain Institute of Healing Arts, Inc.
P.O. Box 563
Dolores, CO 81323
(970) 882-3120   www.instituteofhealingarts.com

CLASSROOM HOURS: 650 (675 including 25-hour community service project)

COST: $6,150.00 (payment plan)—day program

EMPHASIS: relaxation, medical

SCHOOL STATEMENT: Small class sizes where emphasis is placed on the scientific basis of medical massage and the personal and educational development of students.

Silver Sword Academy of Massage Therapy and Spa Services
835 East 2nd Ave., Ste. B5
Durango, CO 81301
(970) 247-5008

Southwest Academy of Natural Therapies
1006 Main St.
Grand Junction, CO 81501
(970) 242-9224   www.southwestacademy.com

CLASSROOM HOURS: 500

COST: $5,000.00 (payment plan)—day/night

EMPHASIS: relaxation, graduate program in structural integration

SCHOOL STATEMENT: Our program focuses on the mastery of hands-on massage skills as well as supporting classes necessary to prepare students to become competent, independent massage practitioners.

Southwest School of Massage
1480 East 2nd Ave., Ste. 8
Durango, CO 81301
(970) 259-6965   www.SWSM.com

CLASSROOM HOURS: 739 (850 total hours)

COST: $6,800.00 (payment plan)—day/night/weekend

EMPHASIS: relaxation, sports, deep tissue, energy, Eastern/Asian

SCHOOL STATEMENT: We provide students with the opportunity to excel beyond current standards, and to represent the field of massage therapy with integrity and professionalism.

CONNECTICUT

Accredited Schools	COMTA	IMSTAC	ABHES	ACCET	ACCSCT
Connecticut Center	•				•

Connecticut Center for Massage Therapy
www.ccmt.com

75 Kitts Lane
Newington, CT 06111
(877) 282-2268

25 Sylvan Road South
Westport, CT 06880
(877) 292-2268

CLASSROOM HOURS (Newington): 525–638 (36–44 credit hours)—day/night/weekend

CLASSROOM HOURS (Westport): 638–1040 (44–73 credit hours)—day/night/weekend

EMPHASIS: relaxation, sports, medical, deep tissue, energy, Eastern/Asian

SCHOOL STATEMENT: Accredited by COMTA and ACCSCT; Over 20 years of educational excellence; financial aid to those who qualify; most courses approved for college credits; holistic orientation; placement assistance.

Galen Institute
1025 Silas Deane Highway
Wethersfield, CT 06109
(860) 721-1904 www.galeninstitute.com
CLASSROOM HOURS: 600
COST: $5,995.00–day/night
EMPHASIS: medical, chair massage
SCHOOL STATEMENT: Class size limited. Programs are mornings and evenings.

DELAWARE

Accredited Schools	COMTA	IMSTAC	ABHES	ACCET	ACCSCT
Dawn Training Center					•
Deep Muscle Therapy Center				•	
Delaware Learning Institute		•			

Dawn Training Center
2400 W. Fourth St.
Wilmington, DE 19805
(302) 575-1322 www.dawntrainingcenter.com
CLASSROOM HOURS: 600
COST: $6,895.00 including books and supplies (grants, no-int. loans, payment plan)–night program
EMPHASIS: relaxation, sports medical, deep tissue
SCHOOL STATEMENT: Dawn is nationally accredited (ACCSCT). Students begin to create a clientele in the school clinic, and the school provides training in allied medical careers.

Deep Muscle Therapy School
5317 Limestone Rd.
Wilmington, DE 19808
(302) 239-1613 www.dmtcmassage.com
CLASSROOM HOURS: 650
COST: $6,500.00 (grants, no-int. loans, payment plan)–day/night
EMPHASIS: relaxation, sports, medical, deep tissue, energy, Eastern/Asian
SCHOOL STATEMENT: We are ACCET-accredited and dedicated to excellence in massage education. Our program emphasizes relaxation and clinical knowledge. We accept Federal Financial Aid and other funding.

Delaware Learning Institute
(888) 663-1121 www.healinghands.net
Country Garden Business Center
Route 113, Box 114-D
Dagsboro, DE 19939
3515 Silverside Road
Clayton Building, Ste 204
Wilmington, DE 19801

Delaware School of Shiatsu and Massage Therapy
2102 A Drummond Plaza, Bldg. 2
Newark, DE 19711
(302) 737-2500 www.QIMYO.com
CLASSROOM HOURS: 600
COST: $4,975.00 including books (payment plan)–night/weekend
EMPHASIS: relaxation, sports, deep tissue, energy, Eastern/Asian, cranial, myofascial
SCHOOL STATEMENT: Founded on the principles of holistic Qi Myo massage and shiatsu; instructors focus on developing sensitive, therapeutic, goal-oriented touch. Separate shiatsu and massage therapy programs.

Holistic Health Enhancement School
5700 Kirkwood Hwy., Ste. 205
Wilmington, DE 19808
(302) 598-0854
CLASSROOM HOURS: 130/500
COST: contact school–day/night/weekend
EMPHASIS: relaxation, sports, deep tissue, energy, Eastern/Asian, reflexology
SCHOOL STATEMENT: We prepare students for state and national certification and offer continuing education. The atmosphere is professional, relaxing, and conducive to the highest quality learning experience.

Karen Carlson's International Academy of Holistic Massage and Science
P.O. Box 3940
Centreville, DE 19807
(302) 777-7307

Polytech Adult Education
P.O. Box 102
Woodside, DE 19980
(302) 697-4545 www.polytech2.k12.de.us

DISTRICT OF COLUMBIA

Accredited Schools	COMTA	IMSTAC	ABHES	ACCET	ACCSCT
Potomac Massage Training Inst	•				

Potomac Massage Training Institute
4000 Albermarle St., NW, 5th floor
Washington, DC 20016
(202) 686-7046 www.pmti.org
CLASSROOM HOURS: 514 (1180 total hours)
COST: $6,000.00 (payment plan)–day/night
EMPHASIS: relaxation, deep tissue, integrative massage, client-centered work

SCHOOL STATEMENT: The massage program is holistic, recognizing each person's unique inner health and growth process, with anatomy, physiology, kinesiology, and skill techniques forming the foundation.

FLORIDA

Accredited Schools	COMTA	IMSTAC	ABHES	ACCET	ACCSCT
Academy of Healing Arts					•
American Institute of Massage Therapy				•	
Core Institute	•				
Educating Hands	•				
Florida College of Natural Health	•				•
Florida School of Massage	•				
High-Tech Institute					•
Humanities Center Institute					•
Institute of Career Education					•
National School of Technology			•		
Sarasota School of Massage Therapy	•				
SE School of Neuromuscular					•
Southeast Inst. of Oriental Medicine			•		
Southeast Institute/Suncoast Center					•

Schools Offering Associate's Degree

Florida College of Natural Health

Academy of Career Training
3501 Vine St., Ste. 111
Kissimmee, FL 34741
(407) 943-8777

Academy of Healing Arts, Massage & Facial Skin Care
3141 S. Military Trail
Lake Worth, FL 33463
(561) 969-0899   www.ahamassage.com

CLASSROOM HOURS: 624

COST: $4,900.00 (payment plan)—day/night

EMPHASIS: relaxation, deep tissue, energy

SCHOOL STATEMENT: The AHA has been in operation under the same owner since 1983. AHA specializes in Aromatherapy, reflexology and neuromuscular training as well as Swedish massage.

Alpha Institute of Spa and Salon Services
910 10th St.
Lake Park, FL 33403
(561) 845-1400

CLASSROOM HOURS: 500 (100-hour additional colon hydrotherapy program)

COST: $3,600.00 (no-int. loans, payment plan)—day/night

EMPHASIS: relaxation massage

Alpha Institute of the Treasure Coast, Inc.
1599 S.E. Port St. Lucie Blvd.
Port St. Lucie, FL 34952
(561) 337-5533   www.alphainstituteoftc.com

CLASSROOM HOURS: 500

COST: $4,345.00 (no-int. loans, payment plan)—day/night (facial specialist program also available)

EMPHASIS: relaxation

SCHOOL STATEMENT: Class emphasis on the non-traditional student with small classes and relaxed, caring atmosphere. Flexible schedules and payment plans. Great Florida weather and attractions nearby.

Alpha School of Massage
4642 San Juan Ave.
Jacksonville, FL 32210
(904) 389-9117

American Institute of Massage Therapy, Inc.
416 E. Atlantic Blvd.
Pompano Bch., FL 33060
(954) 568-6200 or (800) 752-2793   www.aimt.com

CLASSROOM HOURS: 600

COST: $5,000.00 (scholarships, payment plan)—day/night (12-month or 6-month programs)

EMPHASIS: relaxation, sports, medical, deep tissue, nutrition & natural health

SCHOOL STATEMENT: Become highly skilled and successful licensed massage therapists and/or colon therapists with broad background in natural health! Our graduates are eligible for National Certification Exam.

Arlington School of Massage
1239 Rogero Rd.
Jacksonville, FL 32211
(904) 745-1688

A.S.M. Beauty World Academy, Inc.
2556 N. State Rd. 7 (Hwy. 441)
Hollywood, FL 33021
(954) 966-5998

CLASSROOM HOURS: 650

COST: $6,800.00 including books and supplies (scholarships, grants, no-int. loans, payment plan)—day/night

EMPHASIS: relaxation, sports, medical, deep tissue, energy, Eastern/Asian

SCHOOL STATEMENT: We always keep our school updated on the newest thing in the massage therapy industry.

Atlantic Vocational Technical Center
4700 Coconut Creek Pkwy.
Coconut Creek, FL 33063
(954) 977-2000

Bhakti Academy School of Intuitive Massage and Healing
25400 U.S. 19 North, Ste. 116
Clearwater, FL 33763
(813) 724-9727

Boca Raton Institute
5499 N. Federal Hwy
Boca Raton, FL 33487
(561) 241-8105   www.bocaschools.com

Bonita Springs School, Inc.
10915 Bonita Beach Rd., Ste. 2111
Bonita Springs, FL 34135
(941) 495-0714

CLASSROOM HOURS: 500

COST: $3,441.42 including books and materials (grants, no-int. loans, payment plan)—day/night

EMPHASIS: relaxation, sports, medical, deep tissue, energy, Eastern/Asian, chair, aromatherapy, spa, hydrotherapy

SCHOOL STATEMENT: Benefits of Bonita Springs School: flexible attendance policy, half-time programs, first week no cost or obligation, owner is licensed LMT, flexible payment plans, internship clinic.

Broward Community College
3501 Southwest Davie Rd., Bldg. 8
Davie, FL 33314
(954) 475-6735   www.broward.cc.fl.us

Central Florida School of Health Sciences
1318 S. Crystal Lake Dr.
Orlando, FL 32806
(407) 898-8145

Central Florida School of Massage Therapy, Inc.
450 N. Lakemont Ave., Ste. A
Winter Park, FL 32792
(407) 673-6776   www.massagetherapy.cc

CLASSROOM HOURS: 525

COST: $4,575.00 including books and polo shirt (no-int. loans, payment plan)—day/night

EMPHASIS: relaxation, medical, deep tissue, energy

SCHOOL STATEMENT: The school provides a comprehensive education in the art and science of massage therapy, balancing professional expertise with personal growth in a supportive environment.

Coastal School of Massage Therapy
434 Osceola Ave.
Jacksonville Beach, FL 32250
(904) 270-1700

Century School of Massage Therapy
7421 Jefferson Ave.
Century, FL 32535
(850) 256-0775   www.Massagegulfcoast.com

CLASSROOM HOURS: 600/750/1000/1150

COST: $4,900.00/$8,275.00/$9,125.00/10,725.00 includes massage table, books, supplies and uniform (loans and payment plan)—day/night

EMPHASIS: medical, sports, spa

SCHOOL STATEMENT: CSMT's dedicated and experienced staff offer a caring and professional environment to provide you with the most in-depth massage education possible.

Community Technical and Adult Education
1014 SW 7th Rd.
Ocala, FL 34474
(352) 671-7200

Core Institute School of Massage Therapy
223 West Carolina St.
Tallahassee, FL 32301
(850) 222-8673   www.coreinstitute.com

CLASSROOM HOURS: 650

COST: $5,200.00 (scholarships, payment plan)—day/night

EMPHASIS: relaxation, sports, medical, deep tissue, energy, Eastern/Asian, myofascial, structural

SCHOOL STATEMENT: The core institute is dedicated to promoting and modeling wellness through touch; embracing professionalism in education, caring in community service, and knowledge through research and inquiry.

Dade Medical Institute
3401 NW 7th St.
Miami, FL 33125
(305) 644-1171

Daytona Beach Community College
1200 W. International Speedway Blvd.
Daytona Beach, FL 32120-2811
(904) 254-3000 ext. 3052   www.dbcc.cc.fl.us

Daytona Institute of Massage Therapy
1500 Ridgewood Ave., Ste. B
Holly Hill, FL 32117
(386) 267-0565

DG Erwin Technical Center
2010 E. Hillsborough Ave.
Tampa, FL 33610
(813) 231-1800

Educating Hands School of Massage
120 S.W. 8th St.
Miami, FL 33130
(305) 385-6991   www.EducatingHands.com

CLASSROOM HOURS: 624

COST: $5,400.00 (payment plan)—day/night

EMPHASIS: personal growth, eclectic bodywork

SCHOOL STATEMENT: Foundational to our approach is the commitment to students' personal growth, as well as the development of their sensitivity awareness tactile, visual, emotional, energetic.

EduTech Center
18850 U.S. 19 North. Bldg. 5
Clearwater, FL 33764-3135
(727) 535-0608

Emerald Coast Massage School
913-B North Beal Pkwy
Fort Walton Beach, FL 32547
(850) 314-7714   www.Massagegulfcoast.com

CLASSROOM HOURS: 600/750/1000/1150

COST: $5,575.00/$8,950.00/$9,800.00/$11,400.00 including massage table, books, supplies and uniform (loans and payment plan)—day/night/full and part time

EMPHASIS: medical, sports, spa

SCHOOL STATEMENT: ECMS's nurturing and experienced staff strongly emphasize the clinical aspects of massage therapy in the treatment of sports and stress related specific injuries.

Exotica Academy Inc.
6229 Miramar Pkwy.
Miramar, FL 33023
(954) 981-2576

Florida Academy of Massage & Skin Care
8695 College Parkway, Ste. 110
Fort Myers, FL 33919
(941) 489-2282   www.massage-skincare.com

CLASSROOM HOURS: 500 (540 total hours)

COST: $3,575.00 including books and supplies (scholarships, no-int. loans, payment plan)—full-time/part-time

EMPHASIS: relaxation, stress reduction

SCHOOL STATEMENT: Our mission is to prepare our graduates with quality training to enter the field of massage therapy or skin care as competent, skilled professionals.

Florida College of Natural Health
www.fcnh.com

Main Campus: 2001 W. Sample Rd., Ste. 100
Pompano Beach, FL 33064/(800) 541-9299

Branch Campus: 7925 NW 12th St., Ste. 201
Miami, FL 33126/(800) 599-9599

Branch Campus: 887 E. Altamonte Dr.
Altamonte Springs, FL 32701/(800) 393-7337

Branch Campus: 1751 Mound St., Ste. G-100
Sarasota, FL 34236/(800) 966-7117

CLASSROOM HOURS: 624 (diploma)/1149 (Associate's degree)

COST: $6,020.00–$15,610.00 including books and supplies (scholarships, grants, no-int. loans, payment plan)—day/night (classes begin monthly)

EMPHASIS: relaxation, sports, medical, deep tissue, energy, Eastern/Asian

SCHOOL STATEMENT: We offer financial aid to those who qualify. New day and evening classes begin monthly. Job placement assistance upon graduation. Founded in 1986.

Florida Health Academy of Naples
261 Ninth St. S.
Naples, FL 34102
(941) 263-9391

Florida Keys Learning Institute
Hyatt Resort & Marina
601 Front Street
Key West, FL 33040
(800) 264-9835   www.healinghands.net

Florida School of Massage
6421 SW 13th St.
Gainesville, FL 32608
(352) 378-7891   www.massageonline.com

CLASSROOM HOURS: 705

COST: $5,700.00 (payment plan)—day program

EMPHASIS: relaxation, deep tissue

SCHOOL STATEMENT: FSM has 28 years of experience providing massage education as a vehicle for personal growth and empowerment, cultivating compassionate touch in a nurturing community experience.

Florida's Therapeutic Massage School
1300 E. Gadsen St.
Pensacola, FL 32501
(850) 433-8212

CLASSROOM HOURS: 600

COST: $3,450.00 (no-int. loans, payment plan)—day/night

EMPHASIS: relaxation, sports, medical, deep tissue, energy, Eastern/Asian

SCHOOL STATEMENT: We offer a comprehensive, holistic program in medical and stress management massage. We have a dedicated, caring, knowledgeable staff for our day and night programs.

Haney Vocational Technical Center
3016 Highway 77
Panama City, FL 32405
(850) 747-5500   www.bay.k12.fl.us/schools/htc

Heritage Institute
www.heritage-education.com

6831 Palisades Park Court
Ft. Myers, FL 33912
(941) 936-5822 or (800) 887-8556

4130 Salisbury Rd.
Jacksonville, FL 32216
(904) 322-0910 or (800) 339-5599

High-Tech Institute
1000 Woodcock Rd.
Orlando, FL 32803
(888) 326-1985   www.high-techinstitute.com

Humanities Center Institute of Allied Health School of Massage
4045 Park Blvd.
Pinellas Park, FL 33781
(727) 541-5200   www.2touch.com

Institute of Career Education
1750 45th Street
West Palm Beach, FL 33407
(561) 881-0220   www.vocedu.com

International School of Beauty Inc.
7127 US 19
New Port Richey, FL 34652
(727) 848-8415

Lindsey Hopkins Technical Education Center
750 NW 20th St.
Miami, FL 33127
(305) 324-6070   www.dade.k12.fl.us/lindsey

Loraine's Academy, Inc.
1012 58th St. North
St. Petersburg, FL 33710
(727) 347-4247   www.lorainesacademy.com

CLASSROOM HOURS: 600

COST: $6,329.50 including books and massage table (grants, payment plan)—day/night

EMPHASIS: relaxation, sports, Eastern/Asian

SCHOOL STATEMENT: The diverse faculty of Loraine's Academy offers the massage student a wide spectrum view of the field. Our low teacher/student ratio provides individualized attention.

Massage Therapy Institute
2200 N. Ponce DeLeon Blvd., Ste. 4
St. Augustine, FL 32084
(904) 829-1997   www.massage-institute.com

CLASSROOM HOURS: 500+

COST: $3,950.00 including books (no-int. loans, payment plan)—day or night programs, part-time or full-time

EMPHASIS: medical, deep tissue, Eastern/Asian

SCHOOL STATEMENT: Dedicated to educating excellent massage therapists, highly regarded as professional healthcare providers, emphasis is on outcome-oriented massage based on solid assessment skills

National School of Technology, Inc.
4410 W. 16th Ave., Ste. 52
Hialeah, FL 33012
(305) 893-0005   www.nst.cc

National School of Technology, Inc.
9020 SW 137th Ave.
Miami, FL 33186
(305) 893-0006   www.nst.cc

National School of Technology, Inc.
16150 17th Ave.
N. Miami Beach, FL 33162
(305) 893-0007   www.nst.cc

New Concept Massage and Beauty School
2022 S.W. 1st St.
Miami, FL 33135
(305) 642-3020   www.MassageAndBeauty.com

CLASSROOM HOURS: 605

COST: $4,290.00 including books and supplies (scholarships, grants, no-int. loans, payment plan)—day/night

EMPHASIS: relaxation, medical, energy

SCHOOL STATEMENT: We are a school of cosmetology, nails, skin and massage. Students develop the skills and knowledge needed in the modern world of beauty and massage.

Orange Technical Education Centers
Westside Tech. 955 E. Story Rd.
Winter Garden, FL 34787
(407) 905-2000

Palm Beach Community College
4200 Congress Ave.
Lake Worth, FL 33461
(561) 439-7222   www.pbcc.cc.fl.us

Pensacola Junior College
1000 College Blvd.
Pensacola, FL 32504
(850) 484-2200 or (888) 897-3605   www.pjc.cc.fl.us

Pensacola School of Massage Therapy
1730 Creighton Rd.
Pensacola, FL 32504
(850) 474-1330   www.Massagegulfcoast.com

CLASSROOM HOURS: 600/750/1000/1150

COST: $4,900.00/$8,275.00/$9,125.00/$10,725.00 including massage table, books, supplies and uniform (no-int. loans, payment plan)—day/night/full or part time

EMPHASIS: medical, sports, spa

SCHOOL STATEMENT: PSMT's nurturing and experienced staff strongly emphasize the clinical aspects of massage therapy in the treatment of sports and stress related specific injuries.

The Institute
1850 SW 8th st., 4th floor
Miami, FL 33135
(305) 642-4104 or (305) 541-5554
http://theinstitute.com

Ridge Technical Center
7700 State Road 544
Winter Haven, FL 33881
(863) 299-2512, ext. 247 or (863) 419-3060 ext. 247

CLASSROOM HOURS: 750—day/night

EMPHASIS: Basic massage, Eastern/Asian

SCHOOL STATEMENT: Our program advances the art and science of massage in a caring, professional and ethical manner, while promoting self-confidence, personal growth and leadership skills.

Sarasota School of Massage Therapy
1932 Ringling Blvd.
Sarasota, FL 34236
(941) 957-0577   www.sarasotamassageschool.com

CLASSROOM HOURS: 600

COST: $5,500.00 including books (grants, payment plan)–day/night; full-time or part-time

EMPHASIS: relaxation, medical, deep tissue, Eastern/Asian, hydrotherapy

SCHOOL STATEMENT: Prepare for National Certification and Florida licensure in Sarasota, on the beautiful Gulf of Mexico. Transform your life!

Sheridan Vocational Technical Center
5400 Sheridan St.
Hollywood, FL 33021
(954) 985-3220

SNI School of Massage & Allied Therapies
518 N. Federal Highway
Lake Worth, FL 33460
(561) 582-5349

Soothing Arts Massage School
737 Hwy. 98 East, Ste. #2
Destin, FL 32541
(850) 269-0820

CLASSROOM HOURS: 546

COST: $4,250.00 (payment plan)–day/night

EMPHASIS: spa treatments

SCHOOL STATEMENT: Soothing Arts is committed to providing excellent massage therapy education to ensure successful practitioners. The thoroughness and quality of the education makes our school unique.

Southeast Institute/Suncoast Center
4910 West Cypress St.
Tampa, FL 33607
(813) 287-1099

Southeast Institute of Oriental Medicine
10506 N. Kendall Dr.
Miami, FL 33176
(305) 595-9500   www.seiom.com

CLASSROOM HOURS: 500

COST: $6,000.00–day/night

EMPHASIS: relaxation, sports, medical, deep tissue, energy, Eastern/Asian

SCHOOL STATEMENT: SEIOM has a faculty in Oriental bodywork each with over 20 years experience. Shiatsu and Tui-Na. In addition: Qi Kung, Reiki, Cranial and Aroma Therapy.

Southeastern School of Neuromuscular and Massage Therapy, Jacksonville
9088 Golfside Dr.
Jacksonville, FL 32256
(904) 448-9499   www.se-massage.com

Space Coast Health Institute
1070 S. Wickham Rd.
West Melbourne, FL 32904
(321) 722-9000 or (888) 733-3529
www.spacecoasthealth.com

Suncoast Center for Natural Health
4910 W. Cypress St.
Tampa, FL 33607
(813) 287-1099   www.suncoastmassageschool.com

Vocational Institute of Florida
1849 W. Flagler St.
Miami, FL 33135
(305) 269-0772

GEORGIA

Accredited Schools	COMTA	IMSTAC	ABHES	ACCET	ACCSCT
Academy of Somatic Healing Arts		•			
Atlanta School of Massage	•	•			•
Georgia Medical Institute			•		
High-Tech Institute					•
Lake Lanier School of Massage		•			
Medix School			•		
Rising Spirit Institute					•

Academy of Healing Arts
486 New St.
Macon, GA 31201
(478) 746-0025

Academy of Somatic Healing Arts (ASHA)
7094 Peachtree Industrial Blvd., Bldg. 4
Norcross, GA 30071
(404) 315-0394   www.ashamassage.com

CLASSROOM HOURS: 630 (Swedish, NMT)/775 (Swedish, sports, NMT)

COST: $6,000.00/$7,000.00–day/night/weekend

EMPHASIS: Foundational Swedish with advanced clinical certification

SCHOOL STATEMENT: Founded in 1991 by holistic pioneer Jim Gabriel, ASHA was the first US massage school to include advanced clinical certifications in its core curriculum.

Atlanta School of Massage
2300 Peachford Rd., Ste. 3200
Atlanta, GA 30338
(770) 454-7167   www.atlantaschoolofmassage.com

CLASSROOM HOURS: 600 (evenings)/720 (days)

COST: $7,975.00/$8,375.00 (grants)—day/night plus six Saturdays

SCHOOL STATEMENT: The Atlanta School of Massage programs emphasize integrating a variety of techniques with a refined ability to interact meaningfully with each client.

Augusta School of Massage
3512½ Wheeler Rd.
Augusta, GA 30909
(706) 733-2040

Georgia Medical Institute
6431 Tara Blvd.
Jonesboro, GA 30236
(770) 603-0000   www.corinthianschools.com

High-Tech Institute
1090 N. Chase Pkwy., Ste. 200
Marietta, GA 30067
(888) 481-0047   www.high-techinstitute.com

Lake Lanier School of Massage
621 A Green St.
Gainesville, GA 30501
(770) 287-0377   www.school-of-massage.com

CLASSROOM HOURS: 600

COST: $6,600.00 (payment plan)—day/night

EMPHASIS: relaxation, deep tissue, energy, Eastern/Asian, nutrition, acupressure, cranio-sacral, pregnancy massage

SCHOOL STATEMENT: Our excellent curriculum, devotion to individual attention and a committed and loving staff have been the perfect formula to guide our students to success.

Medix School
2108 Cobb Parkway
Smyrna, GA 30080
(770) 980-0002   www.medixschool.com

Rising Spirit Institute of Natural Health
4330 Georgetown Square II, Ste. 500
Atlanta, GA 30338
(770) 457-2021

CLASSROOM HOURS: 750

COST: $8,100.00 (grants, payment plan)—day/night/weekend

EMPHASIS: relaxation, deep tissue, neuromuscular, seated massage, reflexology

SCHOOL STATEMENT: Graduates receive professional, comprehensive curriculum emphasizes the skills necessary for operating a successful massage therapy practice. Financial aid is available to those who qualify.

Savannah School of Massage Therapy
6413 B Waters Ave.
Savannah, GA 31406
(912) 355-3011   www.ssomt.com

CLASSROOM HOURS: 500+

COST: $5,500.00 approximately (grants, payment plan)—day/night/weekend/work-study

EMPHASIS: relaxation, sports, medical, deep tissue, energy

SCHOOL STATEMENT: We are dedicated to promoting excellence in massage therapy education, and committed to ensuring that students gain the necessary skills to excel in this field.

HAWAII

All Hawaiian School of Massage
1750 Kalakaua Ave., Ste. 2301
Honolulu, HI 96826
(808) 946-8878

Aloha Kauai Massage Workshop
Box 622, Hanalei
Kauai, HI 96714
(808) 826-9990

American Institute of Massage Therapy
22 F Oneawa St.
Kailua, HI 96734
(808) 263-2468   www.aimt-hi.com

CLASSROOM HOURS: 600

COST: $2,800.00 including books (payment plan)—weekend program

EMPHASIS: relaxation, sports, energy, advanced therapeutic Swedish

SCHOOL STATEMENT: Integrated massage training—body, mind, emotions, spirit. Mastering the art and science of massage therapy. Check out our awesome website: www.AIMT-HI.com

Big Island Academy of Massage, Inc.
207 Kino'ole St.
Hilo, HI 96720
(808) 935-1405 or (888) 715-5519
www.bigislandmassage.com

CLASSROOM HOURS: 500 (plus 100-hour apprenticeship)

COST: $4,995.00 including books (scholarship, payment plan)—day/night/weekend

EMPHASIS: relaxation, sports, medical, deep tissue, energy, Eastern/Asian, lomilomi

SCHOOL STATEMENT: Founded in 1992, our staff gives you an eclectic array of techniques with style, flavored with island aloha for state licensing or national certification.

The Hawaiian Islands School of Body Therapy & Wellness Center
P.O. Box 300
Captain Cook, HI 96704
(808) 323-3800 or (800) 928-9645
www.hawaiianmassageschool.com

CLASSROOM HOURS: 650/1000/1250

COST: $6,175.00/$8,250.00/$9,250.00 (payment plan)—day/night/weekend

EMPHASIS: relaxation, sports, medical, deep tissue, energy

SCHOOL STATEMENT: We prepare students for the State Board Examinations and educate and prepare students for working in the business world.

Hawaii College of Health Science
1750 Kalakaua Ave., Ste. 2404
Honolulu, HI 96826
(808) 941-8223

Honolulu School of Massage, Inc.
1136 12th Ave., 2nd floor
Honolulu, HI 96816
(808) 733-0000   www.hsmhi.com

CLASSROOM HOURS: 630

COST: $6,750 including books and supplies (payment plan)—day/night (8-week intensive or 16 week program)

EMPHASIS: relaxation, sports, medical, deep tissue, energy, Eastern/Asian

SCHOOL STATEMENT: To meet Hawaii State licensing and National Certification Requirements. Continuing Education. Community involvement. Nationally recognized 200 hour aromatherapy program.

Ho'ola O Lomi Lomi Lapa'au Clinic & School
P.O. Box 6202
Hilo, HI 96720
(808) 961-3118   www.lokahiola.org

Institute of Body Therapeutics
P.O. Box 11634
Lahaina, HI 96761
(808) 667-5058

Kona Hawaii School of Muscular Massage
75-6082 Alii Dr., Ste. 10
Kailua-Kona, HI 96740
(808) 936-9013 or (808) 331-2830
www.muscularmassage.com/khsmm.html

Maui Academy of the Healing Arts
1847 South Kihei Rd., Ste. 103
Kihei, HI 96753
(808) 879-4266 OR (888) 874-4266
www.massageschoolmaui.com

Maui School of Therapeutic Massage
P.O. Box 1891
Makawao, HI 96768
(808) 572-1888

CLASSROOM HOURS: 600

COST: $3,300.00 (payment plan)—day/night/weekend

EMPHASIS: medical, deep tissue, neuromuscular, clinical practice

SCHOOL STATEMENT: Become a licensed massage therapist while enjoying the sun and sea of Hawaii! Seven-month and twelve-month courses begin in September and March.

Pacific Center for Awareness & Bodywork
P.O. Box 672
Kilauea, HI 96754
(808) 828-6797

Spa Luna School for Massage Therapists
810 Haiku Rd., Ste. 209
Haiku, Maui, HI 96708
(808) 575-2440   www.spaluna.com

IDAHO

Accredited Schools	COMTA	IMSTAC	ABHES	ACCET	ACCSCT
Academy of Professional Careers				•	

Academy of Professional Careers
8590 W. Fairview Ave.
Boise, ID 83704
(208) 672-9500   www.academyofhealthcareers.com

COST: contact school—day/night; 1000-hour holistic health practitioner program. Financial aid is available to those who qualify.

EMPHASIS: relaxation, sports, deep tissue, energy, reflexology, shiatsu

SCHOOL STATEMENT: APC offers a year-round 730-hour massage therapy program and a

A Gift of Health School of Massage
445 Marjacq Ave.
Idaho Falls, ID 83401
(208) 524-1696

The American Institute of Clinical Massage Ltd.
780 Pines Rd., No. 105
Post Falls, ID 83854
(208) 457-8909   www.aicmtouch.com

CLASSROOM HOURS: 1250

COST: $7,650.00 including books, supplies, table or chair (no-int. loans, payment plan)—day/night

EMPHASIS: relaxation, sports, medical, deep tissue, Eastern/Asian, Ayurvedic

Canyon School of Massage
629 Lonestar Rd.
Nampa, ID 83651
(208) 461-5427

Center for Health Touch
3915 W. State St.
Boise, ID 83703
(208) 429-0699

Healing Arts Institute
211 W. Jefferson St.
Boise, ID 83702
(208) 336-9134

Idaho Institute of Wholistic Studies
1412 W. Washington
Boise, ID 83702
(208) 345-2704

Idaho School of Massage Therapy
5383 Franklin Rd.
Boise, ID 83705
(208) 343-1847   www.idschoolmassage.com

Moscow School of Massage
S. 600 Main
Moscow, ID 83843
(208) 882-7867

CLASSROOM HOURS: 600 (670 total hours)

COST: $5,100.00 (payment plan)—day program (Tu., Th., plus some weekend hours)

EMPHASIS: relaxation, sports, medical, deep tissue, health sciences

SCHOOL STATEMENT: MSM is dedicated to exceeding existing educational standards for massage therapists. The anatomical and clinical emphasis of our curriculum prepares students for successful massage careers.

New Images Academy
1270 South Vinnell Way
Boise, ID 83709
(208) 375-0190
http://newimagesacademy.uswestdex.com

Razzle Dazzle Massage School
222 Holly
Nampa, ID 83686
(208) 375-0190

Twin Falls Institute of Holistic Studies
P.O. Box 49/3999 Highway 93
Filer, ID 83328
(208) 326-4870

CLASSROOM HOURS: 108 basic class (334-500 total hours)

COST: 108 hours $1,000.00 (payment plan) (advanced courses individually priced)—night/weekend

EMPHASIS: relaxation, medical, energy

SCHOOL STATEMENT: Our school allows students to take the basic course and advanced courses while employed in a full-time employment. Classes limited to 12 students.

ILLINOIS

Accredited Schools	COMTA	IMSTAC	ABHES	ACCET	ACCSCT
Central Illinois School of Massage		•			
Chicago School of Massage Therapy	•				•
Illinois School of Health Careers			•		
Kishwaukee College Massage Program	•				
Northern Prairie Sch. of Ther. Massage		•			

Schools Offering Associate's Degree

Illinois Central College
Wellness & Massage Training Institute

Academy Massage Therapy
1715 5th Ave., Stes. 4 and 5
Moline, IL 61265
(309) 762-8231

CLASSROOM HOURS: 746

COST: $7,437.00 including books and massage table (payment plan)—day program

EMPHASIS: relaxation, sports, medical, deep tissue, energy, Eastern/Asian

SCHOOL STATEMENT: Established in 1987, Academy Massage Therapy offers an experiential learning environment, with the opportunity for limitless gains in knowledge of the body, mind and spirit.

Advanced Anatomy Massage Academy
650 N. Addison
Villa Park, IL 60181
(630) 823-4217 or (888) 832-4232
www.aamaschool.com

Black Hawk College
6600-34th Ave.
Moline, IL 61265
(309) 755-2200   www.bhc.edu

The Body Therapy Center School of Massage
4 Executive Woods
Swansea, IL 62226
(618) 239-6400

Center for Therapeutic Massage & Wellness
2704 Woodridge Dr.
Woodridge, IL 60517
(630) 960-9053
CLASSROOM HOURS: 500
COST: Approx $5,000.00 (varies with electives) (payment plan)—day/night/weekend
EMPHASIS: relaxation, sports, energy

Central Illinois School of Massage Therapy
5111 N. Glen Park Place
Peoria, IL 61614
(309) 692-0123   www.gotbalance.com
CLASSROOM HOURS: 748
COST: $7,000.00 (payment plan)—day/night/weekend
EMPHASIS: relaxation, sports, medical, deep tissue, energy, Eastern/Asian
SCHOOL STATEMENT: Our program is committed to training massage therapists that can integrate into any setting, including medical. We've moved into gorgeous 10,000 sq. ft. health/wellness complex.

Chicago College of Healing Arts
1622 W. Devon Ave.
Chicago, IL 60660
(773) 764-0960   www.livingwithherbs.com

Chicago National College of Naprapathy
3330 N. Milwaukee Ave.
Chicago, IL 60641
(773) 282-2686   www.naprapathy.edu

Chicago School of Massage Therapy
2918 N. Lincoln Ave.
Chicago, IL 60657
(773) 477-9444   www.csmt.com
CLASSROOM HOURS: 612
COST: $8,400.00 including books and materials (scholarships, grants, payment plan)—day program, varied schedule
EMPHASIS: relaxation, sports, medical, deep tissue
SCHOOL STATEMENT: Primary focus is Swedish Massage with other modalities.

College of duPage
425 Fawell Blvd.
Glen Ellen, IL 60137
(630) 942-2800   www.cod.edu

European Healing Center of Massage Therapy
8707 Skokie Blvd., Ste. 112
Skokie, IL 60077
(847) 673-7595

Hallowood
P.O. Box 106/213 N. Prospect
Cambridge, IL 61238
(309) 526-8056 or (866) 425-5696

CLASSROOM HOURS: 750
COST: $4,500.00 including books (payment plan)
EMPHASIS: Swedish/therapeutic, medical, eclectic
SCHOOL STATEMENT: Hallowood's emphasis is on sensitive, compassionate caregiving, realistic and practical ethics, hands-on fluency as well as practical effective business and marketing skills.

Hälsa Hem School of Massage, Inc.
2 Drawbridge Rd., Ste. T
Springfield, IL 62704
(217) 546-9011
CLASSROOM HOURS: 100/400—day/night/weekend
EMPHASIS: relaxation, energy

Illinois Central College
5111 N. Glen Park Pl.
Peoria, IL 61614
(309) 693-PATH   www.icc.cc.il.us
(Associate's Degree offered)

Illinois School of Health Careers
220 S. State St., Ste. 600
Chicago, IL 60604
(312) 913-1230   www.schoolofhealthcareers.com
CLASSROOM HOURS: 600
COST: $5,300.00 (payment plans, federal aid)
EMPHASIS: relaxation, deep tissue, clinical massage, marketing

Illinois Valley Community College
Therapeutic Massage Program, Rm. A-218
815 N. Orlando Smith Ave.
Oglesby, IL 61348
(815) 224-2720

Khepra School of Massage Therapy
1473 Ring Rd.
Calumet City, IL 60409
(708) 868-4686

Kishwaukee College
21193 Malta Rd.
Malta, IL 60150
(815) 825-2086   http://kish.cc.il.us

LifePath School of Massage Therapy
511 N. Glen Park Pl.
Peoria, IL 61641
(309) 693-7284

Marco Polo Massage Therapist School, Inc.
4011 West School St.
Chicago, IL 60641
(773) 205-5400

Midwest College of Cosmetology
755 W. Raab
Normal, IL 61761
(800) 811-2228

Midwest Institute of Massage Therapy
4715 W. Main St.
Belleville, IL 62223
(618) 239-6977

National University of Health Sciences Massage Therapy
200 E. Roosevelt Rd.
Lombard, IL 60148
(800) 826-NATL or (630) 889-6566   www.nuhs.edu

Northern Prairie School of Therapeutic Massage & Bodywork, Inc.
138 N. Fair St.
Sycamore, IL 60178
(815) 899-3382   www.northernprairieschool.com

CLASSROOM HOURS: 600 total hours (classroom hours unspecified)

COST: $7,800.00 ($10,000.00 including books, supplies, massage table)(payment plan)—day/night + some Saturdays

EMPHASIS: relaxation, energy, Eastern/Asian, lymphatic

SCHOOL STATEMENT: This premier holistic private schooling results in grads having a 100% pass rate on national board exams. A supportive environment with individual attention is provided.

Redfern Training Systems
9 S. 531 Wilmette Ave.
Darien, IL 60561
(630) 960-0844

CLASSROOM HOURS: 690

COST: $5,000.00 including books (no-int. loans, payment plan)—day/night

EMPHASIS: relaxation, sports, deep tissue

SCHOOL STATEMENT: We exercise an ongoing enrollment policy with flexible classes (morning, afternoon or evenings available). Classes are kept small for individualized attention, in a friendly environment.

School of Holistic Massage and Reflexology
1040 Ogden Ave.
Downers Grove, IL 60515
(630) 968-7827

Shawnee Community College
8364 Shawnee College Rd.
Ullin, IL 62992
(618) 634-3277   www.shawnee.cc.il.us

CLASSROOM HOURS: 525

COST: $1,800.00 including books and supplies (grants, no-int. loans, payment plan)—3:00 to 9:00 p.m. Tu., Th.

EMPHASIS: relaxation, medical, deep tissue

SCHOOL STATEMENT: Massage therapy program consists of more than 500 hours in three semesters. Graduates qualify to take the National Certification Exam for Therapeutic Massage and Bodywork (NCETMB).

Soma Institute—The National School of Clinical Massage Therapy
14 East Jackson Blvd., Ste. 1300
Chicago, IL 60604
(312) 939-2923   www.thesomainstitute.com

CLASSROOM HOURS: 700

COST: $7,000.00 (scholarships, no-int. loans, payment plan)—day/night/weekend

EMPHASIS: sports, medical, deep tissue

SCHOOL STATEMENT: Soma's unrivaled reputation, acclaimed curriculum, affordable tuition, remarkable financial assistance program, flexible schedules, and convenient location are just some of the reasons to choose Soma.

Waubonsee Community College
Route 47 at Waubonsee Drive
Sugar Grove, IL 60554
(630) 466-2467   www.wcc.cc.il.us

Wellness & Massage Training Institute
1051 Internationale Parkway
Woodridge, IL 60517
(630) 739-9684   www.wmti.com

CLASSROOM HOURS: 770 (Associate's degree through college program)

COST: $9,000.00 including books (scholarships, grants, payment plan)—day/night

EMPHASIS: relaxation, sports, deep tissue, energy, Eastern/Asian

SCHOOL STATEMENT: WMTI is a Private Vocational School approved by the Illinois State Board of Education offering professional training in a variety of complementary health care fields.

Wellspring Centre of Natural Healing Arts
402 East Roosevelt Rd. Ste. 102
Wheaton, IL 60187
(630) 588-1950   www.wellspringcentre.com

INDIANA

Accredited Schools	COMTA	IMSTAC	ABHES	ACCET	ACCSCT
Alexandria School of Scientific Th.	•				
Professional Careers Institute					•

Schools Offering Associate's Degree

Ivy Tech State College

Vibrant Life Resources School of Massage

Academy of Reflexology & Health Therapy Int'l
8397 E. 10th St.
Indianapolis, IN 46219
(317) 897-5111

CLASSROOM HOURS: 200

COST: $1,900.00 (no-int. loans, payment plan)—weekend program

EMPHASIS: relaxation, sports, deep tissue, energy, reflexology, homeopathy

SCHOOL STATEMENT: A state accredited school under the guidelines of the Indiana Commission on Proprietary Education. Established in 1990 and fully accredited.

Alexandria School of Scientific Therapeutics
809 S. Harrison/P.O. Box 287
Alexandria, IN 46001
(765) 724-9152 or (800) 622-8756   www.assti.com

Alternatives for Health, Inc.
1260 Jackson St.
Columbus, IN 47201
(812) 376-9194

American Certified Massage School, Inc
(219) 661-9099 or (888) 662-2585
www.hhgi.net

Locations:

100 S. Main
Crown Point, IN 46307

58 Lincolnway
Valparaiso, IN 46383

CLASSROOM HOURS: 505 (1000 total hours)

COST: $5,900.00 including books (payment plan)—day/night

EMPHASIS: relaxation, sports, medical, deep tissue

SCHOOL STATEMENT: A.C.M.S. was created to provide reasonable priced massage training—from people who love to teach massage—to people who have a great desire.

Aquarian Age Alternatives
301 S. Rangeline Rd.
Carmel, IN 46032
(317) 843-1138

Healing Arts Institute
518 S. Harrison St.
Shelbyville, IN 46176
(317) 392-2389

Healthy Lifestyle School of Massage Therapy
303 N. High St.
Muncie, IN 47305
(765) 281-9019   www.hlsmt.qpg.com

CLASSROOM HOURS: 700

COST: $6,500.00 (payment plan)—day + evening program

EMPHASIS: therapeutic massage, precision neuromuscular

SCHOOL STATEMENT: We focus on the student's well-being, in-depth anatomy, physiology, therapeutic massage, deep tissue, specifics, precision neuromuscular therapy, body movement, relaxation, nutrition and business skills.

Indiana Business College Massage Program
8150 Brookville Rd.
Indianapolis, IN 46239
(317) 375-8000   www.ibcmedical.com

Indiana College of Bodywork Modalities
7801 E. 88th Street
Indianapolis, IN 46256
(317) 841-3840

Indiana University/Purdue University
425 University Blvd.
Indianapolis, IN 46202
(317) 274-5555

Indiana University Kokomo Div. of Continuing Studies
2300 S. Washington
Kokomo, IN 46904
(765) 455-9426   www.IUK.edu/scs

CLASSROOM HOURS: 524

COST: $4,500.00 including books (payment plan)—night program

EMPHASIS: relaxation, sports, medical, deep tissue, Eastern/Asian

SCHOOL STATEMENT: Comprehensive 500-hour program that adheres to the educational standards and guidelines by the American Massage Therapy Association.

Ivy Tech State College
3800 N. Anthony Blvd.
Fort Wayne, IN 46805
(219) 482-9171   www.ivy.tec.in.us

BRANCH CAMPUSES: Anderson, Columbus, Evansville, Elkhart, Ft. Wayne, Indianapolis, Kokomo, Lafayette, Lawrenceburg, Madison, Marion, Michigan City, Muncie, Richmond, Sellersburg, South Bend, Terre Haute

(associate's degree offered)

Lewis School of Massage Therapy
3400 Michigan St.
Hobart, IN 46342
(219) 962-9640

CLASSROOM HOURS: 680

COST: $6,300.00 including books (payment plan)—weekend program

EMPHASIS: relaxation, sports, medical, deep tissue, energy, Eastern/Asian

SCHOOL STATEMENT: Our school focuses on developing the "practitioner in the student"; people skills, community stewardship, perfect practice, empathetic methods are instilled with philosophy/medical ethics studies.

Merrillville Beauty College
48 W. 67th Pl.
Merrillville, IN 46410
(219) 769-2232

Midwest Academy of Healing Arts
Office: 5447 Spring Creek Circle
Indianapolis, IN 46254
(317) 293-8076

Classsroom: 44 W. Main St.
Brownsburg, IN 46112
(317) 858-4263

Midwest Institute of Massage and Natural Therapeutics
150 Lincolnway, Ste. 2003
Valparaiso, IN 49383
(219) 465-0906

CLASSROOM HOURS: 650

COST: $5,300.00 plus $500.00 supply and material fee (payment plan)—2 evenings per week + 3 Saturdays per month for 10 months

EMPHASIS: relaxation, sports, deep tissue, energy, Western and Eastern herbs, nutrition, homeopathic first aid, counseling skills

SCHOOL STATEMENT: MIMNT prepares the massage therapist who desires holistic training. Graduates are a "step ahead", able to address mind and spirit as well as body.

Professional Careers Institute
7302 Woodland Dr.
Indianapolis, IN 46278
(317) 299-6001

Regional College of Massage Therapy
1415 Director's Row, Ste. 10a
Fort Wayne, IN 46808
(219) 482-6593   www.rcmtinc.com

Sawyer College
www.sawyercollege.com

3803 E. Lincoln Hwy.
Merrillville, IN 46410
(219) 945-1511

6040 Hohman Ave
Hammond, IN 46320
(219) 931-0436

CLASSROOM HOURS: 584

COST: approx. $7,000.00 (scholarships, grants, no-int. loans, payment plan)—day/night

EMPHASIS: relaxation, sports, medical, deep tissue, energy, Eastern/Asian

SCHOOL STATEMENT: Our program is clinically based and covers all information and hours to encourage National Certification. Students receive assistance in employment and financial aid.

Therapeutic Bodyworks School of Massage
8944 St. Peter's Street.
Indianapolis, IN 46227
(317) 888-3008

Vibrant Life Resources School of Massage & Wholistic Health
6109 W. Jefferson Blvd.
Ft. Wayne, IN 46804
(260) 436-8807   www.vibrantliferesources.com

CLASSROOM HOURS: 705/759/1116 (Associate's degree)

COST: $6,280.00/$6,820.00/$10,915.00 (payment plan, limited scholarships)—day program/Sundays plus evenings

EMPHASIS: relaxation, sports, medical, deep tissue, energy, Eastern/Asian, MFR, cranio-sacral

SCHOOL STATEMENT: VLR offers Certificate, Diploma, or associate of applied science in Therapeutic Massage and Bodywork. Weekend/evening or Daytime classes, full or part-time. Ohio approved.

IOWA					
Accredited Schools	COMTA	IMSTAC	ABHES	ACCET	ACCSCT
Capri College					•
Carlson College	•	•			

Bio-Chi Institute
1925 Geneva
Sioux City, Iowa 51103
(712) 252-1157

Body Wisdom Massage Therapy School
P.O. Box 1206
Ankeny, IA 50021
(800) 457-7339   www.bodywisdomschool.com

CLASSROOM HOURS: 25–1000

COST: $375.00–$11,920.00 (scholarships, grants, no-int. loans, payment plan)—day program (tailored schedules available)

EMPHASIS: relaxation, sports, medical, deep tissue, neuromuscular, energy, Eastern/Asian, myofascial, lymphatic, pre-natal, infant, animal massage

SCHOOL STATEMENT: Specializing in top quality education, expert teachers fly in from any US location. Programs are flexible and meet state requirements nationwide. Single courses, CEU available.

Capri College
www.capricollege.com

315 2nd Ave. S.E.
Cedar Rapids, IA 52401
(800) 397-0612

425 E. 59th St.
Davenport, IA 52807
(800) 728-1336

395 Main St.
Dubuque, IA 52001
(800) 728-0712

Carlson College of Massage Therapy
11809 County Road, Box 28
Anomosa, IA 52205
(319) 462-3402   www.carlsoncollege.com

CLASSROOM HOURS: full-time 650; part-time 525

COST: $6,000.00 including books, supplies, massage table or chair (no-int. loans, payment plan)—day/night/weekend

EMPHASIS: relaxation, sports, medical, deep tissue, energy, Eastern/Asian, herbology

SCHOOL STATEMENT: We offer a thorough comprehensive program located in a safe beautiful retreat like country environment with walking trails, basketball court, fruit trees and herb garden.

College of Massage and the Healing Arts Center
3601 Douglas Ave.
Des Moines, IA 50310
(515) 277-2126

CLASSROOM HOURS: 500

COST: $5,500.00 including books, massage table and accessories—night/evening & weekend

EMPHASIS: relaxation, energy, holistic massage therapy

SCHOOL STATEMENT: Get more than you expect! Plan for success in your career and life with innovative teaching style, individualized mentoring, and wholistic approach to maximize healing.

Eastwind School of Holistic Healing
209 E. Washington, Ste. 305
Iowa City, IA 52240
(319) 351-3262   www.eastwindschool.com

CLASSROOM HOURS: 500–600

COST: $5,370.00 including books (payment plan)—day program (Mon. and Tu.)

EMPHASIS: relaxation, medical, energy, Eastern/Asian, shiatsu, cranio-sacral

SCHOOL STATEMENT: Eastwind School emphasizes a holistic approach to bodywork providing many modalities with extensive elective offerings. Visit our website, or call us for details.

Holistic Horizons
200 Jefferson, Ste. 303
Burlington, IA 52601
(319) 752-0175

CLASSROOM HOURS: 515

COST: $5,665.00 (pay per module)—day/night/weekend

EMPHASIS: relaxation, deep tissue, energy, Eastern/Asian

SCHOOL STATEMENT: Holistic Horizons is a learning institute to foster the study of the Healing Arts. Send a SASE for more information to the above address.

Institute of Therapeutic Massage & Wellness
516 W. 35th St.
Davenport, IA 527806
(877) 445-4869 or (319) 445-1055
www.learntomassage.com

Iowa College of Natural Health
1932 SW 3rd Rd.
Ankeny, IA 50021
(515) 965-2991

Iowa Massage Institute
3017 Indianola Rd.
Des Moines, IA 50315
(515) 280-7611

CLASSROOM HOURS: 500

COST: $5,000.00 including books and supplies (no-int. loans, payment plan)—weekend program

EMPHASIS: relaxation, sports, medical, deep tissue, Eastern/Asian, reflexology, A&P, pregnancy/infant, MFR, seated

SCHOOL STATEMENT: Fundamental education in the art of massage therapy in a comfortable, safe and "hands-on" environment

La'James College
227 East Market St.
Iowa City, IA 52245
(319) 337-2109   www.lajames.net

CLASSROOM HOURS: 625 total hours (in-class hour not specified)

COST: $5,000.00 (payment plan)—day/weekend

EMPHASIS: relaxation, sports, medical, deep tissue, energy, Eastern/Asian

SCHOOL STATEMENT: The massage therapy course is an intensive study of body massage and the treatments as well as applications associated with the practice of massage therapy.

La'James College
512 Central Avenue
Fort Dodge, IA 50501
(888) 880-2106   www.lajames.net

La'James College
24 2nd St. N.E.
Mason City, IA 50401
(515) 424-2161   www.lajames.com

The Shiatsu Clinic & School
1025 N. Summit St.
Iowa City, IA 52245
(319) 338-4300   www.focusedtouchshiatsu.com

Windemere Institute of Healing Arts
1014 S. Mill St.
Decorah, IA 52101
(800) 874-0905 or (563) 382-8495   www.windemere.org

CLASSROOM HOURS: 684

COST: $7,250.00 including books and supplies (payment plan)—4-day intensives Sat-Tues once per month for 18 months

EMPHASIS: relaxation, medical, deep tissue, energy, Eastern/Asian, spa, other

SCHOOL STATEMENT: Windemere prepares the Healing Arts Practitioner for a professional healing career, integrating Eastern philosophies, energy concepts, Western bodywork methods and principles of nutrition and detoxification.

KANSAS

BMSI Institute
8665 W. 96th St., Ste. 300
Overland Park, KS 66212
(913) 649-3322   www.bsmi-institute.com

CLASSROOM HOURS: 550

COST: $5,775.00 (scholarships, payment plan)—night/weekend

EMPHASIS: relaxation, sports, medical, deep tissue

SCHOOL STATEMENT: BMSI is known for our quality instructors, variety of techniques, solid business and science curriculum, and our student clinic, which is open to the public.

Johnson County Community College
Massage Therapy Program
9780 W. 87th St., Overland Park, KS 66212
(913) 469-4422   www.jccc.net

Kansas College of Chinese Medicine
9235 E. Harry, Bldg. 100, Ste. 1A
Wichita, KS 67207
(316) 691-8822   www.kccm.edu

Kansas Massage Institute
4525 S.W. 21st
Topeka, KS 66604
(785) 273-4747   www.kansasmassage.ohgolly.com

Lunaria Bodywork Institute
1103 Massachusetts Street
Lawrence, KS 66044
(785) 841-1587   www.lunaria.net

CLASSROOM HOURS: 500

COST: $5,000.00 (grants, payment plan)—day/night (full-time or part-time)

EMPHASIS: Swedish massage

SCHOOL STATEMENT: Heal with your heart and hands. LBI's 500 hour program offers: Swedish, deep tissue, acupressure, reflexology, aromatherapy, anatomy, physiology, pathology, yoga, student clinic and more.

Total Health Works Massage Therapy School
138 S. Hydraulic
Wichita, KS 67211
(316) 262-8400

CLASSROOM HOURS: 100–200 (600 total hours)

COST: $8.00 per hour (payment plan)—night/weekend/seminars

EMPHASIS: relaxation, sports, deep tissue, aromatherapy, pregnancy massage

SCHOOL STATEMENT: Total Health Works will utilize the highest standards possible to provide the professional skills and training which will inspire the utmost confidence in our graduates.

KENTUCKY

Advanced Massage Therapeutics
2700 Bardstown Rd.
Louisville, KY 40205
(502) 895-3500

Blue Grass Professional School of Massage Therapy
501 Darby Creek Rd., Ste. 14
Lexington, KY 40509
(859) 264-1450 or (800) 731-6031

Kentucky Academy of Medical Massage
5016 Main St., Box 10
May's Lick, KY 41055
(606) 763-6334

Lexington Healing Arts Academy
630 South Broadway
Lexington, KY 40508
(859) 252-5656

CLASSROOM HOURS: 600

COST: $4,700.00 including books (payment plan)—day/night

EMPHASIS: relaxation, sports, deep tissue, energy, Eastern/Asian

SCHOOL STATEMENT: We are state-licensed and NCBTMB-approved. Our program provides strong base in anatomy and physiology as well as integrating Western medicine and Eastern methods of healing.

Louisville School of Massage
7410 New LaGrange Rd., Ste. 320
Louisville, KY 40222
(502) 429-5765

Natural Health Institute of Western Kentucky
950 Stonebrook Lane
Paducah, KY 42003
(270) 442-7377   www.natural-health-inst.com

CLASSROOM HOURS: 500

COST: $6,212.00 (includes massage table)(scholarships, payment plan)—night/weekend

EMPHASIS: relaxation, sports, medical, deep tissue, energy

SCHOOL STATEMENT: We promote quality education and services in natural health therapies and support appropriate bridging between natural health and conventional medicine to promote wellness.

Sun Touch Massage School
914 W. Broadway
Mayfield, KY 42066
(270) 247-8923   www.suntouch.org

CLASSROOM HOURS: 500

COST: $4,800.00 including books and supplies (no-int. loans, payment plan)—day/night

EMPHASIS: relaxation, sports, deep tissue, energy, Easter/Asian, reiki, connective tissue, prenatal

SCHOOL STATEMENT: Our courses qualify a student to take the national certification exam, and/or become licensed in Tennessee, Missouri, or other states requiring 500 hours.

LOUISIANA

Accredited Schools	COMTA	IMSTAC	ABHES	ACCET	ACCSCT
Blue Cliff College					•
King's Career College			•		

Blue Cliff School of Therapeutic Massage
New Orleans, LA (800) 975-5405
Lafayette, LA (877) 269-0615
Shreveport, LA (877) 437-1222
Gulfcoast, MI (228) 896-9727

Career Technical College
1611 Louisville Ave.
Monroe, LA 71201-6027
(318) 323-2889   www.careertc.com

Central Louisiana School of Therapeutic Massage
2901 Highway 28 East, Ste. C
Pineville, LA 71360
(318) 445-5433

Delta College
2401 N. Highway 190
Covington, LA 70433
(985) 892-6651

In Touch Bodyworks
11224 Boardwalk Dr., Ste. c-1
Baton Rouge, LA 70816
(504) 293-8556

King's Career College
141 Ocean Dr.
Baton Rouge, LA 70806
(225) 926-5535   www.kings.edu

Louisiana Institute of Massage Therapy
1108 Lafitte St.
Lake Charles, LA 70601
(318) 474-9435   www.massagecafe.com/LIMT.htm

CLASSROOM HOURS: 500

COST: $39,000.00 including books (grants, payment plan)—weekend program

EMPHASIS: relaxation, sports, medical, deep tissue

SCHOOL STATEMENT: In-hospital internship, affordable tuition, program director is author of textbook, Massage Therapy: Principles and Practice—Susan G. Salvo

Medical Training College
10525 Plaza Americana
Baton Rouge, LA 70816
(225) 926-5820

CLASSROOM HOURS: 674

COST: $6,000.00 (grants, no-int. loans, payment plan)—day/night

EMPHASIS: relaxation, sports, deep tissue, Eastern/Asian, anatomy, physiology

South Louisiana Institute of Massage
1799 Stumpf Blvd., Bldg. 2, Ste. 1
Gretna, LA 70056
(504) 368-4263   www.therapeuticmassageschool.com

MAINE

Accredited Schools	COMTA	IMSTAC	ABHES	ACCET	ACCSCT
Downeast School of Massage	•				
New Hampshire Institute	•				
Polarity Realization Institute		•			

Downeast School of Massage
P.O. Box 24/99 Moose Meadow Lane
Waldoboro, ME 04572
(207) 832-5531   www.downeastschoolofmassaage.com

CLASSROOM HOURS: 613 (sports)/715 (shiatsu)/607 (body-mind)—day/night; part-time or full-time

EMPHASIS: relaxation, sports, medical, deep tissue, energy, Eastern/Asian, geriatric, pregnancy, reflexology, pediatric massage, Swedish massage

SCHOOL STATEMENT: We train individuals in the art and science of therapeutic massage for an entry-level professional career, for continuing education, and for personal growth.

Fuller Circles School for Therapeutic Massage
5 Kimball St.
Waterville, ME 04901
(207) 877-5650

New Hampshire Institute for Therapeutic Arts, School of Massage
39 Main St.
Bridgton, ME 04009
(207) 647-3794

Poland Spring Health Institute School of Massage & Natural Therapy
32 Summit Spring Rd.
Poland Spring, ME 04274
(207) 998-2894   www.pshi.org

CLASSROOM HOURS: 600

COST: $3,500.00 (payment plan)day program

EMPHASIS: relaxation, hydrotherapy, exercise therapy

SCHOOL STATEMENT: PSHI promotes physical, mental, emotional and spiritual well-being through lifestyle enhancement and education. Our program emphasizes anatomy and physiology, diseases, lifestyle factors and massage techniques.

Polarity Realization Institute—Portland, ME
222 St. Johns St., Ste. 301
Portland, ME 04101
(800) 262-8530   www.holisticcareers.com

Therapeutic Bodywork Learning Center
185 Harlow St., Ste. 2
Bangor, ME 04401
(207) 947-7078

EMPHASIS: relaxation, medical, deep tissue, energy

SCHOOL STATEMENT: Small classes with individual attention. Classes become communities helping each other learn.

Ann Arundel Community College
101 College Pkwy
Arnold, MD 21012
(410) 647-7100   www.aacc.cc.md.us

Baltimore School of Massage
6401 Dogwood Rd.
Baltimore, MD 21207
(410) 944-8855 or (877) 944-8855   www.bsom.com

Community College of Baltimore County
7201 Rossville Blvd
Baltimore, MD 21237
(410) 682-6000   www.ccbc.cc.md.us

CLASSROOM HOURS: 750 (Associate's Degree offered)

COST: $4,500.00 including books and supplies (no-int. loans, payment plan)—day/night/weekend

EMPHASIS: relaxation, sports, medical, deep tissue, energy, Eastern/Asian

SCHOOL STATEMENT: Curriculum is designed to graduate massage therapists who think analytically along with a highly developed client sensitivity in a holistic approach to therapeutic massage.

Garrett County Community College
687 Mosser Rd./P.O. Box 151
McHenry, Maryland 21541
(301) 387-3000   http://garrett.gcc.cc.md.us

Holistic Massage Training Institute
1 E. University Parkway, Ste. 110
Baltimore, MD 21218
(410) 243-4688   www. holisticmassagetraining.org

MARYLAND

Accredited Schools	COMTA	IMSTAC	ABHES	ACCET	ACCSCT
The Baltimore School of Massage	•				•

Schools Offering Associate's Degree

Allegany College of Maryland
Community College of Baltimore County

Allegany College of Maryland, Massage Program
12401 Willowbrook Rd. SE
Cumberland, MD 21502
(301) 784-5191   www.alleganycollege.com

CLASSROOM HOURS: 70 college credits (Associate's degree)

COST: $6,020.00 in-county tuition (scholarships, grants, payment plans)—day program

MASSACHUSETTS

Accredited Schools	COMTA	IMSTAC	ABHES	ACCET	ACCSCT
Bancroft School of Massage					•
Healing Touch Institute		•			
Muscular Therapy Institute				•	
Polarity Realization Institute		•			
Stillpoint Program	•				

Schools Offering Associate's Degree

Springfield Technical Community College

Bancroft School of Massage Therapy
333 Shrewsbury St.
Worcester, MA 01604
(508) 757-7923   www.bancroftsmt.com

CLASSROOM HOURS: 822.5

COST: $13,325.00—day/weekend

EMPHASIS: relaxation, sports, medical, deep tissue, energy, Eastern/Asian, reflexology

SCHOOL STATEMENT: Bancroft prepares students to work professionally in the allied health field of massage therapy. Federal Stafford loans, tuition payment plans, supplemental loans, placement assistance available.

The Central Mass School of Massage and Therapy, Inc.
200 Main St.
Spencer, MA 01562
(800) 766-6572   www.centralmassschool.com

CLASSROOM HOURS: 600

COST: $8,995.00 including books and supplies (grants, no-int. loans, payment plan)—day/night

EMPHASIS: relaxation, sports, medical, deep tissue, Eastern/Asian

SCHOOL STATEMENT: A Medically Oriented program designed for adult learners. Hands-on learning in a friendly family-like environment. Classes meet Monday, Tuesday and Wednesday. Call Today.

DoveStar Institute
120 Court St.
Plymouth, MA 02360
(508) 830-0068   www.dovestar.edu

Healing Touch Institute
37 Water St.
Wakefield, MA 01880
(781) 246-2449

Kripalu Bodywork Certification Training Program
Kripalu Center for Yoga and Health
P.O. Box 793
Lenox, MA 01240
(413) 448-3217   www.kripalu.org

CLASSROOM HOURS: 200/500

COST: $1,290.00/$4,200.00 plus accommodation costs—room and meals are approx. 90% of tuition fee (scholarships available) residential intensives, 10–200 hours of continuing education also offered

EMPHASIS: relaxation, energy, Eastern/Asian, medical

SCHOOL STATEMENT: Kripalu offers a beautiful retreat setting and a transformative lifestyle. Credit considered for 1000 hours of previous professional bodywork experience and bodywork and science courses.

Massage Institute of Cape Cod
www.capecod-massage-school.com
(508) 240-5372 or (508) 247-9412

P.O. Box 2183, 57 Rte. 6
Orleans, MA 02653

461 Main St.
Hyannis, MA 02601

Massage Institute of New England
22 McGrath Hwy., Ste. 11
Somerville, MA 02143
(617) 666-3700   www.mine.baweb.com

Muscular Therapy Institute
122 Rindge Ave.
Cambridge, MA 02140
(617) 576-1300   www. mtinstitute.com

CLASSROOM HOURS: 612/900

COST: $9,300.00/$13,500.00—day program/weekend program/ 1 day + 1 eve. weekly

EMPHASIS: relaxation, sports, medical, deep tissue, energy, muscular therapy

SCHOOL STATEMENT: Accredited school with a national reputation for excellence. Offers a dynamic curriculum and extensive job placement services. Financial aid available for those who qualify.

Palmer Institute of Massage & Bodywork
10 Jefferson Ave.
Salem, MA 01970
(978) 740-0044 or (866) 740-0055
www.palmerinstitute.com

Polarity Realization Institute
www.holisticcareers.com

Administrative offices:

126 High St., Ipswich, MA 01938
(978) 356-0980 or (800) 262-8530

Additional locations:

Plymouth (508) 747-4333
Westboro (508) 836-8864

Solidago School of Massage
10 School St.
Amesbury, MA 01913
(978) 388-8800   www.amesburyctrforhealing.com

Springfield Technical Community College
One Armory Square
Springfield, MA 01105
(413) 755-4885   www.stcc.mass.edu

(Associate's degree offered)

StillPoint Program at
Greenfield Community College
270 Main St., Greenfield, MA 01301
(413) 775-1620   www.gcc.mass.edu

MICHIGAN

Accredited Schools	COMTA	IMSTAC	ABHES	ACCET	ACCSCT
Ann Arbor Institute of Massage Th.	•				•
Carnegie Institute					•
Health Enrichment Center					•
Irene's Myomassology Institute			•		
Kalamazoo Center of Healing Arts		•			
Olympia Career Tr. Inst				•	

Schools Offering Associate's Degree

Kirtland Community College
Oakland Community College

Alternative Healing & State Licensed School
1725 Auburn Rd.
East Rochester Hills, MI 48307
(248) 852-3044

CLASSROOM HOURS: 500

COST: $3,6750.00 (no-int. loans, payment plan)—day/night/weekend electives

EMPHASIS: relaxation, sports, medical, deep tissue, energy, reflexology, Thai, chair, laStone

SCHOOL STATEMENT: We adhere to the highest ethical standards. We offer an accelerated 16-week therapeutic massage and bodywork program. Small classes, personal instruction. Practical, well-rounded education.

Ann Arbor Institute of Massage Therapy
2835 Carpenter Rd.
Ann Arbor, MI 48108
(734) 677-4430   www.aaimt.com

CLASSROOM HOURS: 750

COST: $7,300.00 including books and massage table—day/night/weekend workshops

EMPHASIS: relaxation, sports, medical, deep tissue, Eastern/Asian

SCHOOL STATEMENT: Our program is founded on the most sound and ethical clinical and educational experience required to produce excellence in the field of massage therapy.

Baker College
www.baker.edu

1020 S. Washington, Owosso, MI 48867
(800) 879-3797 or (989) 729-3350

1050 W. Bristol Rd, Flint, MI 48507
(800) 964-4299 or (810) 766-4000

2800 Springport, Jackson, MI 49202
(888) 343-3683 or (517) 788-7800

Blue Heron Academy of Clinical Massage Therapy
2020 Raybrook S.E., Ste. 104
Grand Rapids, MI 49546
(616) 285-9999   www.blueheronacademy.com

Body Wise, Inc.
7125 Ridgewood Rd.
Clarkston, MI 48346
(248) 922-1353

Carnegie Institute
550 Stephenson Hwy., Ste. 100
Troy, MI 48083
(248) 589-1078   www.carnegie-institute.com

Creative Health Arts School of Natural Health
12901 Fort Custer
Galesburg, MI 49053
(616) 665-7797

CLASSROOM HOURS: 561

COST: $5,610.00 (payment plan)—day/night/weekend

EMPHASIS: relaxation, deep tissue, energy, Eastern/Asian

SCHOOL STATEMENT: In a peaceful county setting learn ancient massage arts within wise woman traditions. Innovative, creative and individualized approach. Small classes.

Flint School of Therapeutic Massage
8240 Embury Road
Grand Blanc, MI 48439
(810) 953-4811   www.fstm.com

Health Enrichment Center
204 E Nepessing Street
Lapeer, MI 48446
(810) 667-9453   www.healthenrichment.com

Institute of Natural Therapies
P.O. Box 222
Hancock, MI 49930
(906) 482-2222

CLASSROOM HOURS: 500 (806 total hours)

COST: $5,200.00 includes books and massage table (grants, payment plan)—weekend program

EMPHASIS: medical, Eastern/Asian, multilevel program

SCHOOL STATEMENT: Graduates become innovators and developers of the massage therapy profession as a whole.

Irene's Myomassology Institute
26061 Franklin Rd.
Southfield, MI 48075
(248) 350-1400   www.myomassology.com

CLASSROOM HOURS: 600

COST: $5,896.00 (scholarships, payment plan)—day/night/ electives offered on weekends

EMPHASIS: relaxation, sports, deep tissue, energy, Eastern/Asian, therapeutic and holistic health

SCHOOL STATEMENT: Irene's Myomassology Institute is committed to providing the best therapeutic bodywork and holistic health program, promoting physical, emotional and spiritual health of individuals and society.

Kalamazoo Center for the Healing Arts
4528 West "KL" Ave.
Kalamazoo, MI 49006
(616) 373-0910   www.KCHA.com

CLASSROOM HOURS: 520

COST: $5,440.00 (no-int. loans, payment plan)—day/weekend

EMPHASIS: relaxation, sports, deep tissue, energy, Eastern/ Asian

SCHOOL STATEMENT: Focus is on inner growth as students become practitioners. Instruction is client-centered, and the product of 15 years of running a large professional clinic.

Kirtland Community College
10775 N. St. Helen Rd.
Roscommon, MI 48653
(517) 275-5000   www.kirtland.cc.mi.us

(Associate's Degree offered)

Lakewood School of Therapeutic Massage
1102 6th St.
Port Huron, MI 48060
(810) 987-3959   www.lakewoodschool.com

CLASSROOM HOURS: 500 (800 total hours)

COST: $3,900.00 (scholarships, grants, payment plan)—day/ night

EMPHASIS: relaxation, sports, medical, deep tissue, energy

SCHOOL STATEMENT: We embrace the art and science of massage by integrating relaxation techniques with therapeutic applications while honoring the personal growth process of each student.

Lansing Community College
2100 HHS/P.O. Box 40010
Lansing, MI 48901
(517) 483-1410   www.lcc.edu

CLASSROOM HOURS: 576

COST: $1,800.00 (scholarships, grants, no-int. loans, payment plan)—day/night/weekend

EMPHASIS: relaxation, medical, energy

SCHOOL STATEMENT: Community college located downtown in Michigan's capital city with a satellite campus in Howell.

Marquette School of Therapeutic Massage
125 Washington
Marquette, MI 49855
(906) 225-1700

Michigan Institute of Healing Arts & Sciences
492 Capital Ave. SW
Battle Creek, MI 49015
(616) 660-8515

Michigan Institute of Massage Therapy
3518 Apple Valley Rd.
Okemos, MI 48864
(517) 347-2547

Michigan Institute of Therapeutic Massage
370 Country Club Road
Holland MI 49423
(616) 494-9055
http://school.mlive.com/school/michiganinstitute

Michigan School of Myomassology
3270 Greenfield Rd.
Berkley, MI 48072
(248) 542-7228   www.therapeutic-touch.com/msm

Naturopathic Institute of Therapies and Education
1410 S. Mission St.
Mt. Pleasant, MI 48858
(989) 773-1714

CLASSROOM HOURS: 240 (600 total hours)

COST: $4,995.00 includes books and massage table (no-int. loans, payment plan)—weekend program

EMPHASIS: relaxation, deep tissue, energy, reflexology, cranial sacral, aromatherapy

SCHOOL STATEMENT: A unique massage and naturopathic school offering weekend classes and a 4-year Naturopathic Doctor program and a 2-year Homeopathic program.

Oakland Community College
Highland Lakes Campus
7350 Cooley Lake Rd.
Waterford, MI 48327
(248) 942-3100   www.occ.cc.mi.us

(Certificate or Associates Degree offered)

Olympia Career Training Institute
1750 Woodworth NE
Grand Rapids, MI 49525
(616) 364-8464

Somerset School of Massage Therapy
4290 Miller Rd.
Flint, MI 48507
(810) 230-0353   www.somersetsalon.com

CLASSROOM HOURS: 500

COST: $1,700.00 including manual (payment plan)—day/night

EMPHASIS: relaxation, deep tissue, energy, Eastern/Asian, reflexology, maternity, ethics, hot rock massage, reiki

SCHOOL STATEMENT: Dedicated to total mind and body wellness. Student/teacher ratio 6/1. Features spa techniques for students wishing to work in a spa environment.

Spring Renewal
3493 Washington
Saugatuck, MI 49453
(616) 857-2602   www.springrenewal.com

CLASSROOM HOURS: 600

COST: $4,500.00 (grants, payment plan)—day/night/weekend

EMPHASIS: relaxation, deep tissue, energy

SCHOOL STATEMENT: Fun, professional, comprehensive approach to massage. Experiential in nature.

Stressage Massage Institute
16587 Wyoming
Detroit, MI 48221
(313) 864-8355

Wellspring Institute For Therapeutic Massage and Bodywork
20312 Chalon
St. Clair Shores, MI 48080
(810) 772-8520

CLASSROOM HOURS: up to 1000

COST: 500 hours $4,250.00 (payment plan)—nights, afternoons and weekends

EMPHASIS: relaxation, sports, medical, deep tissue, energy, Eastern/Asian

SCHOOL STATEMENT: The most important factor in choosing a massage school is how your class hours are spent. We feel that hands-on training best prepares you for this work.

MINNESOTA

Accredited Schools	COMTA	IMSTAC	ABHES	ACCET	ACCSCT
High Tech Institute					•
Minneapolis School of Massage		•			•
Sister Rosalind Gefre Schools		•			

Schools Offering Associate's Degree

Minneapolis School of Business—*Brooklyn Ctr.*
Minneapolis School of Business—*Richfield*

CenterPoint
1313 5th Street S.E., Ste. 336
Minneapolis, MN 55414
(612) 617-9090 or (800) 738-0795
www.centerpointmn.com

College of St. Catherine Minneapolis
Massage Education Program
220 Lowery Ave., NE
Minneapolis, MN 55408
(651)-690-7836 or (800) 945-4599
http://paradox.stkate.edu

Globe College
7166 10th St. North
Oakdale, MN 55128
(651) 730-5100   www.globecollege.com

CLASSROOM HOURS: 600—day/night/on-line program

EMPHASIS: relaxation, sports, medical, deep tissue, energy, Eastern/Asian

SCHOOL STATEMENT: Basics of massage and introduction to other styles

Healing Touch Therapeutic Massage School
Office: 20 SW 2nd Ave., S-14, Rochester, MN 55902
Classroom: 41/2 First Ave. SE, Rochester
(507) 287-6162 or (800) 305-6162
http://members.aol.com/HEALTUCH

High Tech Institute
5701 Shingle Creek Pkwy.
Brooklyn Center, MN 55430
(888) 324-9700   www.hightechschools.com

Lake Superior College
2101 Trinity Rd.
Duluth, MN 55811-3399
(800) 432-2884 or (218) 733-7600   www.lsc.cc.mn.us

Minneapolis School of Massage and Bodywork, Inc.
81 Lowry Ave. NE.
Minneapolis, MN 55418
(612) 788-8907   www.mplsschoolofmassage.org

CLASSROOM HOURS: 626

COST: $5,900.00 (scholarships, grants, no-int. loans, payment plan)—day/night

EMPHASIS: relaxation, sports, deep tissue

SCHOOL STATEMENT: MSMB is the oldest and largest school of massage in Minnesota. Institutionally accredited by ACCSCT; program accredited by IMSTAC.

Minnesota School of Business—Brooklyn Ctr
5910 Shingle Creek Pkwy
Brooklyn Ctr, MN 55430
(763) 566-7777   www.globecollege.com

(Associate's Degree offered)

Minnesota School of Business—Richfield
1401 W. 76th St.
Richfield, MN 55423
(612) 861-2000 www.globecollege.com
(Associate's Degree offered)

**Minnesota State College—Southeast
Technical—Red Wing Campus**
308 Pioneer Rd. & Hwy 58
Red Wing, MN 55066
(651) 385-6300 www.southeasttech.mnscu.edu

**Minnesota State College—Southeast
Technical—Winona Campus**
1250 Homer Rd. P.O. Box 409
Winona, MN 55987-0409
(507) 453-2700 www.southeasttech.mnscu.edu

Northern Lights School of Massage Therapy
1313 S.E. Fifth St., Ste. 209
Minneapolis, MN 55414
(800) 738-0795 or (612) 379-3822 www.nlsmt.com

**Northwestern Health Sciences University
Massage Program**
2501 W. 84th St.
Bloomington, MN 55431
(800) 888-4777 or (952) 888-4777 www.nwhealth.edu

**Sister Rosalind Gefre's School of
Professional Massage**
www.sisterrosalind.org

Main Campus: 149 E. Thompson Ave., Ste. 150
West St. Paul, MN. 55118
(651) 554-3010

Additional Locations:

300 Elton Hills Dr., Rochester, MN 55901
(507) 286-8608

165 W. Lind Ct., Mankato, MN 56001
(507) 344-0220

CLASSROOM HOURS: 750

COST: $6,531.00 (no-int. loans, payment plan)—day/night

EMPHASIS: relaxation, sports, medical, deep tissue, energy, Eastern/Asian, spirituality

SCHOOL STATEMENT: The Schools of Massage are based on Christian principles and seek to work in harmony with God's plan for spiritual, psychological and physiological well being.

St. Paul Technical College
235 Marshall Ave.
St. Paul, MN 55102
(651) 846-1314 or (651) 846-1600 www.sptc.mnscu.edu
CLASSROOM HOURS: 600 (30 credits)
COST: $2,600.00 (grants, payment plan)—day program
EMPHASIS: relaxation, sports, medical
SCHOOL STATEMENT: St. Paul Technical College's Massage Therapy Certificate Program meets the minimum requirement of

600 technical hours of study required by the American Massage Therapy Association.

Tao Institute Inc.
919 West St. Germain
St. Cloud, MN 56301
(320) 253-8028 www.taoinstituteinc.com

Touch of Life School of Massage
574 Prairie Center Dr., Ste. 155
Eden Prairie, MN 55344
(952) 996-9655

MISSISSIPPI

Accredited Schools	COMTA	IMSTAC	ABHES	ACCET	ACCSCT
Blue Cliff College					•
Mississippi School of Ther. Massage	•				

Blue Cliff School of Therapeutic Massage
942 E. Beach Dr.
Gulf Coast, MS 39507
(228) 896-9727

Healing Touch School for Massage
4700 Hardy St.
Hattiesburg, MS 39402
(601) 261-0111

Mississippi School of Therapeutic Massage
5120 Galaxie Dr.
Jackson, MS 39206
(601) 362-3624 or (888) 284-3054

**The Natural Healing Arts School of
Massage Therapy**
1303 Sunset Dr., Ste. B
Grenada, MS 38901
(662) 229-0010 www.web-sarasota.com/nhasmt
CLASSROOM HOURS: 700
COST: $4,900.00 (grants, no-int. loans, payment plan)—night program
EMPHASIS: relaxation, sports, medical, deep tissue, energy, Eastern/Asian
SCHOOL STATEMENT: School founded in Sarasota, FL in 1978. There are three schools in Mississippi. Grenada Campus, Tupelo Campus, Southaven (Memphis) Campus. Main phone (662) 229-0010.

Wellness Therapies Massage School
330 Kerr St.
Long Beach, MS 39560
(877) 544-6677 www.WellnessTherapies.org

CLASSROOM HOURS: 700

COST: $4,500.00 (scholarships, grants, payment plan)—day program

EMPHASIS: relaxation, sports, medical

SCHOOL STATEMENT: A Non-Profit Christian Massage School focused on providing healthcare in the spirit of love.

MISSOURI

Accredited Schools	COMTA	IMSTAC	ABHES	ACCET	ACCSCT
Allied Medical College			•		
Massage Therapy Training Institute		•			
Midwest Inst. for Medical Assistants			•		
Missouri College					•
Professional Massage Training Center					•
St. Louis College of Health Careers			•		

A Gathering Place—Wellness Education Center
3391 N. Hwy. 67
Florissant, MO 63033
(314) 831-4558

CLASSROOM HOURS: 520

COST: $5,000.00 (payment plan)—day/night

EMPHASIS: relaxation, sports, medical, deep tissue, energy, Eastern/Asian

SCHOOL STATEMENT: State-approved; Nationally Certified Category "A" CEUs; Class sizes create a family-like atmosphere; Students learn bodywork for the mind-body-soul in our 520-hour program.

Allied Medical College
500 Northwest Plaza Tower, Ste. 400
St. Louis, MO 63074
(314) 739-4450   www.alliedmedicalcollege.com

Healing Arts Center
7405 Manchester Rd. Ste. 120
St. Louis, MO 63143
(314) 647-8080

Kaleidoscope School of Massage
7645 Delmar Blvd.
St. Louis, MO 63130
(314) 862-7442

Massage Therapy Institute of Missouri
5 South Ninth St., Ste. 205
Columbia, MO 65201
(573) 875-7905

Massage Therapy Training Institute
9140 Ward Parkway, Ste. 100
Kansas City, MO 64114
(816) 523-9140   www.mtti.net

CLASSROOM HOURS: 500 (massage)/250 (wellness consultant)/300 (energy therapy)

COST: $6,195.00/$3,095.00/$4,295.00 (payment plan)—day/night/weekend

EMPHASIS: relaxation, sports, medical, deep tissue, energy, Eastern/Asian, wellness

SCHOOL STATEMENT: Since 1988, MTTI has led the way in bodywork and wellness careers, locally and nationally. MTTI is dedicated to creating a better world through wellness education.

The Midwest Institute of Bodywork & Somatic Therapy
5518 N. Antioch Rd.
Kansas City, MO 64119
(816) 453-3577   www.body-somatics.com

CLASSROOM HOURS: 558 (1058 total hours)

COST: $8,445.00 (payment plan)—night/weekend

EMPHASIS: sports, medical, deep tissue, energy, Eastern/Asian

SCHOOL STATEMENT: Our programs are designed to embrace wholeness through integration of body, mind, spirit and the perception of health as a balance among the three.

Midwest Institute for Medical Assistants
4260 Shoreline Dr., Ste. 100
Earth City, MO 63045
(314) 965-8363

Missouri College
10121 Manchester Rd.
St. Louis, MO 63122
(314) 821-7700 or (800) 216-6732
www.missouricollege.com

Professional Massage Training Center
229 E. Commercial
Springfield, MO 65803
(417) 863-7682   www.skilledtouch.com

CLASSROOM HOURS: 600

COST: $6,500.00 (no-int. loans, payment plan)—day/night/weekend

SCHOOL STATEMENT: PMTC is an accredited massage program that emphasizes wellness massage as well as giving students experience in hospital settings.

School of Massage Arts
3322 S. Campbell, Ste. A
Springfield, MO 65807
(888) 886-0256 or (417) 886-0256

St. Charles School of Massage Therapy
2440 Executive Dr., Ste. 100
St. Charles, MO 63303
(636) 498-0777   www.spastcharles.com

CLASSROOM HOURS: 600

COST: $5,600.00 (payment plan)—day/night

EMPHASIS: relaxation, sports, deep tissue, energy, Eastern/Asian

SCHOOL STATEMENT: Our school is committed to providing an environment conducive to learning and skill building and achieving excellence in instruction and practice.

St. Louis College of Health Careers
www.stlouiscollege.com

4044 Butler Hill Rd., St. Louis, MO 63129
(314) 845-6100

4484 West Pine Blvd., St. Louis, MO 63108
(314) 652-0300

Wholistic Life Center School of Massage
Rt. 1, Box 1783
Washburn, MO 65772
(417) 435-2216   www.wholisticlifecenter.org

CLASSROOM HOURS: 600

COST: $3,750.00 (scholarships, payment plan)—day program

EMPHASIS: relaxation, sports, medical, energy, Eastern/Asian

SCHOOL STATEMENT: Health reflects a balance of mind, body, spirit and emotions. These four parts are nurtured for the individual to become a healer. Residence program offered.

MONTANA

Asten Center for Natural Therapeutics
121 W. Legion
Whitehall, MT 59759
(406) 287-5670   www.astencenter.com

Big Sky Somatic Institute
1802 11th Ave., Ste. A
Helena, MT 59601
(406) 442-8998 or (866) 442-8273
www.bigskysomatic.com

Health Works Institute
111 South Grand, Annex 3
Bozeman, MT 59715
(406) 582-1555   www.healthworksinstitute.com

CLASSROOM HOURS: 775

COST: $7,750.00 (payment plan)—day/weekend/summer programs

EMPHASIS: relaxation, sports, medical, deep tissue, energy, Eastern/Asian, neuromuscular, myofascial, mind/body

SCHOOL STATEMENT: Health Works Institute enhances the physical and spiritual health of individuals and society, by providing experiential learning programs that foster personal and professional development.

Montana School of Massage
1220 W. Broadway
Missoula, MT 59802
(406) 549-9244   www.montanamassage.com

Rocky Mountain School of Masage
1509 13th St. West
Billings, MT 59102
(406) 652-2633

School of Good Medicine Massage
404 E. 1st Ste. C
Whitefish, MT 59937
(406) 862-3603

Serenity Center
P.O. Box 4822
Whitefish, MT 59937
(888) 487-4453 or (406) 862-3808

NEBRASKA

Accredited Schools	COMTA	IMSTAC	ABHES	ACCET	ACCSCT
Myotherapy Institute					•
Omaha School of Massage Therapy					•

Gateway College of Massage Therapy
2607 Dakota Ave.
South Sioux City, NE 68776
(402) 494-8390

Midwest School of Massage
10159 J St.
Omaha, NE 68127
(402) 331-8383

Myotherapy Institute
6020 South 58th St., Bldgs. A, B and C
Lincoln, NE 68516
(402) 421-7410

Omaha School of Massage Therapy
9748 Park Dr.
Omaha, NE 68127
(402) 331-3694   www.osmt.com

CLASSROOM HOURS: 1000

COST: $7,925.00 including books and massage table (grants, payment plan)—day/night

EMPHASIS: relaxation, Eastern/Asian

SCHOOL STATEMENT: Our focus is to teach and encourage natural and holistic health through massage and bodywork along with complementary alternative therapies.

Universal College of Healing Arts
Non-Profit School of Massage Therapy
4922 Dodge St.
Omaha, NE 68132
(402) 556-4456   www.UCHA.com

CLASSROOM HOURS: 500–1000

COST: $7,650.00 (scholarships, payment plan)—day/night/weekend

EMPHASIS: relaxation, sports, medical, deep tissue, energy, Eastern/Asian

SCHOOL STATEMENT: Descriptions by our graduates: "Caring", "Holistic", "small and respectful classes", "Effective massage routine", "reviewed a variety of modalities", "solid preparation for nationals and state boards".

NEVADA

Accredited Schools	COMTA	IMSTAC	ABHES	ACCET	ACCSCT
Acad. of Medical & Business Careers					•
Dahan Institute of Massage Studies					•
Nevada School of Massage Therapy	•				•

Academy of Medical and Business Careers
901 Rancho Lane, Ste. 190
Las Vegas, NV 89106
(800) 684-6301   www.AcademyLV.com

Baum Healing Arts Center
1800 Hwy. 50 E., Ste. 14
Carson City, NV 89701
(775) 884-1145

CLASSROOM HOURS: 600

COST: $6,000.00 including books and supplies (payment plan)—day/night/weekend

EMPHASIS: relaxation, sports, medical, deep tissue, energy, Eastern/Asian

SCHOOL STATEMENT: We provide comprehensive programs in massage therapy for beginners and licensed therapists seeking continuing education. We are licensed by the Commission on Postsecondary Education.

Community College of Southern Nevada
6375 W. Charleston Blvd., #W 1-A
Las Vegas, NV 89146
(702) 651-5690 or (702) 651-5015   www.ccsn.nevada.edu

Dahan Institute of Massage Studies
(702) 434-1338   www.dahanmassage.com

3320 East Flamingo Rd. Ste. Ste. 32
Las Vegas, NV 89121

2911 N. Tenaya Way Ste. 205
Las Vegas, NV, 89128

Nevada Career Institute
3025 E. Desert Inn Rd., Ste. 11
Las Vegas, NV 89121
(702) 893-3300

Nevada School of Massage Therapy
2381 E. Windmill Lane
Las Vegas, NV 89123
(702) 456-4325 or (800) 750-HEAL   www.nevadasmt.com

Northwest Health Careers
2701 N. Tenaya Way, Ste. 120
Las Vegas, NV 89128
(702) 254-7577   www.nwhealthcareers.com

CLASSROOM HOURS: 550

COST: $5,720.00 including books and uniforms (payment plan)—day/night

EMPHASIS: relaxation, sports, deep tissue

SCHOOL STATEMENT: NW Health Careers is proud to announce the addition of their Module System Advanced Massage Program. This program will allow for more diversity in student scheduling.

Ralston School of Massage
at Washoe Medical Center, 77 Pringle Way
Reno, NV 89502
(775) 982-5450   www.ralstonmassage.com

CLASSROOM HOURS: 560 (total hours 710)

COST: $3,495.00 (payment plan)—day/night

EMPHASIS: relaxation, sports, medical

SCHOOL STATEMENT: Located inside a major medical hospital working with staff and patients in addition to local university athletes—offers our students a uniquely progressive massage education.

Truckee Meadows Community College
7000 Dandini Blvd.
Reno, NV 89512
(775) 829-9010   www.tmcc.edu

NEW HAMPSHIRE

Accredited Schools	COMTA	IMSTAC	ABHES	ACCET	ACCSCT
New Hampshire Inst. for Ther. Massage	•				

DoveStar Institute
50 Whitehall Road
Hooksett, NH 03106
(603) 669-9497 or (888) 222-5603   www.dovestar.edu

New England Academy of Therapeutic Sciences
127 Goldmine Rd.
Peterborough, NH USA 03458
(603) 563-7760   www.neats.com

New Hampshire Community Technical College
www.nhctcs.tec.nh.us

505 Amherst St., Nashua, NH 03061
(603) 882-7022   www.nashua.tec.nh.us

One College Drive, Claremont, NH 03743
(603) 542-7744   www.claremont.tec.nh.us

New Hampshire Institute for Therapeutic Arts
153 Lowell Rd.
Hudson, NH 03051
(603) 882-3022

North Eastern Institute of Whole Health
22 Bridge St.
Manchester, NH 03101
(603) 623-5018

CLASSROOM HOURS: 750

COST: $6,500.00 (payment plan)—day/night/weekend

EMPHASIS: relaxation, sports, medical, deep tissue, energy, Eastern/Asian

SCHOOL STATEMENT: Eastern and Western techniques, day, evening, Saturday programs. Spring and Fall enrollment. 60 Elective hours. NH Postsecondary Education Commission approved. NCBTMB and ABMP accredited.

NEW JERSEY

Accredited Schools

Accredited Schools	COMTA	IMSTAC	ABHES	ACCET	ACCSCT
Academy of Massage Therapy	•				•
Healing Hands Institute	•				
Helma Institute of Massage Therapy					•
Institute for Health Education					•
Institute for Therapeutic Massage	•				•
Philadelphia School of Massage	•				
Somerset School of Massage	•			•	

Schools Offering Associate's Degree

Lourdes Institute of Wholistic Studies

Academy of Massage Therapy
401 South Van Brunt St.
Englewood, NJ 07631
(888) AMT-7898   www.academyofmassage.com

CLASSROOM HOURS: 500-1062

COST: $5,400.00–$12,000.00 (grants, no-int. loans, payment plan)—day/night/weekend

EMPHASIS: relaxation, sports, medical, deep tissue, energy, Eastern/Asian, spa

SCHOOL STATEMENT: Financial aid to those who qualify. Accredited by COMTA and ACCSCT.

Academy of Natural Health Sciences
102 Green St.
Woodbridge, NJ 07095
(732) 634-2155

Academy of Therapeutic Massage & Healing Arts
206 N. High St.
Millville, NJ 08332
(856) 327-7797

American Institute of Alternative Medicine
105 Old Matawan Rd., Ste. 2C
Old Bridge, NJ 08857
(732) 651-6060

Atlantic County Healing Arts Institute
800 Route 50, Ste. 2F
Mays Landing, NJ 08330
(609) 625-7500 or (866) LEARN-MT
www.achaimassage.com

CLASSROOM HOURS: 500   day/night/weekend

Bergen Healing Arts Institute for Massage
207 Kinderkamack Rd.
Emerson, NJ 07630
(201) 967-7833

bodyConcepts Wellness Institute
196 Paterson Ave., 2nd Floor
East Rutherford, NJ 07073
(201) 635-1099   www.bcwellness.com

Body, Mind & Spirit Learning Alliance
917-2 N. Main St. (166)
Toms River, NJ 08753
(732) 349-7153   www.bmslearning.com

CLASSROOM HOURS: 550

COST: $4,800.00 (payment plan)—day/night

EMPHASIS: relaxation, sports, medical, deep tissue, energy, Eastern/Asian

SCHOOL STATEMENT: Our holistic program includes a wide variety of bodywork styles, personal development, and professionalism, providing graduates with the skills for success in this exciting field.

Center for Therapeutic Massage, Inc.
963 Holmdel Rd.
Holmdel, NJ 07733
(732) 332-0333

CLASSROOM HOURS: 550

COST: $5,500.00 (no-int. loans, payment plan)—day/night

EMPHASIS: sports, medical, deep tissue

SCHOOL STATEMENT: Small classes—student teacher ratio 3:1. Gaining the reputation "Marine Corps of Massage Training". Devoted, outstanding instructors who are the best at what they do.

Dahn Healing and Massage Institute, Inc.
111 Homans Ave.
Closter, NJ 07624
(201) 784-0820

The Essex Group Institute for Massage and Bodywork
21 Grove Avenue
Verona, NJ 07044
(973) 571-9801   www.egimassage.com

CLASSROOM HOURS: 420 (550 total hours)

COST: $5,900.00 (payment plan)—night program

EMPHASIS: relaxation, deep tissue

Gentle Healing School of Massage
1274 Cranbury/South River Road
Cranbury, NJ 08512
(609) 409-2700
www.gentlehealingspa.com/GH/School.htm

Gloucester County College
Lifelong Learning Center
1400 Tanyard Rd.
Sewell, NJ 08080
(856) 468-5000   www.gccnj.edu

Healing Hands Institute for Massage Therapy
41 Bergenline Ave.
Westwood, NJ 07675
(201) 722-0099   www.healinghandsinstitute.com

Healing Hands School of Massage
515 White Horse Pike
Haddon Heights, NJ 08035
(856) 546-7471 or (215) 676-9891
www.webhostcorp.com/members/healinghands

Health Choices Holistic Massage School
170 Township Line Rd.
Hillsborough, NJ 08844
(908) 359-3995   www.health-choices.com

Helma Institute of Massage Therapy
101 Rt. 46 West
Saddle Brook, NJ 07663
(201) 226-0056   www.Helma.com

CLASSROOM HOURS: 550—day/night

EMPHASIS: Swedish, sports, medical, Eastern/Asian, reflexology, lymph drainage

SCHOOL STATEMENT: Formed in 1981, Helma offers years of experience and dedication. The school is committed to continuous renewal, and offers an advanced continuing education program.

The Institute for Health Education
7 Spielman Road
Fairfield, NJ 07004
(973) 808-1666   www.healthed-nj.com

CLASSROOM HOURS: 629

COST: $5,300.00 including books and supplies (scholarships, payment plan)—day/night

EMPHASIS: relaxation, sports, medical, deep tissue, energy, Eastern/Asian

SCHOOL STATEMENT: The Institute is committed to providing programs the will serve to enhance your professionalism and skill level to help serve your clients better.

Institute for Therapeutic Massage
www.massageprogram.com

125 Wanaque Ave.
Pompton Lakes, NJ 07442
(973) 839-6131

1 Sheila Dr.
Tinton Falls, NJ 07724
(732) 936-9111

Campus at UMDNJ
150 Bergen St., E-325
Newark, NJ 07103
(973) 839-6131

JSG School of Massage Therapy, Inc.
676 Winters Ave.
Paramus, NJ 07652
(201) 394-9200   www.Jsgmassage.org

CLASSROOM HOURS: unspecified; total hours 550

COST: $5,900.00 includes all supplies except table (no-int. loans, payment plan)—night program with weekends

EMPHASIS: relaxation, sports, medical, Eastern/Asian, prenatal, geriatric, chair

SCHOOL STATEMENT: "Small and personal", maximum 10 students. Comprehensive curriculum, extensive audio-visual aids and extern practicum and volunteer hours. Meets NCTMB requirements, AMTA approved massage school.

Lourdes Institute of Wholistic Studies
900 Haddon Ave., Ste. 100
Collingswood, NJ 08108
(856) 869-3134   www.lourdeswellnesscenter.org

CLASSROOM HOURS: 650 (700 total hours)

COST: $5,400.00 (scholarships, grants, no-int. loans, payment plan)—day/night/weekend

EMPHASIS: relaxation, deep tissue, Eastern/Asian, myofascial release, reflexology, shiatsu

SCHOOL STATEMENT: Together, Lourdes Institute and Camden County College offer an Associates Degree and Certification in Massage Therapy. Also offered: Certifications in shiatsu, reflexology, yoga teacher training.

Morris Institute of Natural Therapeutics
3108 Route 10 West, Mareen Building
Denville, NJ 07834
(973) 989-8939

North Jersey Massage Training Center
Parsippany Medical Complex
3699 Route 46
Parsippany, NJ 07054
(973) 263-2229   www.newjerseymassage.com

Omega Institute
7050 Route 38 East
Pennsauken, NJ 08109
(856) 663-4299   www.omegacareers.com

CLASSROOM HOURS: 600

COST: $6,710.00 including books and supplies (scholarships, grants, payment plan)—day/night

EMPHASIS: relaxation, sports, medical

SCHOOL STATEMENT: Coursework is geared to prepare the learner for a career in massage. Introductory courses in popular modalities are included in the curriculum.

Onyx Massage Institute
25 Broad Ave., 2nd Floor
Palisades Park, NJ 07650
(201) 943-7211

Philadelphia School of Massage Therapy
(856) 227-8363   www.healinghands.net:

108-L Greentree Road
Turnersville, NJ 08012

6712 Washington Avenue, Ste. 309
Egg Harbor, NJ 08234

Rizzieri Institute for Healing Arts
3001C West Lincoln Dr.
Marlton, NJ 08053
(856) 988-8600 ext. 207   www.Rizzieri.com

CLASSROOM HOURS: 670 full-time/600 part-time

COST: $5,900.00 full-time/$5,400.00 part-time (scholarships, payment plan)—full-time days/part-time nights and weekends

EMPHASIS: relaxation, sports, deep tissue, energy

SCHOOL STATEMENT: Rizzieri Institute for Healing Arts offers programs in massage therapy, shiatsu and yoga teacher training. Continuing education classes are also available.

Seashore Healing Arts Center
505 New Road, Ste. 7
Somers Point, NJ 08244
(609) 601-9272   www.seashorehealingartscenter.com

Somerset School of Massage Therapy
www.ssmt.org

7 Cedar Grove Lane, Somerset, NJ 08873
(732) 356-0787

1985 Highway 34, Wall Township, NJ 07719
(732) 282-0100

CLASSROOM HOURS: 550

COST: $5,700.00 (no-int. loans, payment plan)—day/night

EMPHASIS: relaxation, sports, medical, deep tissue

SCHOOL STATEMENT: SSMT is the largest and most credentialed school of massage in NJ. Flexible and convenient hours; approved for Title IV federal funds and student loans.

South Jersey School of Muscle Therapy
1400 Chews Landing Rd.
Laurel Springs, NJ 08021
(856) 227-8090

Therapeutic Massage Training Center
560 Springfield Ave.
Westfield, NJ 07090
(908) 789-2288   www.MassageTrainingCenter.com

CLASSROOM HOURS: 512

COST: $4,500.00 including books—night/weekend

EMPHASIS: relaxation, medical, deep tissue, energy, Eastern/ Asian

SCHOOL STATEMENT: Small classes, personalized, attentive training. Since 1988, T.M.T.C. has trained students in the art of massage/ bodywork as well as the profession.

Tighina Institute
99 Montgomery St., Jersey City, NJ 07302
P.O. Box 3582, Jersey City, NJ 07303
(201) 434-3544

CLASSROOM HOURS: 550 (NJ)/1056 (NY)/500 (advanced)— morning/afternoon/evening

EMPHASIS: relaxation, sports, medical, deep tissue, Eastern/ Asian, reflexology, hot stone massage

SCHOOL STATEMENT: Tighina Institute offers three complete curriculums: New Jersey State Program of Education; New York State program of Education; Additional education for NJ State program graduates.

Warren County Community College (CCPD)
475 Route 57 West
Washington, NJ 07882
(908) 689-7613

NEW MEXICO

Accredited Schools	COMTA	IMSTAC	ABHES	ACCET	ACCSCT
New Mexico Sch. of Nat. Therapeutics		•			
Southwest Health Career Inst., the			•		
Universal Therapeutic Massage Inst.					•

Schools Offering Associate's Degree

The Medicine Wheel

Body Dynamics School of Massage Therapy
3901 Georgia, NE Ste. B-4
Albuquerque, NM 87110
(505) 881-1314

Crystal Mountain Massage Therapy School & Clinic
4125 Carlisle NE
Albuquerque, NM 87107
(505) 872-2030

CLASSROOM HOURS: 550 (700 total hours)—day/night

EMPHASIS: sports, deep tissue, energy, hospital rehab. patient internship

SCHOOL STATEMENT: We cultivate each student's ability to provide a magnificent massage by teaching excellence in essentials, like compassion and ethics, as well as fabulous massage techniques.

Eastern New Mexico School of Massage Therapy
PO Box 2142
Clovis, NM 80102
(505) 763-0551

Massage Therapy Training Institute
2701 Picacho Plaza, Ste. 4
Las Crusas, NM 88005
(505) 523-6811   www.zianet.com/mmti

The Medicine Wheel—A School of Holistic Therapies
1243 West Apache
Farmington, NM 87401
(505) 322-1914   www.medicinewheelonline.com

CLASSROOM HOURS: 750/840/1200 (Associate's degree)

COST: $7,500.00/$8,310.00/$12,675.00 (grants, payment plan)—day program

EMPHASIS: medical, energy, Eastern/Asian

SCHOOL STATEMENT: Our accredited programs are designed for the serious student of medical/therapeutic massage and Chinese medicine. Includes classes in nutrition, herbology and mind-body connection.

Mesilla Valley School of Therapeutic Arts
P.O. Box 1277
Mesilla, NM 88046
(505) 527-1239   www.massagetherapyschoolsnm.com

CLASSROOM HOURS: 700

COST: $3,700.00 (payment plan)—day/night/weekend

EMPHASIS: relaxation, sports, medical, deep tissue, energy, Eastern/Asian, special populations, MFR, NMT, lymphatic, therEx, reflexology

SCHOOL STATEMENT: MVSTA, open for 15 years, offers quality, holistic education. Comprehensive teaching methods emphasize relaxation, repetition and "circular learning" to enhance information retention.

Muscle Therapy Center
1711 N. Jefferson St.
Hobbs, NM 88240
(505) 393-3425

New Mexico Academy of Healing Arts
P.O. Box 932
Santa Fe, NM 87504
(505) 982-6271 or (888) 808-5188
www.nmhealingarts.org

New Mexico College of Natural Healing
310 W. 6th St.
Silver City, NM 88062
(505) 538-0050 or (888) 813-8311
www.newmexicohealing.com

CLASSROOM HOURS: 800

COST: $5,900.00 (scholarships, payment plan)

EMPHASIS: deep tissue, energy, structural integration

New Mexico School of Natural Therapeutics
202 Morningside SE
Albuquerque, NM 87108
(505) 268-6870   www.nmsnt.org

CLASSROOM HOURS: 750

COST: $4,800.00 (scholarships, payment plan)—day/night

EMPHASIS: Swedish massage, polarity therapy

SCHOOL STATEMENT: Our goal is to graduate highly skilled holistic practitioners dedicated to helping others and themselves experience increased physical, mental and emotional health and well-being.

Northern New Mexico Comm. Coll.
921 Paseo de Onate
Espanola, NM 87532
(505) 747-2100   www.nnm.cc.nm.us

Scherer Institute of Natural Healing
1091-A Siler Rd./P.O. Box 5737
Santa Fe, NM 87502
(505) 982-8398   www.schererinstitute.com

Southwest Health Career Institute
5981 Jefferson Rd NE, Ste A
Albuquerque, NM 87109
(505) 345-6800   www.swhci.com

Taos School of Massage
7418 NDCBU
Taos, NM 87571
(505) 758-2725

CLASSROOM HOURS: 650

COST: $4,400.00 (payment plan)—day program

EMPHASIS: relaxation, sports, deep tissue, energy, Eastern/Asian

SCHOOL STATEMENT: This school specializes in BodyMind Clearing, a unique synthesis of deep tissue, applied kinesiology and body-centered facilitation skills within the self-expression model of healing.

Universal Therapeutic Massage Institute, Inc.
3410 Aztec Rd. NE
Albuquerque, NM 87107
(800) 557-0020 or (505) 888-0020

White Mountain School of Applied Healing
1204 Mechem Ste. 10
Ruidoso, NM 88345
(505) 258-3046

CLASSROOM HOURS: 655

COST: $4,480.00 including books and supplies (payment plan)—weekend program

EMPHASIS: relaxation, sports, medical, deep tissue, energy, Eastern/Asian

SCHOOL STATEMENT: Dedicated to providing comprehensive instruction in massage therapy and physical wellness to provide Southern New Mexico with successful, highly-skilled and qualified professional massage therapists.

NEW YORK

Accredited Schools	COMTA	IMSTAC	ABHES	ACCET	ACCSCT
New York Institute of Massage					•
Swedish Institute					•

Schools Offering Associate's Degree

Finger Lakes Community College
Orange County Community College
Rockland Community College
Swedish Institute
Trocaire College

Center for Natural Wellness
School of Massage Therapy
62 Washington St.
Rensselaer, NY 12144
(518) 449-2737   www.cnwsmt.com

CLASSROOM HOURS: 1020

COST: $9,300.00 (payment plan)—day (full-time)/nights plus 1 Saturday per month (part-time)

EMPHASIS: relaxation, sports, medical, deep tissue, energy, Eastern/Asian, NYS exam preparation

Columbia-Greene Community College
4400 Rt. 23
Hudson, NY 12534
(518) 828-4181   www.sunycgcc.edu

Finger Lakes Community College
4355 Lakeshore Drive
Canandaigua, NY 14424
(716) 394-3500   www.fingerlakes.edu

CLASSROOM HOURS: 64 credit hours (Associate's degree)

COST: $5,000.00 including books and supplies (scholarships)—day/night

EMPHASIS: relaxation, sports, medical, deep tissue, energy, Eastern/Asian, yoga, tai chi, oriental healing arts

SCHOOL STATEMENT: Program develops skills necessary for the practice of massage therapy while preparing students in the life sciences and alternative therapies along with general education courses.

Finger Lakes School of Massage
1251 Trumansburg Rd.
Ithaca, NY 14850
(607) 272-9024

CLASSROOM HOURS: 1000

COST: $10,100.00 (scholarships, payment plans)—6 month day program/6-weekend aromatherapy program

EMPHASIS: relaxation, sports, medical, deep tissue, energy, Eastern/Asian, aromatherapy

SCHOOL STATEMENT: Our intensive program emphasizes professional development and the integration of body, mind and spirit—in an atmosphere of respect and compassion. "A Journey Worth Taking"

Hudson Valley School of Massage Therapy
7-9 Cummings Ln., Ste. A
Highland, NY 12528
(845) 691-2547   www.hvsmassagetherapy.com

New York College for Wholistic Health
Education & Research
6801 Jericho Turnpike
Syosset, NY 11791
(800) 922-7337   www.nycollege.edu

New York Institute of Massage
4701 Transit Rd./PO Box 645
Buffalo, NY 14231
(716) 633-0355   www.nyinstituteofmassage.com

North Country Community College
20 Winona Ave., P.O. Box 89
Saranac Lake, NY 12983
(888) 879-6222 or (518) 891-2915   www.nccc.edu

Onondaga School of Therapeutic Massage
302 N. Goodman St., Ste. 200
Rochester, NY 14607
(716) 241-0070   www.massage-school.com

CLASSROOM HOURS: 1000

COST: $9,800.00 (grants, payment plan)–day/night

EMPHASIS: relaxation, medical

SCHOOL STATEMENT: To provide training in the science of massage with the intent of graduating exceptionally trained, high quality massage therapists.

Onondaga School of Therapeutic Massage
220 Walton St.
Syracuse, NY 13202
(315) 424-1159   www.massage-school.com

CLASSROOM HOURS: 1000

COST: $9,800.00 (grants, payment plan)–day/night

EMPHASIS: relaxation, medical

SCHOOL STATEMENT: To provide training in the science of massage with the intent of graduating exceptionally trained, high quality massage therapists.

Orange County Community College
115 South St.
Middletown, NY 10940
(845) 341-4291   www.sunyorange.edu
(Associate's degree offered)

Rockland Community College
145 College Rd.
Suffern, NY 10901
(845) 574-4000   www.sunyrockland.edu
(Associate's Degree offered)

Swedish Institute
226 West 26th St., 5th floor
New York, NY 10001
(212) 924-5900, ext. 0   www.swedishinstitute.com

CLASSROOM HOURS: 1226 (Associate's degree)

COST: $15,990.00 (scholarships, grants, payment plan)–day/night/weekend

EMPHASIS: relaxation, sports, medical, deep tissue, energy, Eastern/Asian, anatomy/physiology, neurology, pathology.

SCHOOL STATEMENT: In-depth training in Western and Eastern massage offering the knowledge, hands-on techniques, assessment tools, communication skills and clinical experience necessary for developing a satisfying career.

Trocaire College
360 Choate Avenue
Buffalo, NY 12422
(716) 826-1200   www.trocaire.edu

CLASSROOM HOURS: 1073 (Associate's degree)

COST: $20,000.00 (approx.) including books and supplies (scholarships, grants)–day/night

EMPHASIS: medical with holistic perspective, energy, Eastern/Asian, relaxation, wellness massage

SCHOOL STATEMENT: Trocaire College is a Mercy institution where knowledge and caring come together

NORTH CAROLINA

Accredited Schools	COMTA	IMSTAC	ABHES	ACCET	ACCSCT
Body Therapy Institute	•				
Medical Arts Massage School				•	
Southeastern Sch. of Neuromuscular					•

Schools Offering Associate's Degree

Carteret Community College
Lenoir Community College
Sand Hills Community College

Blue Ridge Healing Arts Academy
175 Furr Ave., NW
Concord, NC 28777
(704) 795-7478   www.blueridgemassage.com

Body Therapy Institute
300 South Wind Road
Siler City, NC 27344
(888) 500-4500   www.massage.net

CLASSROOM HOURS: 650

COST: $8,500.00 (payment plan)–day/night

EMPHASIS: relaxation, deep tissue, energy

SCHOOL STATEMENT: BTI offers an integrative approach to massage and bodywork therapy in a spectacular natural environment for learning and healing.

Caldwell Community College
2855 Hickory Blvd.
Hudson, NC 28638
(882) 726-2200

Carteret Community College
3505 Arendell St.
Morehead City, NC 28557
(252) 222-6000   http://gofish.carteret.cc.nc.us
(Associate's degree offered)

Center for Massage and Natural Health
2 Eagle Street, PO Box 888
Asheville, NC 28802
(828) 252-0058   www.centerformassage.com

Coastal Carolina Institute
2520 Independence Blvd.
Wilmington, NC 28412
(910) 792-0844

Edmund Morgan School of Neuromuscular & Massage Therapy
20605 N. Main St.
Cornelius, NC 28031
(704) 896-3656   www.edmundcenter.com

Forsyth Technical Community College
2100 Silas Creek Pkwy.
Winston-Salem, NC 27103
(336) 723-0371   www.forsyth.tec.nc.us

CLASSROOM HOURS: 660 hours plus 15 college credits

COST: $1,350.00 (grants)—day/night

EMPHASIS: relaxation, sports, medical, NMT

SCHOOL STATEMENT: FTCC focuses on outcome-based massage. The students graduate with good education in massage and bodywork. FTCC has a 92% pass rate with NCB exam.

Gloria's Asthenic Therapy School
1309 Morganton Rd.
Fayetteville, NC 28305
(910) 484-6827   www.myncmassageschool.com

CLASSROOM HOURS: 500

COST: $4,000.00 (payment plan)—day/night

EMPHASIS: relaxation, sports, medical, deep tissue, energy, Eastern/Asian

SCHOOL STATEMENT: Our school provides students with an environment where sharing of ideas, acceptance of different personalities, respect for others, individual ideas and beliefs are granted.

Guilford Technical Community College
901 S. Main St.
High Point, NC 27260
(336) 454-1126, ext. 4133   http://technet.gtcc.cc.nc.us

Lenoir Community College
231 Highway 58 South/P.O. Box 188
Kinston, NC 28502
(252) 527-6223   www.lenoir.cc.nc.us

diploma and associates degree programs

evenings & weekends

EMPHASIS: relaxation, medical, deep tissue

Medical Arts Massage School
6541 Meriden Dr.
Raleigh, NC 27616
(919) 872-6386

Miller-Motte Technical College
606 S. College Rd.
Wilmington, NC 28403
(800) 784-2110   www.miller-motte.com

Natural Touch School of Massage Therapy
Greensboro, NC 27407
(336) 808-0178   www.NaturalTouchSchool.com

CLASSROOM HOURS: 500

COST: $4,500.00 (payment plan)—day/night

EMPHASIS: Relaxation, deep tissue, energy

SCHOOL STATEMENT: Our goal is to awaken each person so they might reach out into the world and aid others in the return to wholeness and wellness.

North Carolina School of Natural Healing
20 Battery Park Ave., Room 510
Asheville, NC 28801
(828) 252-7096   www.higherself.com

CLASSROOM HOURS: 625

COST: $5,200.00 (payment plan)—night/weekend

EMPHASIS: relaxation, deep tissue, energy, Eastern/Asian

SCHOOL STATEMENT: Professional training with a focus on spirit, meditation and the heart. Grounded, sound technical training emphasizing awareness, sensitivity and tools for success.

The North Carolina School of the Healing Arts
400 Oberlin Rd., Ste. 140
Raleigh, NC 27605
(919) 821-1444   www.healthecology.com

CLASSROOM HOURS: 560

COST: $8,300.00 (payment plan)—day/weekend

EMPHASIS: relaxation, energy, Eastern/Asian, lymphatic massage

SCHOOL STATEMENT: Holistic health care embraces the individual as well as the family. The healing arts accounts for all stages and ages of health and prevention.

Sand Hills Community College
3395 Airport Rd.
Pinehurst, NC 28387
(910) 695-3966   www.sandhills.cc.nc.us

CLASSROOM HOURS: 1008/2500 (Associate's degree)

COST: $1,500.00 (scholarships, grants)—day/night

EMPHASIS: relaxation, sports, medical, deep tissue, energy, Eastern/Asian

SCHOOL STATEMENT: The massage program is limited to 20 participants each year. Classes begin in the fall. The college offers a one-year diploma and a two-year associates degree.

Southeastern School of Neuromuscular and Massage Therapy of Charlotte, Inc.
4 Woodlawn Green, Ste. 200
Charlotte, NC 28217
(704) 527-4979 or (800) 420-HAND
www.se-massage.com

CLASSROOM HOURS: 500

COST: $6,325.00 including books and supplies (payment plan)—day/night

EMPHASIS: Neuromuscular Massage Therapy

SCHOOL STATEMENT: Offering the two most marketable skills: Swedish massage and neuromuscular therapy in 6 months! You can build your career with the right foundation.

Therapeutic Massage Training Institute
726 East Blvd.
Charlotte, NC 28203
(704) 338-9660

The Whole You School of Massage & Bodywork
143 Woodview Dr.
Rutherfordton, NC 28139
(828) 287-0955   www.wholeyou.com

CLASSROOM HOURS: 525 (plus 67.5 hours supervision)

COST: $4,800.00 (payment plan)—weekend program

EMPHASIS: relaxation, sports, medical, deep tissue, energy, Eastern/Asian

SCHOOL STATEMENT: An eclectic approach that combines Eastern and Western practices. Our program includes 19 modalities.

NORTH DAKOTA

Schools Offering Associate's Degree

Williston State College

Institute of Myofascial Studies
1003 E. Interstate Avenue
Bismarck, ND 58501
(701) 221-2725

Professional Institute of Massage Therapy
4720 7th Ave. SW, Ste. E
Fargo, ND 58103
(701) 281-5078   www.pimtfargo.com

CLASSROOM HOURS: year one 1100, year two 1100

COST: year one $6,250.00, year two $6,250.00 (payment plan)—day program

EMPHASIS: relaxation, sports, medical, deep tissue

SCHOOL STATEMENT: PIMT uses the Canadian standard of massage therapy; assessment and treatment following medical principles and proven science. PIMT has campuses in Saskatchewan, Manitoba, and BC, Canada.

Sister Rosalind Gefre's School of Professional Massage
1519 First Ave. S., Ste. A
Fargo, ND 58103
(701) 297-5993

Williston State College
1410 University Ave.
Williston, ND 58802
(701) 774-4200   www.wsc.nodak.edu

CLASSROOM HOURS: 850/1240 (Associate's degree)

COST: $3,000.00/$6,000.00 including books and supplies (scholarships, grants, payment plan)—day program

EMPHASIS: relaxation, sports, medical, deep tissue

SCHOOL STATEMENT: This program is designed to prepare the student to work in the clinical environment with less emphasis on spa work.

OHIO

Accredited Schools	COMTA	IMSTAC	ABHES	ACCET	ACCSCT
American Institute of Alternative					•
National Institute of Massotherapy				•	
Ohio College of Massotherapy					•
Professional Skills Institute			•		
Tri-State College of Massotherapy					•
Youngstown College					•

Schools Offering Associate's Degree

Cuyahoga Community College Eastern Campus

Ohio College of Massotherapy

Stark State College of Technology

American Institute of Alternative Medicines
6685 Doubletree Ave.
Columbus, OH 43229
(614) 825-6278   www.massageaway.com

CLASSROOM HOURS: 720/1080/2018

COST: $8,000.00/$11,200.00/$22,000.00 (grants, no-int. loans, payment plan)—day/night/weekend

EMPHASIS: relaxation, sports, medical, deep tissue, energy, Eastern/Asian, acupressure

SCHOOL STATEMENT: AIAM is accredited by ACCSCT, approved by Ohio Medical Board, eligible for federal financial aid, veterans benefits. High quality programs. Your success is our success.

American Institute of Massotherapy
96 S. Washington St.
Tiffin, OH 44883
(419) 448-1355   www.tiffinohio.com/aim

Blanchard Valley Academy of Massage Therapy
1655 A Tiffin Ave.
Findlay, OH 45840
(419) 423-2628   www.bvamt.com

Carnegie Institute of Integrative Medicine & Massotherapy
1292 Waterloo Rd.
Suffield, OH 44260
(330) 630-1132   www.CIMASSOTHERAPY.org

CLASSROOM HOURS: 600/800

COST: $3,900.00 (scholarships, no-int. loans, payment plan)—day/night/weekend

EMPHASIS: relaxation, sports, medical, deep tissue, energy, Eastern/Asian

SCHOOL STATEMENT: Career based diploma program approved by Ohio Medical Board and State Board of Proprietary Schools. Accredited by ABHES.

Central Ohio School of Massage
1120 Morse Rd., Ste. 250
Columbus, OH 43229
(614) 841-1122   www.cosm.org

Cleveland School of Massage
8027-B Darrow Rd. (Rte. 91)
Twinsburg, OH 44087
(330) 405-1933   http://home.neo.rr.com/massageschool

Columbus State Community College
550 E. Spring St.
Columbus, OH 43216
(614) 287-5353 or (800) 621-6407   www.cscc.edu

Cuyahoga Community College Eastern Campus
4250 Richmond Rd.
Highland Hills, OH 44122
(216) 987-2000   www.ccc.interactivetour.com/eastern

(Associate's degree offered)

EHOVE Career Center
316 W. Manson Rd.
Milan, OH 44846
(419) 499-4663   www.ehove-jvs.k12.oh.us

Harmony Path College of Massage Therapy
20950 Center Ridge Rd., Ste. 201
Rocky River, OH 44116
(440) 333-6633   www.harmonypath.org

CLASSROOM HOURS: 528 (614 total hours)

COST: $6,600.00 (payment plan)—day/night

EMPHASIS: relaxation, medical, deep tissue, energy

SCHOOL STATEMENT: We develop caring, ethical, balanced massage therapists who understand the interconnection of mind, body and spirit, and use their skills and knowledge to support wellness.

Healing Arts Institute
340 Three Meadows Dr.
Perrysburg, OH 43551
(419) 874-4496   www.haiohio.com

CLASSROOM HOURS: 700

COST: $6,825.00 (payment plan)—day/night (full-time or part-time)

EMPHASIS: relaxation, sports, medical, deep tissue, energy, Eastern/Asian

Hocking Technical College
3301 Hocking Pkwy.
Nelsonville, OH 45764
(740) 753-3591   www.hocking.edu

Institute of Therapeutic Massage, Inc.
9508 State Rt. 65, P.O. Box 350
Ottawa, OH 45875
(419) 523-9580

Knox County Career Ctr.
306 Martinsburg Rd.
Mt. Vernon, OH 43050
(740) 397-5820   www.kccc.k12.oh.us

Lakeland Community College
7700 Clock Tower Dr.
Kirtland, OH 44094
(440) 953-7000 or (800) 589-8520
www.lakeland.cc.oh.us

National Institute of Massotherapy
2110 Copley Rd.
Akron, OH 44320
(330) 867-1996

National Institute of Massotherapy (Cleveland Branch)
12684 Rockside Rd.
Garfield Hts., OH 44125
(216) 662-6955

CLASSROOM HOURS: 607

COST: $6,900.00 (scholarships, grants, payment plan)—day/night/weekend (full-time or part-time)

EMPHASIS: relaxation, sports, medical, deep tissue, Eastern/Asian

SCHOOL STATEMENT: NIM is dedicated to helping students achieve proficiency in therapeutic skills and developing the personal awareness necessary for a successful practice in bodywork.

North Central State College
2441Kenwood Circle
Mansfield, OH 44901
(419) 755-4800 or (419) 755-4805
www.ncstate.tec.oh.us

Northwest Academy of Massotherapy
1910 Indian Wood Circle, Ste. 301
Maumee, OH 43566
(419) 893-6464

Oakes Massage Therapy College
330 Fourth St., S.E.
Massillon, OH 44646
(330) 832-2002   www.infowire.net/oakes

Ohio Academy of Holistic Health
2380 Bellbrook Ave.
Xenia, OH 45385
(800) 833-8122 or (937) 708-3232   www.oahh.com

Ohio College of Massotherapy
225 Heritage Woods Dr.
Akron, OH 44321
(330) 665-1084   www.ocm.edu

CLASSROOM HOURS: 730/1600 (Associate's degree)—day/night/weekend/on-line program

EMPHASIS: relaxation, sports, medical, deep tissue

SCHOOL STATEMENT: Ohio College of Massotherapy created a subsidiary called OCM Online which has the first online program in Massage Therapy. The school has an extensive bookstore.

Professional Skills Institute
20 Arco Dr.
Toledo, OH 43607
(419) 531-9610 or (888) 531-9610   www.proskills.com

School of Transformational Massage Therapy
1901 Selma Rd.
Springfield, OH 45505
(937) 836-7925

S.H.I. Integrative Medical Massage School
www.shimassage.com

North Dayton Campus:
8132 N. Main St., Dayton, OH 45415
(888) 414-5600 or (937) 454-0914

South Campus:
130 Cook Rd., Lebanon, OH 45036
(888) 335-4283 or (513) 932-8712

Stark State College of Technology
6200 Frank Rd. NW
Canton, OH 44720
(330) 966-5458   www.stark.cc.oh.us

CLASSROOM HOURS: 844 (certificate)
                    1288 (Associate's degree)

COST: $89.00 per credit hour (scholarships, grants)—weekend program

EMPHASIS: relaxation, medical, deep tissue

SCHOOL STATEMENT: Our program is designed to prepare students for the State Medical Board of Ohio Exams in anatomy & physiology and in massage theory.

Tri-State College of Massotherapy
9159 Market St., Ste. 26
North Lima, OH 44452
(330) 629-9998   www.tristatemasso.com

CLASSROOM HOURS: 602

COST: $6,500.00 (grants, payment plan)—day/night/weekend

EMPHASIS: relaxation, medical

SCHOOL STATEMENT: Basic Swedish massage taught. Exposure to Trager(r), CranioSacral Therapy, Ortho-Bionomy(r), Zero Balancing, Visceral Massage Techniques, Neuromuscular Massage, Entergy Integration, and Hot Stone Massage. Small/personal.

Youngstown College of Massotherapy
14 Highland Ave.
Struthers, OH 44471
(330) 755-1406 or (800) 454-1406   www.yocm.com

OKLAHOMA					

Accredited Schools	COMTA	IMSTAC	ABHES	ACCET	ACCSCT
Community Care College			•		
Oklahoma Health Academy					•

Body Business School of Massage Therapy
615 W. Evergreen
Durant, OK 74701
(580) 924-2309

CLASSROOM HOURS: 300

COST: $2,500.00 (scholarships, grants, payment plan)—night/weekend

EMPHASIS: relaxation, sports, medical, deep tissue, energy

SCHOOL STATEMENT: Located in Southeastern Oklahoma we are Durant's premiere massage training facility. Over 25 years experience in massage therapy and marketing. Let us help you achieve your dream!

Central State Massage Academy
8494 NW Expressway, OKC Mkt. Sq.
Oklahoma City, OK 73162
(405) 722-4560   www.centralstateacademy.com

Community Care College
5810 E. Skelly Dr., 1st Floor
Tulsa, OK 74135
(918) 610-0027

Massage Therapy Institute of Oklahoma
9433 East 51st Ste. H
Tulsa, OK 74145
(918) 622-6644   www.mtio.org

Me Ke Akua Health Center
6600 S. Yale Ave. Ste. 1307
Tulsa, OK 74136
(918) 496-1888

Oklahoma Health Academy
1939 N. Moore Ave.
Moore, OK 73160
(405) 943-8800

Oklahoma School of Natural Healing
1660 E. 71st St., Ste. 2-0
Tulsa, OK 74136
(918) 496-9401

Praxis College of Health Arts and Sciences
8900 N. Western Ave.
Oklahoma City, OK 73114
(405) 879-0224

Southern Oklahoma School of Massage Therapy
6000 State Road 22, P.O. Box 624
Bokchito, OK 74726
(580) 295-3158

CLASSROOM HOURS: 250 (300 total hours)

COST: $1,200.00 (payment plan)—day/weekend

EMPHASIS: relaxation, sports, medical, deep tissue

SCHOOL STATEMENT: We are a licensed and bonded private vocational school teaching Swedish Massage Level I and a variety of continuing education classes.

OREGON					

Accredited Schools	COMTA	IMSTAC	ABHES	ACCET	ACCSCT
East-West College	•				

Schools Offering Associate's Degree

Central Oregon Community College

Ashland Massage Institute
P.O. Box 1233
Ashland, OR 97521
(541) 482-5134
http://schools.naturalhealers.com/ashland

CLASSROOM HOURS: 570

COST: $5,600.00 (payment plan)—night program

EMPHASIS: relaxation, deep tissue, energy, Eastern/Asian

SCHOOL STATEMENT: Quality training in small-school community emphasizes Swedish, Eastern and Western techniques, health science foundation, and competent professional entry. Fall retreat. Movement and stillness themes.

Ashmead College School of Massage, Vancouver, WA
120 N.E. 136th Ave.
Portland Area, OR 98684
(360) 885-3152   www.ashmeadcollege.com

Central Oregon Community College—Massage Therapy Program
2600 NW College Way
Bend, OR 97701
(541) 617-1407   www.cocc.edu/massage

CLASSROOM HOURS: 1107 (2 years; associates degree)

COST: $9,763.00 (scholarships, grants)—day/night (some weekends second year)

EMPHASIS: sports, medical, deep tissue

SCHOOL STATEMENT: Our program is committed to training our students to 1) become successful licensed Massage Professionals and 2) complement health care providers by treating soft tissue dysfunctions.

East-West College of the Healing Arts
4531 S.E. Belmont St.
Portland, OR 97215
(503) 231-1500 or (800) 635-9141   www.ewcha.com

Lane Community College
4531 Willamette St.
Eugene, OR 97401
(541) 726-2252   www.lanecc.edu

Massage U
314 Jersey St.
Silverton, OR 97381
(800) 757-6257 or (503) 873-9030

Oregon School of Massage
www.oregonschoolofmassage.com

9500 SW Barbur Blvd., Ste. 100
Portland, OR 97219
(503) 244-3420 or (800) 844-3420

Branch campus:
440 Ferry St. SE, Salem, OR 97302
(503) 844-3420

Rogue Community College
3345 Redwood Hwy.
Grants Pass, OR 97527
(541) 956-7500   www.rogue.cc.or.us

PENNSYLVANIA

Accredited Schools	COMTA	IMSTAC	ABHES	ACCET	ACCSCT
Acad. of Medical Arts and Business					•
Allied Medical and Technical Careers					•
Baltimore School of Massage					•
Berks Technical Institute					•
Career Training Academy	•	•			•
Computer Learning Network					•
East West School		•			
Great Lakes Institute of Technology					•
Massage Therapy Program	•				
Pennsylvania Institute of Massage	•	•			
Pennsylvania Sch. of Muscle Therapy	•	•			

Schools Offering Associate's Degree

Academy of Medical Arts and Business (AMAB)

Allied Medical & Technical Careers

Pennsylvania School of Muscle Therapy

Academy of Medical Arts and Business (AMAB)
2301 Academy Drive
Harrisburg, PA 17112
(717) 545-4747   www.acadcampus.com

CLASSROOM HOURS: 755 (diploma)/1540 (Associate's degree)

COST: $8,400.00/$17,590.00 ($3,800.00 per semester) (scholarships, grants, no-int. loans, payment plan)—day/night/Saturday

EMPHASIS: relaxation, sports, medical, deep tissue, energy, Eastern/Asian, lymphatic, cranial-sacral, pregnancy, pediatric, spa, geriatric

SCHOOL STATEMENT: AMAB is located in the foothills of the Blue Mountains, near Harrisburg. On-site child care center, café. Personal attention. Nearby attractions include Hershey, sporting events.

Allied Medical Careers, Inc.
517 Ash St.
Scranton, PA 18509
(570) 342-8000 or (570) 558-1818

Allied Medical & Technical Careers
166 Slocum St.
Forty Fort, PA 18704
(570) 288-8400

(Associate's Degree offered)

Alternative Conjunction Clinic and School of Massage Therapy
716 State Street
Lemoyne, PA 17043
(717) 737-6001   www.alternativeconjunction.com

CLASSROOM HOURS: 604/900

COST: $6,795.00/$9,625.00 including books, supplies, table (grants, no-int. loans, payment plan)—day/night/weekend

EMPHASIS: relaxation, sports, medical, deep tissue, Eastern/Asian

SCHOOL STATEMENT: Our massage therapy programs are medically and clinically based. Eastern and Western knowledge is taught to give students the most balanced base

Baltimore School of Massage—York Campus
170 Red Rock Rd.
York, PA 17402
(717) 268-1881   www.bsmyork.com

CLASSROOM HOURS: 637

COST: $6,680.00 (grants, payment plan)—day/night

EMPHASIS: relaxation, deep tissue, myofascial release

SCHOOL STATEMENT: This is a vocational training program to prepare students to be professional massage therapists and have a successful and rewarding career.

Berks Technical Institute
2205 Ridgewood Rd.
Wyomissing, PA 19610
(800) 821-4662   www.berkstechnical.com

Career Training Academy
www.careerta.com/programs.html

950 Fifth Avenue
New Kensington, PA 15068
(724) 337-1000

Expomart, 105 Mall Blvd., Ste. 300 W
Monroeville, PA 15146
(412) 372-3900

1500 North Way Mall
Pittsburgh, PA 15237
(412) 367-4000

Central PA School of Massage
336 S. Fraser St.
State College, PA 16801
(814) 234-4900 or (888) 649-3337
www.schoolofmassage.com

Community College Of Allegheny County
8701 Perry Hwy.
Pittsburgh, PA 15237-5353
(412) 369-3737   www.ccac.edu

Computer Learning Network
401 E. Winding Hill Rd., Ste. 101
Mechanicsburg, PA 17055
(800) 338-8038   www.clntraining.net

CLASSROOM HOURS: 960

COST: $10,735.00 including books, uniforms, supplies, massage table (scholarships, grants, no-int. loans, payment plan)—day/night

EMPHASIS: relaxation, sports, deep tissue

SCHOOL STATEMENT: Do you like to help people and earn great money? CIN's extensive Massage Therapy program is for you! Learn how to wipe people's stresses away.

East-West School of Massage Therapy
504 Park Rd. North
Wyomising, PA 19610
(610) 375-7520   www.ewsmt.com

Empire Beauty School
Knights Road Shopping Ctr.
4026 Woodhaven Rd
Philadelphia, PA 19154
(800) 295-8390 or (215) 637-3700
www.empirebeauty.com

Franklin Academy
324 N. Centre St.
Pottsville, PA 17901-2505
(570) 622-6060 or (570) 622-8370

Great Lakes Institute of Technology
5100 Peach St.
Erie, PA 16509
(800) 394-4548 or (814) 864-6666   www.glit.org
CLASSROOM HOURS: 900—day/night

Health Options Institute, Inc.
1410 Main St.
Northampton, PA 18067
(610) 261-0880   www.healthoptionsinstitute.com

CLASSROOM HOURS: 524

COST: $6,400.00 (payment plan)—day/night/weekend

EMPHASIS: relaxation, sports, deep tissue, energy, Eastern/Asian

SCHOOL STATEMENT: Outstanding quality of classes in Deep Muscle Massage, Reflexology, Shiatsu, Nutrition and Holistic Health, Sports Massage, Polarity, Neuromuscular Therapy, Stretch Rehab, Therapeutic Touch and more

Lancaster School of Massage
1210 Willow St. Pike
Lancaster, PA 17603
(717) 293-9698   www.LancasterSchoolOfMassage.com
CLASSROOM HOURS: 520

COST: $5,250.00 (payment plan)—day/night

EMPHASIS: relaxation, sports, medical, deep tissue, energy

Lehigh Valley Healing Arts Academy, Inc.
5412 Shimerville, Rd.
Emmaus, PA 18049
(610) 965-6165   www.LVHAA.com

CLASSROOM HOURS: 620 (bodywork)/500 (shiatsu)/200 (reflexology)

COST: $6,280.00 (bodywork) (no-int. loans, payment plan)—day/night/weekend

EMPHASIS: relaxation, sports, medical, deep tissue, energy, Eastern/Asian, herbs, polarity, aromatherapy, sound vibrational healing

SCHOOL STATEMENT: We are a progressive healing arts school with a unique spirit that embraces the whole being and the web in which we live. Come meet us!

Massage Arts & Sciences Center of Philadelphia
1515 Locust St., 2nd Floor
Philadelphia, PA 19102
(215) 985-0674   www.massagearts.com

Massage Therapy Program
10050 Roosevelt Blvd.
Philadelphia, PA 19116
(215) 969-1170 or (800) 264-9835
www.healinghands.net

Mt. Nittany Institute of Natural Health
301 Shiloh Rd.
State College, PA 16801
(814) 238-1121   www.mtnittanyinstitute.com
CLASSROOM HOURS: 540 (675 total hours)

COST: $6,500.00 (payment plan)—day/weekend

EMPHASIS: relaxation, sports, deep tissue, energy, Eastern/Asian, elder massage, cancer massage, professional development

SCHOOL STATEMENT: Mt. Nittany Institute's holistic approach to massage education, business preparation and developing a healing presence prepares students well for meaningful, rewarding work.

Pennsylvania Center for Holistic Studies
2938 Ridge Pike
Eagleville, PA 19403
(610) 635-0666   www.pachs.org
CLASSROOM HOURS: 545

COST: $5,895.00 including books and supplies (grants, payment plan)—day/night/weekend/combination

EMPHASIS: relaxation, sports, energy, Eastern/Asian, aromatherapy, personal development

SCHOOL STATEMENT: Pennsylvania Center for Holistic Studies embraces the holistic approach to health and learning by considering the mind, body, emotions and environment of students and clients.

Pennsylvania Institute of Massage Therapy
93 S. Westend Blvd., Ste 103
Quakertown, PA 18951
(215) 538-5339   www.PAmassage.com
CLASSROOM HOURS: 525

COST: $5,250.00 (payment plan)—day/night/weekend

EMPHASIS: relaxation, medical, deep tissue

SCHOOL STATEMENT: PIMT has beautiful facilities, including a student lounge. There is a working student clinic. Free tutoring is available. A massage supply store is on-site.

Pennsylvania Learning Institute
210 Montage Mountain Rd.
Moosic, PA 18507
(800) 264-9835　www.healinghands.net

Pennsylvania School of Muscle Therapy
1173 Egypt Rd./P.O. Box 400
Oaks, PA 19456
(610) 666-9060　www.psmt.com

CLASSROOM HOURS: 629 to 1043 (Associate's degree)

COST: $6,500.00 to $11,500.00 (scholarships and grants for degree candidates, payment plan)—day/night/weekend (full-time or part-time)

EMPHASIS: relaxation, sports, medical, deep tissue, Eastern/Asian

SCHOOL STATEMENT: Nationally recognized for over 20 years, PSMT is an educational leader with COMTA & IMSTAC accreditation, college credit recommendations, various program options and an associates degree.

Pittsburgh School of Massage Therapy
10989 Frankstown Rd.
Pittsburgh, PA 15235
(412) 241-5155　www.pghschmass.com

CLASSROOM HOURS: 616

COST: $4,600.00 (scholarships, payment plan)—day/night/weekend/custom schedules available

EMPHASIS: relaxation, sports, medical, deep tissue

SCHOOL STATEMENT: We are a student-centered organization committed to promoting the art, science and profession of massage therapy through excellence in education and training.

Professional School of Massage
131 E. Maple Ave.
Langhorne, PA 19047
(215) 750-0700　www.TeachTouch.com

CLASSROOM HOURS: 500

COST: $4,750.00 (payment plan)—day/night/weekend

EMPHASIS: relaxation, sports, medical, deep tissue, energy, Eastern/Asian

SCHOOL STATEMENT: Our intention is to ensure that our graduates have the necessary knowledge technically, practically, and compassionately to manifest their destinies.

School of Body Therapies
807 Floralvalle Rd.
Yardley, PA 19047
(215) 752-7666　www.body-therapies.com

Synergy Healing Arts Center and Massage School
13593 Monterey Lane
Blue Ridge Summit, PA 17214
(717) 794-5778

CLASSROOM HOURS: 550

COST: $5,600.00 including books (payment plan)—day/night

EMPHASIS: relaxation, sports, deep tissue, energy

The Valley School of Healing Arts
RR Ste. 2, Box 901
Port Trevorton, PA 17864
(570) 374-2222

CLASSROOM HOURS: massage 600; reflexology 325; alt. healing 325

Students may enroll and pay for one course at a time day/night/weekend

EMPHASIS: relaxation, medical, energy, shiatsu, MFR, reflexology

RHODE ISLAND

Arthur Angelo School of Cosmetology and Hair Design
151 Broadway
Providence, RI 02903
(401) 272-4300　www.arthurangelo.com

Community College of Rhode Island
400 East Avenue
Warwick, RI 02886
(401) 825-1000　www.ccri.cc.ri.us

SOUTH CAROLINA

Accredited Schools	COMTA	IMSTAC	ABHES	ACCET	ACCSCT
Charleston School of Massage				•	
Southeastern Sch. of Neuromuscular					•

Aiken Technical College
P.O. Box 696
Aiken, SC 29802
(803) 593-9231 or (800) 246-6198　www.aik.tec.sc.us

Alpha School of Massage
499 Pleasantburg Dr.
Greenville, SC 29607
(864) 232-1818

Charleston School of Massage

778 Folly Rd.
Charleston, SC 29412
(843) 762-7722   www.charlestonmassage.com

CLASSROOM HOURS: 500/600

COST: $5,225.00/$7,225.00 including books (grants, no-int. loans, payment plan)—day/night

EMPHASIS: relaxation, sports, medical, deep tissue, energy, Eastern/Asian, spa

SCHOOL STATEMENT: An ACCET accredited massage school offering programs of study in clinical massage therapy. We offer a broad preparation in massage technique for the professional.

Dovestar   www.dovestar.edu

20 Palmetto Pkwy
Hilton Head Island, SC 29928
(843) 342-3361

912 South Cashua Rd
Florence, SC 29501
(843) 678-9902

Dovestar/Camelot
611 17th Ave. North
Myrtle Beach, SC29577
(843) 293-7785

Greenville School of Therapeutic Massage

1 Chick Springs Rd., Ste. 214
Greenville, SC 29609
(864) 370-2030   www.greenvillemassage.com

Greenville Technical College

P.O. Box 5616
Greenville, SC 29606
(864) 250-8111   www.greenvilletech.com

Horry Georgetown Technical College

P.O.Box 261966
Conway, SC 29528
(843) 349-3186   www.hor.tec.sc.us

Miller-Motte Technical College

8058 Rivers Ave.
Charleston, SC 29418
(877) 617-4740   www.miller-motte.com

South Carolina Massage Therapy Institute

4720-B Hwy. 17 Bypass South
Myrtle Beach, SC 29577
(843) 293-2225

1607 Augusta Rd.
West Columbia, SC 29169
(803) 739-8934

CLASSROOM HOURS: 500

COST: $5,300.00 including books (payment plan)—day/night (part-time, full-time)

EMPHASIS: relaxation, sports, medical, deep tissue, energy, Eastern/Asian

SCHOOL STATEMENT: We teach the art of massage therapy, including numerous body therapies and sound business practices which prepare the student for success in the marketplace.

Southeastern School of Neuromuscular and Massage Therapy

4600 Goer Dr., Ste. 105
N. Charleston, SC 29406
(843) 747-1279   www.charleston.se-massage.com

CLASSROOM HOURS: 500 (including 40 hours in student clinic)

COST: $5,100.00 (grants, payment plan)—day/night

EMPHASIS: relaxation, medical, deep tissue, neuromuscular therapy

SCHOOL STATEMENT: The Southeastern School of Charleston is committed to providing the most effective educational environment and course content for the study of massage therapy possible.

Southeastern School of Neuromuscular and Massage Therapy

3007 Broad River Rd.
Columbia, SC 29210
(803) 798-8800   www.columbia.se-massage.com

Southeastern School of Neuromuscular and Massage Therapy

850 S. Pleasantburg Dr., Ste. 105
Greenville, SC 29607
(864) 421-9481   www.greenville.se-massage.com

Technical College of the Low Country

Continuing Education Division
921 Ribaut Road/P.O. Box 1288
Beaufort, SC 29901
(843) 525-8205

Trident Technical College, Allied Health Division

P.O. Box 118067
Charleston, SC 29423
(877) 349-7184 or Infoline: (843) 574-6262
www.trident.tec.sc.us

SOUTH DAKOTA

Schools Offering Associate's Degree

National American University

"Carrie's Kadesh" and School of Massage

622 W. 6th Ave.
Mitchell, SD 57301
(605) 996-3916

CLASSROOM HOURS: 860 (1100 total hours)

COST: $4,600.00—day program

EMPHASIS: relaxation, sports, medical, deep tissue, energy

SCHOOL STATEMENT: We are a private school. Our program is intense, yet relaxed—open—and without political intervention. Our goal is to produce outstanding, knowledgeable, reliable massage therapists.

Headlines Academy of Massage
508 6th St., Ste. 305
Rapid City, SD 57701
(605) 388-3645

CLASSROOM HOURS: 600

COST: $5,400.00 (scholarships, grants, in-int. loans, payment plan)—day program

EMPHASIS: relaxation, sports, medical, deep tissue, energy, Eastern/Asian

SCHOOL STATEMENT: Our faculty further the knowledge of our students and participate in the learning process of technical and management skills to prepare them for their career.

National American University
321 Kansas City, St.
Rapid 57701
(605) 394-4800   www.national.edu

(Associate's degree offered)

South Dakota School of Massage Therapy
902 W. 22nd. St.
Sioux Falls, SD 57105
(605) 334-4422

TENNESSEE					
Accredited Schools	COMTA	IMSTAC	ABHES	ACCET	ACCSCT
High-Tech Institute					•
Roane State Community College	•				
Tennessee Institute of Healing Arts	•				•

Bodyworks School of Massage
541 Carriage House Drive
Jackson, TN 38305
(731) 664-4891

Center Of Rehabilitative Education (C.O.R.E.)
9220 Park West Blvd.
Knoxville, TN 37923
(865) 694-4220

CLASSROOM HOURS: 550

COST: $6,200.00 (scholarships, grants, payment plan)—day/night

EMPHASIS: sports, medical, deep tissue

SCHOOL STATEMENT: A short drive from the Great Smokeys National Park, our curriculum trains students in orthopedic rehabilitation techniques for use in medical or athletic oriented careers.

Cumberland Institute for Wellness Education
500 Wilson Pike Circle, Ste. 121
Brentwood, TN 37027
(615) 370-9794   www.cumberlandinstitute.com

CLASSROOM HOURS: 500

COST: $7,290.00 including books and supplies (payment plan)—day/night

EMPHASIS: relaxation, sports, medical, deep tissue, energy, Eastern/Asian

SCHOOL STATEMENT: Our superior massage therapy education instills the skill, compassion, self-awareness and professionalism that leads beyond certification to a fulfilling, financially successful vocation in massage therapy.

East Tennessee School of Massage Therapy
777 New Hwy. 68
Sweetwater, TN 37874
(423) 337-3221

High-Tech Institute
2710 Old Lebanon Rd., Ste. 12
Nashville, TN 37214
(888) 616-6549   www.high-techinstitute.com

Holston Institute of Healing Arts
208 Suncrest St., Gray, TN
Mailing: 105 Brookfield Dr. Ste. 2, Kingsport, TN 37663
(423) 239-5043   www.kingsport.com/holstoninstitute

Institute of Therapeutic Massage and Movement
1161 Murfreesboro Rd., Ste. 405
Nashville, Tn 37217
(615) 360-8554   www.itmm.citysearch.com

The Massage Institute of Memphis
3445 Poplar Ave., Ste.s 3 & 4
Memphis, TN 38111
(901) 324-4411   www.themassageinstitute.com

Miller Motte Technical College
1820 Business Park Dr.
Clarksville, TN 37040
(800) 558-0071   www.miller-motte.com

Natural Health Institute
209 10th Ave. South, Ste. 212
Nashville, TN 37203
(615) 242-6811   www.natural-health-inst.com

CLASSROOM HOURS: 500

COST: $6,212.00 (scholarships, payment plan)—night/weekend

EMPHASIS: relaxation, sports, medical, deep tissue, energy, Eastern/Asian

SCHOOL STATEMENT: Comprehensive and diverse curriculum offers several areas of specialization. Students eligible for licensure and to sit for national certification board.

Natural Touch Institute, LLC
931 Spring Creed Rd., Ste. 101
East Ridge, TN 37421
(423) 892-5513

CLASSROOM HOURS: 550—day/night

EMPHASIS: relaxation, sports, medical, deep tissue, spa therapy, insurance billing

SCHOOL STATEMENT: Excellence in education. Specializing in medical, sports and deep tissue massage. 12 Faculty members including nurse, physical therapist, sports trainer, Doctor of Chiropractic, and MBA.

Roane State Community College
276 Patton Lane
Harriman, TN 37748
(423) 481-3496   www.rscc.cc.tn.us
Oak Ridge Branch Campus (865) 481-2000

Southern Massage Institute
253 S. Center St.
Collierville, TN 38017
(901) 854-9095

COST: $5,000.00 (no-int. loans, payment plan)—day/night

EMPHASIS: relaxation, sports, medical, deep tissue, energy, Eastern/Asian

SCHOOL STATEMENT: We provide the highest quality massage education., instilling professionalism, competence, skills and self-confidence so each student will achieve success, happiness and a rewarding career.

Tennessee Institute of Healing Arts
7010 Lee Highway, Ste. 712
Chattanooga, TN 37421
(800) 735-1910   www.tiha.com

CLASSROOM HOURS: 1000

COST: $9,270.00 including books (grants, payment plan)—day/night (full-time or part-time)

EMPHASIS: relaxation, medical, neuromuscular therapy

SCHOOL STATEMENT: Twelve-month, 1,000 hour Massage and Neuromuscular Therapy Program, offering a variety of courses. Accredited by ACCSCT and COMTA. Federal financial aid to those who qualify.

Tennessee School of Massage
556 Colonial Rd.
Memphis, TN 38117
(901) 767-8484   www.tsom.net

CLASSROOM HOURS: 750

COST: $7,125.00 (payment plan)—day/night

EMPHASIS: relaxation, sports, deep tissue, energy, spa

SCHOOL STATEMENT: Spaology. What if you could lose yourself and find yourself at the same time? Learn our body treatments while you learn massage therapy—spaah!

Tennessee School of Therapeutic Massage
4704 Western Ave.
Knoxville, TN 37921
(865) 588-7878   www.tennesseeschoolofmassage.com

TEXAS

Accredited Schools	COMTA	IMSTAC	ABHES	ACCET	ACCSCT
Academy of Professional Careers				•	
Lauterstein-Conway School	•				
New Beginning School of Massage		•			•
Western Technical Institute					•

The Academy for Massage Therapy Training
(866) 268-2688   www.academyformassage.com

1039 W. Hildebrand Ave.
San Antonio, TX 78201
(210) 224-8111

Rock Creek Plaza 2132 N. Mays, Ste. 900
Round Rock, TX 78664
(512) 828-0488

2109 Cornerstone Blvd.
Edinburg, TX 78539
(956) 630-3363

Academy of Healing Arts
531 Londonderry Lane, Ste. 132
Denton, TX 76205
(940) 566-1880

Academy of Professional Careers
2201 S. Western, Ste. 102-103
Amarillo, TX 79109
(806) 353-3500   www.academyofhealthcareers.com

day program

EMPHASIS: relaxation, deep tissue

SCHOOL STATEMENT: APC offers a year-round 300-hour massage therapy basic registration program.

Acutech Massage Therapy School
6009 Richmond Ave.
Houston, TX 77057
(713) 783-6797   www.acutechms.com

Alvin Community College
3110 Mustang
Alvin, TX 77511
(281) 756-3502   www.alvin.cc.tx.us

Asten Center for Natural Therapeutics
990 N. Bowser Ste. 860
Richardson, TX 75081
(927) 669-3245   www.astencenter.com

Austin Community College
5930 Middle Fiskville Road
Austin, TX 78752
(512) 223-7000   www2.austin.cc.tx.us

Austin School of Massage Therapy
2600 W. Stassney Lane
Austin, TX 78745
(512) 462-3004 or (800) 276-2768   www.asmt.com

Satellite locations:

619 Kentucky, Ste. 560-E
Amarillo, TX 79102

1300 George Bush Drive
College Station, TX 77842

2636 Walnut Hill Lane, Building 2, Ste. 265
Dallas, TX 75229

6791 Montana
El Paso, TX 79925

1400 8th Avenue
Fort Worth, TX 76104

3602 Slide Road, Ste. B-14
Lubbock, TX 79414

117 West Wall
Midland, TX 79701

2021 North Bryant Blvd.
San Angelo, TX 76903

5225 McCullough
San Antonio, TX 78212

4005 Lake Shore Drive
Waco, TX 76714

Brazosport College
500 College Dr.
Lake Jackson, TX 77566
(979) 230-3000   www.brazosport.cc.tx.us

Christian Associates
1915 N. Frasier, Ste. 101
Conroe, TX 77301
(936) 441-6511

El Paso Community College
215 Francis St./P.O. Box 20500
El Paso, TX 79998
(915) 831-2000   www.epcc.edu

Energistics Institute
2506 Westminister
Pearland, TX 77581
(281) 997-7555
CLASSROOM HOURS: 300

COST: $2,500.00—day/night/weekend

EMPHASIS: relaxation, sports, medical, deep tissue, energy, Eastern/Asian, ortho-bionomy, zen shiatsu

SCHOOL STATEMENT: Understanding human body and effects of massage therapy. Proper movements for safety and injury prevention. Skill for successfully planning, beginning and operating a massage business.

European Institute
33 East Shady Ln.
Houston, TX 77063
(713) 783-1446

European Massage Therapy Institute
7220 Louis Pasteur, Ste. 140
San Antonio, TX 78229
(210) 615-8207

Fort Worth School of Massage
2929 Cleburne Rd.
Fort Worth, TX 76110
(817) 923-9944

Frank Phillips College
P.O. Box 5118
Borger, TX 79008
(806) 274-5311

Giving Tree Cottage
1808 South St.
Nacogdoches, TX 75964
(936) 560-6299

CLASSROOM HOURS: 300

COST: $2,600.00 including books and supplies (no-int. loans, payment plan)—night program, occasional workshops

EMPHASIS: therapeutic Swedish massage

SCHOOL STATEMENT: We believe in creating a challenging and exciting learning environment, encouraging students to become their best—as massage therapists and as individuals.

Guild for Therapeutic Bodywork
3930-H Bee Cave Rd.
Austin, TX 78746
(512) 327-9107

Hands On Approach
2880 LBJ Freeway, Ste. 501
Dallas, TX 75234
(972) 484-8180 or (888) 453-6428
www.handsonapproach.com

Hands-On Therapy School of Massage
410 Ed Carey Dr.
Harlingen, TX 78550
(956) 365-4916

Hands-On Therapy School of Massage
1804 N. Galloway Ave.
Mesquite, TX 75149
(972) 285-6133

Healing Arts Inst. School of Massage Therapy
5601 Aberdeen Ave., Ste. G
Lubbock, TX 79414
(806) 797-0034

**Health Quest Foundation of
Integrative Therapies**
2828 Central Dr., Ste. 400
Bedford, TX 76021
(817) 267-4716

Health Masters School of Massage Therapy
101 Franklin
Houston, TX 77002
(713) 228-8499

CLASSROOM HOURS: 300

COST: $2,700.00 including books & oils (scholarships, payment plan)—day/night/weekend

EMPHASIS: Swedish massage

HFE & Massotherapy School
3930 Kirby Dr.,Ste. 205
Houston, TX 77098
(713) 528-2097

Houston Massage Institute
13932 Westheimer
Houston, TX 77077
(281) 497-4503

Institute of Bodywork Studies
1565 W. Main Ste. 154
Lewisville, TX 75067
(972) 353-8989 or (800) 640-9146
www.bodyworkstudies.com

CLASSROOM HOURS: 300 basic/200 advanced

COST: $2,200.00 including books and supplies

Institute of Cosmetic Arts
1105 Airline
Corpus Christi, TX 78411
(361) 991-8868

Institute of Cosmetology & Esthetics
7011 Harwin Ste. 100
Houston, TX 77036
(713) 783-9988

CLASSROOM HOURS: 300—day program

EMPHASIS: relaxation

SCHOOL STATEMENT: School offers training leading to Texas Department of Health issued license. Massage is taught as part of a total wellness curriculum.

Institute of Natural Healing Sciences
4100 Felps Dr., Ste. E
Colleyville, TX 76034
(817) 498-0716   www.Body-Mind-Spirit.com/INHS

CLASSROOM HOURS: 300 basic/290 advanced

COST: $2,250.00—day/night/weekend

EMPHASIS: relaxation, sports, medical, deep tissue, energy, Eastern/Asian, chair massage, reflexology, cranial/sacral

SCHOOL STATEMENT: Health is the product of the successful inter-relationship between body, mind, spirit, and environment. We aim to help develop personal growth and professionalism.

Lamar State College—Orange
410 Front St.
Orange, TX 77630
(409) 883-7750   www.orange.lamar.edu

**The Lauterstein-Conway Massage School
and Clinic**
4701-B Burnet Road
Austin, TX 78756
(512) 374-9222   www.tlcschool.com

CLASSROOM HOURS: 300/550/750

COST: $2,850.00/$5,700.00/$8,200.00 (scholarships, payment plan)—day/night/weekend programs

EMPHASIS: relaxation, sports, deep tissue, energy, Eastern/Asian, integrative

SCHOOL STATEMENT: Our mission is "to run the school in a manner as healing as the subjects we teach". We emphasize integrity, heartfulness, and clinical expertise.

Lubbock Professional Massage Therapy School
4920 S. Loop 289
Lubbock, TX 79414.
(806) 795-7795   www.schoolofmassagetherapy.com

Massage Education Institute
3195 Calder
Beaumont, TX 77702
(409) 832-3020

Massage Institute and Healing Arts Center
3626 N. Hall, Ste. 826
Dallas, TX 75219
(214) 443-0060   www.massageinst.com

CLASSROOM HOURS: 300 (basic)/600 (advanced)

COST: basic $2,900.00 (most advanced classes $10.00 per hour)(no-int. loans, payment plan, work-study)—day/night/weekend

EMPHASIS: relaxation, sports, medical, deep tissue, energy, Eastern/Asian, prenatal, somatic-emotional integration, reflexology

SCHOOL STATEMENT: Massage Institute and Healing Arts Center is registered with the Texas Department of Health, TX Rehabilitation Commission, Veterans Administration and Texas Commission of the Blind.

Midland College of Health Sciences Continuing Education
3600 N. Garfield, HS 228
Midland, TX 79705
(915) 685-6440

CLASSROOM HOURS: 300

COST: $1,000.00 (scholarships)—night program

SCHOOL STATEMENT: Program meets Texas Department of Health criteria, and includes anatomy and physiology, health and hygiene, hydrotherapy, Swedish massage, business and ethics, clinical setting.

Mind Body Naturopathic Institute
10911 West Ave.
San Antonio, TX 78213
(210) 342-7444 or (800) 939-1110
www.colon-hydrotherapy.com/mindbody.html

MRC School of Massage
6200 Tarnef Dr.
Houston, TX 77074
(713) 522-1423

The Myopractic Institute
5644 Westheimer Ste 217
Houston, TX 77056
(713) 869-5151 or (888) 696-9898   www.myopractic.com

Neuromuscular Concepts School of Massage
8607 Wurzbach Rd., Bldg. Q, Ste. 101
San Antonio, TX 78240
(210) 558-3112   www.frizzellwellness.com

CLASSROOM HOURS: 300 basic/2100 advanced

COST: $2,200.00 basic (payment plan)—night program/weekend workshops

EMPHASIS: relaxation, sports, medical, deep tissue, energy, Eastern/Asian, aromatherapy, stretching, hydrotherapy, advanced workshops

SCHOOL STATEMENT: Paul Frizzell has been in practice for over 30 years, is a licensed acupuncturist, N.D., Ph.D., O.M.D. and an independent instructor. Please call for information.

New Beginning School of Massage
2525 Wallingwood Dr., Ste. 1501
Austin, TX 78746
(512) 306-0975   www.nbegin.com

COST: $2,150.00 (no-int. loans, payment plan)—day/night/ evening + weekend

EMPHASIS: relaxation, deep tissue, energy, Eastern/Asian

North Texas Institute of Therapeutic Massage & Structural Bodywork
1310 S. Stemmons Freeway
Lewisville, TX 75067
(972) 221-7717

North Texas School of Swedish Massage
2335 Green Oaks Blvd. West
Arlington, TX 76016
(817) 446-6629

Odessa College
201 W. University
Odessa, TX 79764
(915) 335-6400   www.odessa.edu

Phoenix School of Massage and Holistic Health
www.themassageschool.com

Main campus: 6610 Harwin, Ste. 256
Houston, TX 77036
(713) 974-5976

Branch campus: 2611 FM 1950 W, Ste. H100
Houston, TX 77068

Power of Touch
2171 Gilmer Rd.
Longview, TX 75604
(903) 295-8090

The Relax Station School of Massage Therapy
1409 Kingwood Dr.
Kingwood, TX 77339
(281) 358-0600

CLASSROOM HOURS: 300

COST: $2,750.00 (payment plan)—day/night

EMPHASIS: relaxation, sports, deep tissue

SCHOOL STATEMENT: The Relax Station offers a thorough basic program. Test results in the state exam are typically higher than state average. Our students are employed frequently upon graduation.

Royal Beauty Careers
5020 FM 1960 W. Ste. A-12
Houston, TX 77069
(281) 580-2554

School of Natural Therapy
4309 N. 10th, Stes. A,B,C
McAllen, TX 78504
(956) 630-0928

St. Philips College—Continuing Education
1801 Martin Luther King Dr.
San Antonio, TX 78203
(210) 531-3200   www.accd.edu

Star Institute School of Therapeutic Massage
1426 Toomey Road
Austin, TX 78704
(512) 479-9977
www.doorway.com/thestarinstitutecom/school.html

Sterling Health Center Massage School
15070 Beltwood Parkway
Addison (Dallas), TX 75001
(972) 991-9293   www.sterlinghealthcenter.com

CLASSROOM HOURS: 300 to 1200

COST: basic $2,250.00, advanced $10.00 per hour (no-int. loans, payment plan)—day/night/weekend

EMPHASIS: relaxation, sports, medical, deep tissue

SCHOOL STATEMENT: Sterling Health Center is approved by Texas Department of Health to provide massage therapy training. Sterling Health Center is also approved to train veterans.

Texas Healing Arts Institute (THAI)
2704 Rio Grande, Ste. 11
Austin, TX 78705
(512) 236-8424   www.texashealingarts.com

CLASSROOM HOURS: 300

COST: $2,350.00 (payment plan)—day/night/accelerated day and summer classes available

EMPHASIS: relaxation, deep tissue, Eastern/Asian

SCHOOL STATEMENT: THAI provides training in the healing arts of massage therapy, Asian bodywork, Zen Shiatsu, and continuing education in bodywork and massage. Small classes . . . exceptional faculty.

Texas Massage Institute
www.TexasMassageInstitute.com

6301 Airport Freeway, Fort Worth, TX 76117
(817) 838-3800

915 W. Parker Rd., Plano, TX 75023
(972) 881-1496

6102 Mockingbird Ln., Ste. 300, Dallas, TX 75214
(214) 828-4000

CLASSROOM HOURS: 300

COST: $2,685.00 including books and supplies (no-int. loans, payment plan)—day/night/weekend

EMPHASIS: relaxation, sports, medical, deep tissue, energy, Eastern/Asian

Therapeutic Body Concepts School of Massage Therapy
6128 Wurzbach
San Antonio, TX 78238
(210) 684-6563   www.massageservices.org

CLASSROOM HOURS: 300

COST: $2,400.00 including books (payment plan)—day/night/weekend

EMPHASIS: relaxation

SCHOOL STATEMENT: State Registered school of massage therapy. Over 11,000 square feet, featuring an indoor heated pool for the hydrotherapy training.

Wellness Skills Two
6301 Airport Freeway
Fort Worth, TX 76117
(817) 838-3800   www.WellnessSkillsTwo.com

CLASSROOM HOURS: 300

COST: $2,685.00 including books and supplies (no-int. loans, payment plan)—day/night/weekend

EMPHASIS: relaxation, sports, medical, deep tissue, energy, Eastern/Asian

Western Technical Institute
9451 Diana Dr.
El Paso, TX 79924
(915) 566-9621   www.wti-ep.com

West Texas Massage Institute
3515 Wolflin Ave.
Amarillo, TX 79102
(806) 354-8840

Williams Institute Massage Therapy, Inc.
810 S. Mason, Ste. 290
Katy, TX 77450
(281) 392-9212

CLASSROOM HOURS: 300

COST: $2,760.00 (estimated) (payment plan)—day program

EMPHASIS: relaxation, Swedish massage

SCHOOL STATEMENT: Modalities and subjects—history of massage, personal development, guided relaxation techniques, medical terminology, hydrotherapy, business practices and professional ethics, human health and hygiene and internship.

World School of Massage and Bodywork
3617 Red Bluff
Pasadena, TX 77503
(713) 472-0383

Independent Massage Instructors

Connor, Joanna P.
Pecan Creek Ranch
Concan, TX 78838
(830) 232-6384

Free, Terry L.
302 N. Raquet Rd.
Lufkin, TX 75904
(936) 634-8085

Frizzell, Paul M.
8607 Wurbach Rd., Bldg. R, Ste. 150
San Antonio, TX 78240
(210) 863-5052

Magee, Harlin Lloyd
1910 Justin Ln.
Austin, TX 78757
(512) 451-3888

UTAH

Accredited Schools	COMTA	IMSTAC	ABHES	ACCET	ACCSCT
Healing Mountain Massage School			•		
Myotherapy College of Utah					•
Provo College					•
Utah Coll. of Massage Therapy	•			•	

Schools Offering Associate's Degree

Provo College

Healing Mountain Massage School
455 South 300 East 103
Salt Lake City, UT 84111
(801) 573-2230   www.healingmountain.org

Myotherapy College of Utah
1174 E. 2700 So. Ste. 19
Salt Lake City, UT 84106
(801) 484-7624   www.MyotherapyCollegeOfUtah.com

CLASSROOM HOURS: 780

COST: $7,785.00 including supplies and massage table (grants, payment plan)—day/night

EMPHASIS: relaxation, sports, medical, deep tissue, energy, Eastern/Asian

SCHOOL STATEMENT: We are a small school specializing in a more clinical approach. Class sizes run from 12 to 20 students for more personal attention.

Myotherapy Institute of Massage
1174 E. 2700 South—Ste. 14 & 15
Salt Lake City, UT 84106
distance education
(800) HEAL YOU   www.myomassage.net

Ogden Institute of Massage Therapy
3500 Harrison Blvd.
Ogden, UT 84403
(801) 627-8227   www.OIMT.net

CLASSROOM HOURS: 610

COST: $7,500.00 (payment plan)—night program

EMPHASIS: sports, medical, deep tissue, Eastern/Asian

SCHOOL STATEMENT: We prepare students for a positive profession.

Provo College
1450 West 820
North Provo, UT 84601
(801) 375-1861
(Associate's Degree offered)

Renaissance School of Massage Therapy
450 S. 400 E., Ste. 190
Bountiful, UT 84010
(801) 292-8515

Sensory Development Institute
1871 W. Canyon View Dr.
St. George, UT 84770
(435) 652-9003   www.sdischool.com

Utah College of Massage Therapy
25 S. 300 East
Salt Lake City, UT 84111
(800) 617-3302   www.ucmt.com

Additional Campuses
in Layton and Utah Valley

VERMONT

Schools Offering Associate's Degree

Community College of Vermont

Community College of Vermont
P.O. Box 120
Waterbury, VT 05676
(802) 222-5490 or (802) 828-4060   www.ccv.vsc.edu
(Associate's degree offered)

Green Mountain Institute for Integrative Therapy
368 Lamb Rd.—Grandview Farm
North Bennington, VT 05257
(802) 442-3886   www.internationalbodywork.com

CLASSROOM HOURS: 500–750—2002 Portugal 500 hr. program
$5,800.00—day program/Portugal intensive

EMPHASIS: relaxation, energy, transformational bodywork

SCHOOL STATEMENT: Programs in Vermont and Portugal integrating physical, emotional and energetic understandings of bodywork. Focus on developing the ability to be truly present. Small classes, individual attention.

Touchstone Healing Arts School of Massage
205 Dorset Street, 2nd Floor
South Burlington, VT 05403
(802) 658-7715

CLASSROOM HOURS: 600

COST: $5,000.00 including books and supplies (grants, payment plan)—day/night (introductory)

EMPHASIS: relaxation, medical, deep tissue, introduction to other modalities

SCHOOL STATEMENT: We provide an environment that honors and empowers individuals to trust in their innate ability to heal themselves and facilitate the healing process of others.

Vermont Institute of Massage Therapy
10 Cottage Grove Ave.
Burlington, VT 05403
(802) 862-1111
http://homepages.together.net/~massage/institute.html

Vermont School Of Professional Massage
14 Merchant St.
Barre, VT 05641
(800) 287-8816

VIRGINIA

Accredited Schools	COMTA	IMSTAC	ABHES	ACCET	ACCSCT
Cayce/Reilly School	•				
Potomac Academy of Hair Design					•
Virginia Learning Institute	•				
Virginia School of Massage	•				•

Advanced Fuller School of Massage
195 S. Rosemont, No. 105
Virginia Beach, VA 23452
(757) 340-3080

CLASSROOM HOURS: 500/700

COST: $3,150.00 (payment plan)—day/night

EMPHASIS: relaxation, sports, medical, deep tissue, energy, Eastern/Asian

SCHOOL STATEMENT: Our proven program challenges students to be the best. After the 250-hour basic, you receive $20 per massage intern pay while completing certification requirements.

AKS Massage School
462 Herndon Parkway, Ste. 208
Herndon, VA 20170
(703) 464-0333   www.AKSmassageschool.com

CLASSROOM HOURS: 602

COST: $4,650.00 (payment plan)—day/night

EMPHASIS: relaxation, sports, deep tissue, energy, wide variety of electives

SCHOOL STATEMENT: AKS believes education and respect for students and staff is vital for the healthy growth that makes AKS graduates personally and professionally responsible in their careers.

American Institute of Massage
2226 West Main St.
Richmond, VA 23220
(804) 254-3977

American Spirit Institute
1601 Willow Lawn Drive, Ste. 614
Richmond, Va. 23230;
(804) 673-1002

473 McLaws Circle, Ste. 1-A
Williamsburg, VA 23185
(757) 220-8000

Ana Visage Academy
10130-B Colvin Run Rd.
Great Falls, VA 22066
(703) 759-2700   www.anaVisage.com

CLASSROOM HOURS: 100 (500 total hours)

COST: $4,500.00 (payment plan)—day/ night/weekend

EMPHASIS: relaxation, sports, deep tissue, energy, Eastern/Asian

SCHOOL STATEMENT: Our objective is for each student to be achieve the highest professional standards within the industry, and attain vocational competencies established by the governing state.

Blue Ridge School of Massage and Yoga
2605-A Ramble Road
Blacksburg, VA 24060
(540) 552-2177   www.amritherapy.com/BRSMY.htm

CLASSROOM HOURS: 500

COST: $4,500.00 (interest-free payment plan)—day/night

EMPHASIS: relaxation, medical, deep tissue, energy, Eastern/Asian, myofascial release

SCHOOL STATEMENT: Quality instruction supportive of personal wellness and transformation. Small class size aids mastery of knowledge and techniques. Program meets state and national certification requirements.

Bodyworks Institute
350 S. Washington Street
Falls Church, VA 22046
(703) 532-5050   www.bodyworksinstitute.com

Career Training Solutions
4343 Plank Rd., Ste. 115
Fredericksburg, VA 22407
(540) 785-2000   www.careertrainingsolutions.com

Cayce Reilly School of Massotherapy
215 67th St.
Virginia Beach, VA 23452
(757) 457-7270   www.are-cayce.com/crsm

Daniels Institute for Holistic Health
2329 Franklin Rd.
Roanoke, VA 24014
(540) 344-3538
www.justwebit.com/members/37049/index.shtml

The Greater Washington Institute of Massage
5587 Guinea Rd.
Fairfax, VA 22032
(703) 425-8686
www.greaterwashingtoninstituteofmassage.com

Kee Business College
825 Greenbriar Circle
Chesapeake, VA 23320
(757) 361-3900   www.keecollege.com

Miller Motte Technical College
1912 Memorial Ave.
Lynchburg, VA 24501
(877) 333-6622   www.miller-motte.com

Natural Touch School of Massage Therapy
291 Park Circle
Danville, VA 24541
(804) 799-0060

Natural Touch School of Massage Therapy
1202 Main St.
Lynchburg, VA 24504
(804) 845-3003

The Piedmont School of Professional Massage
12712 Directors Loop
Woodbridge, VA 22192
(703) 492-2024   www.pspmassage.com

CLASSROOM HOURS: 530

COST: $5,000.00 (grants, payment plan)—day/night

EMPHASIS: relaxation, sports, deep tissue, seated on-site

SCHOOL STATEMENT: Our program provides high quality, individualized instruction in small classes in a relaxed, nurturing environment. We emphasize scientific principles as well as mind/body interaction.

Potomac Academy of Hair Design—Bodyworkers
500 W. Annandale Rd.
Falls Church, VA 22046
(703) 532-5050   www.naccas.org/potomacacademy

Richmond Academy of Massage
2004 Bremo Rd., Ste. 102
Richmond, VA 23226
(804) 282-5003

Richmond School of Health and Technology
1601 Willow Lawn Dr., Ste. 320
Richmond VA 23230
(804) 288-1000

Virginia Academy of Massage Therapy
739 Thimble Shoals Blvd., Ste. 105
Newport News, VA 23606
(757) 595-7757   www.virginiaacademy.com

Virginia Learning Institute
7115 Leesburg Pike, Ste. 315
Fallschurch, VA 22043
(703) 538-0800   www.healinghands.net

Virginia School of Massage
2008 Morton Dr.
Charlotte, VA 22903
(804) 293-4031 or (888) 599-2001   www.vasom.com

Virginia School of Technology
www.vaschooloftech.com

100 Constitution Dr., Ste. 101
Virginia Beach, VA 23462
(757) 499-5447

1001 Boulders Pkwy., Ste. 305
Richmond, VA 23225
(804) 323-1020

WASHINGTON					

Accredited Schools	COMTA	IMSTAC	ABHES	ACCET	ACCSCT
Ashmead College				•	
Brenneke School of Massage	•			•	
Brian Utting School of Massage	•			•	

Acorn Apprenticeship Program
2839 Grant St.
Bellingham, WA 98225
(360) 671-4489

Alexandar School of Natural Therapeutics
4026 Pacific Avenue
Tacoma, WA 98418
(253) 473-1142   www.secretsofisis.com

CLASSROOM HOURS: 650

COST: $8,995.00 (payment plan)—day/night

EMPHASIS: relaxation, medical, deep tissue, energy, spa treatments

SCHOOL STATEMENT: The Alexandar School provides an innovative and creative program in the natural health care field, specifically in the instruction of massage bodywork and spa certification.

Ancient Arts Massage School & Clinic
1111 Jadwin
Richland, WA 99352
(509) 943-9589

Ashmead College
www.ashmeadcollege.com

3019 Colby Ave., Everett, WA 98201
(425) 339-2678

5005 Pacific Hwy. E., Ste. 20, Fife, WA 98424
(253) 926-1435

2111 N. Northgate Way, Ste. 218, Seattle, WA 98133
(206) 527-0807

120 NE 136th St., Ste. 220, Vancouver, WA 98684
(360) 885-3152

CLASSROOM HOURS: 242-1048.75 (805.5 for prof. licensing program)

COST: $3,053.00–$14,285.00 including books (scholarships, grants, payment plan)—day/night

EMPHASIS: relaxation, sports, deep tissue, Eastern/Asian

SCHOOL STATEMENT: Ashmead provides an interactive, learner-centered environment resulting in a firm foundation in practical and theoretical education. Our objective is to prepare students to become successful practitioners.

Bellevue Massage School
16301 N.E. 8th St., Ste. 106
Bellevue, WA 98008
(425) 641-3409

Bodymechanics School of Myotherapy & Massage
3920 Capital Mall Drive SW, Ste. 404
Olympia, WA 98502
(800) 615-5594   www.bodymechanics.net

CLASSROOM HOURS: 900

COST: $10,500.00 including books (payment plan)—day/night

EMPHASIS: relaxation, sports, medical, deep tissue, postural

SCHOOL STATEMENT: The Bodymechanics School is a hospital-based program. This advanced massage therapy program prepares the student for a future as a bodyworker with multiple specialties.

Bodymind Academy
1247 120th Ave NE, Ste. K
Bellevue, WA 98005
(425) 635-0145   www.bodymind-academy.com

CLASSROOM HOURS: 552 (639 total hours)

COST: $7,557.00 including books (scholarship, grant, payment plan)—day, night and weekend programs

EMPHASIS: relaxation, sports, medical, deep tissue, energy, integration

SCHOOL STATEMENT: A state licensed massage school and so much more! Offering these integrative programs: massage, shiatsu, meridian cranial-sacral, counseling hypnotherapy, fitness and nutrition, expressive arts, breathwork

Boulder College of Massage Therapy
6255 Longbow Drive
Boulder CO 80301
(800) 442-5131 or (303) 530-2100   www.bcmt.org

Brenneke School of Massage
160 Roy St.
Seattle, WA 98109
(206) 282-1233 or 1-866-BRENNEKE
www.brennekeschool.com

CLASSROOM HOURS: 650/1000

COST: $7,645.00/$10,950.00 (Payment plan)—day/night (some weekends required)

EMPHASIS: relaxation, sports, deep tissue, energy, treatment techniques

SCHOOL STATEMENT: We believe in the profound, healing power of touch as a tool for integrating body, mind, spirit and emotions.

Brian Utting School of Massage
900 Thomas St., Ste. 200
Seattle, WA 98109
(206) 292-8055 or (800) 842-8731   www.busm.com

CLASSROOM HOURS: 1000+

COST: $10,700.00 (scholarships, payment plan)—day/night (each includes some weekends)

EMPHASIS: Swedish, medical, deep tissue, NMT

SCHOOL STATEMENT: Our mission is to develop outstanding massage therapists with a deeper sense of their humanity.

Cedar Mountain Center For Massage
5601 N.E. St. Johns Rd.
Vancouver, WA 98661
(360) 696-2210

Clover Park Technical College
4500 Steilacoom Blvd. SW
Lakewood, WA 98499-4098
(253) 589-5800   www.cptc.ctc.edu
Massage Program 4021 100th Street S.W
Scott Miller (253) 984-6680

Columbia Massage Institute
712 Swift Blvd., Ste. 2
Richland, WA 99352
(509) 943-1083

ICUR (ME)
726 NE 2nd Ave.
Camas, WA 98607
(360) 833-9899

Inland Massage Institute, Inc.
111 E. Magnesium Rd., Ste. F
Spokane, WA 99208
(509) 465-3303   www.InlandMassage.com

CLASSROOM HOURS: 685

COST: $6,100.00 including books and supplies (scholarships, payment plan)—night program

EMPHASIS: relaxation, sports, medical, deep tissue

SCHOOL STATEMENT: IMI has been the leader in massage education in Eastern Washington since 1986. We provide excellent education and prepare students for viable, exciting careers.

Institute of Structural Medicine
03027 NW 59th St.
Seattle, WA 98107
(206) 784-8504

Northwest Noetic School Of Massage
P.O. Box 8487
Spokane WA 99203
(509) 835-4000

Peninsula College Massage Therapy Program
1502 East Lauridsen Blvd.
Port Angeles, WA 98362
(360) 452-9277   www.pc.ctc.edu

Port Townsend School of Massage
P.O. Box 78
Port Townsend, WA 98368
(360) 379-4066   www.massageeducation.com

CLASSROOM HOURS: 600

COST: $7,140.00 including books—day/weekend

EMPHASIS: relaxation, medical, deep tissue, Eastern/Asian, professional practice

SCHOOL STATEMENT: PTSM's areas of emphasis are: the best traditional/innovative massage techniques; extensive holistic knowledge of the human body; and embodiment of the highest professional integrity.

Renton Technical College Massage Program
3000 NE 4th St.
Renton, WA 98056
(425) 235-2352   www.renton-tc.ctc.edu

Sakie International
Yakima College of Massage & Bodywork
1731 S. 1st St.
Yakima, WA 98901
(509) 457-2773

Soma Institute
730 Klink Rd.
Buckley, WA 98321
(360) 829-1025   www.soma-institute.com

Spectrum Center School of Massage
1001 N. Russell Rd.
Snohomish, WA 98290
(425) 334-5409   www.spectrumschool.com

CLASSROOM HOURS: 684

COST: $7,000.00 (payment plan)—day/night

EMPHASIS: medical massage

SCHOOL STATEMENT: Spectrum offers excellent technical training in a warm personal setting. Class size limited to 18, all hands-on courses include teaching assistants for efficient, individualized learning.

Tri-City School of Massage
26 E. 3rd Ave.
Kennewick, WA 99336
(509) 586-6434
http://members.aol.com/tcschoolmassage

CLASSROOM HOURS: 570

COST: $5,100.00 including books—night program

EMPHASIS: relaxation, sports, medical, deep tissue, energy, Eastern/Asian

SCHOOL STATEMENT: Our focus is on therapeutic massage, presenting a comprehensive set of principles and tools for the student to choose from when dealing with client problems.

Apprenticeship Programs:

Denton Apprenticeship Program
Mary Rose Denton
12506 18th St NE
Lake Stevens, WA 98258
(425) 334-2154

Mary Pat Marshall Apprenticeship Program
143 McCleary Rd.
McCleary, WA 98607
(360) 495-3729

Stanger Apprenticeship Program
Billie Stanger
3802 10th Southeast
East Wenatcee, WA 98802
(509) 884-2516

Wellness Education Center Apprenticeship Program
Dylan Patterson
W. 3511 5th Ave
Spokane, WA 98224
(509) 624-8608

WEST VIRGINIA

Beckley School of Massage Therapy
600 S. Oakwood Ave.
Beckley, WV 25801
(304) 250-0005

Clarksburg Beauty Academy
120 South 3rd St.
Clarksburg, WV 26301
(304) 624-6475

Mountain State School of Massage
601 50th St. SE
Charleston, WV 25304
(304) 926-8822   www.mtnstmassage.com

CLASSROOM HOURS: 800

COST: $6,200.00 (grants, payment plan)—day/weekend

EMPHASIS: relaxation, sports, medical, deep tissue, energy, Eastern/Asian, chair massage, hydrotherapy

New River Holistic Training
3700 Poplar St., Ste. 100
Parkersburg, WV 26101
(304) 422-4111

WISCONSIN

Accredited Schools	COMTA	IMSTAC	ABHES	ACCET	ACCSCT
Lakeside School of Massage	•				•

Balanced Touch Institute
N 7576 Timber Dr.
Rib Lake, WI 54470
(715) 427-3369

Blue Sky Educational Foundation
www.BlueSkyEdu.org

Main Campus: 220 Oak St.
Grafton, WI 53024
(262) 376-1011 or (877) 387-1011

Branch campus: 1640-A Fire Lane Dr.
Green Bay, WI 54311, (920) 406-9770

Branch campus: 2122 Luann Lane
Madison, WI 53713, (608) 270-5241

East West Healing Arts Institute
1902 East Washington Ave.
Madison, WI 53704
(608) 236-9000   www.acupressureschool.com

Fox Valley School of Massage
526 W. Wisconsin Ave., Appleton, WI
Mailing: P.O. Box 615, Neenah, WI 54957
(920) 993-8660   www.fvsm.org

CLASSROOM HOURS: 652/675/700

COST: $5,500.00 (scholarships, no-int. loans, payment plan)—day/night (part-time, full-time)

EMPHASIS: relaxation, sports, medical, deep tissue, energy, Eastern/Asian, many modalities

SCHOOL STATEMENT: Fox Valley School of Massage offers a high value education at the most affordable rates in the state. Classes start in September and February.

Institute of Beauty & Wellness
342 N. Water St.
Milwaukee, WI 53202
(414) 227-2889   www.skininstitute.com

Institute of Natural Therapies
P.O. Box 222
Hancock, WI 49930
(906) 482-2222

Lakeside School of Massage Therapy
www.lakesideschoolmassage.org

1726 N. First St., Milwaukee, WI 53212
(414) 372-4345

6121 Odana Rd, Madison, WI 53719
(608) 274-2484

CLASSROOM HOURS: 750

COST: $7,270.00 including books (no-int. loans, payment plan)—day/night/weekend

EMPHASIS: relaxation, sports, medical, deep tissue, Eastern/Asian

SCHOOL STATEMENT: Lakeside School operates the only schools in Wisconsin accredited by the Commission on Massage Therapy Accreditation. Financial is aid available for those who qualify.

Madison Area Technical College
3550 Anderson St.
Madison, WI 53704
(800) 322-6282 or (608) 246-6100
www.madison.tec.wi.us

Milwaukee School of Massage
830 E. Chambers St.
Milwaukee, WI 53212
(414) 263-1179   www.milwaukeeschoolofmassage.com

CLASSROOM HOURS: 600

COST: $5,900.00 including books and massage table—day/night

EMPHASIS: relaxation, sports, energy, chair, CST, MFR, reflexology

SCHOOL STATEMENT: Unique curriculum—small class size.

Professional Hair Design Academy/ Massage Therapy
3408 Mall Drive
Eau Claire, WI 54701
(715) 835-2345

CLASSROOM HOURS: 580 (630 including clinical)

COST: $6,800.00 including books, massage table and supplies (grants, payment plan) day/night

EMPHASIS: relaxation, sports, deep tissue, Eastern/Asian

St. Croix Center for the Healing Arts
411 County Hwy. UU
Hudson, WI 54016
(715) 381-1402   www.sccha.com

Therapeutic Bodyworks Institute
2345 Silvernail Rd.
Pewaukee, WI 53072
(262) 896-0100

Transformational Intuitive Bodywork In Action (TIBIA)
6225 University Avenue, Ste. 202
Madison, WI 53705
(608) 442-9390   www.reclaiming-the-bliss.org

CLASSROOM HOURS: 600 (650 total hours)

COST: $6,000.00 (payment plan)—one day & evening per week plus 9 weekends

EMPHASIS: relaxation, energy, transformational bodywork

SCHOOL STATEMENT: The Transformational Bodywork Program teaches bodywork as a modality for the shifting of consciousness and the integration of body, mind and spirit.

Wisconsin Institute of Natural Wellness
6211 Durand Ave.
Racine, WI 53406
(262) 554-8722   www.wimassageschool.com

CLASSROOM HOURS: 611

COST: $5,800.00 (scholarships)—night program/day + night program + 11 weekends

EMPHASIS: relaxation, medical, Eastern/Asian

SCHOOL STATEMENT: The Institute is a non-profit school of massage therapy, combining treatment principles of Chinese medicine with Western massage modalities. Small classes in a professional setting.

WYOMING

Sheridan College
3059 N. Coffeen Ave.
Sheridan, WY 82801
(307) 674-6446 ext. 6237   www.sc.cc.wy.us

CLASSROOM HOURS: 715

COST: $3,000.00 (scholarships, grants, no-int. loans, payment plan)—day program

EMPHASIS: Swedish, neuromuscular, medical, sports, relaxation, deep tissue

SCHOOL STATEMENT: Mission Statement of Sheridan College— "Building Student Success Through Educational Leadership"

Index

Massage Schools

To have your information included in future editions, send a brief note on your school letterhead to:

Enterprise Publishing
P.O. Box 179
Carmel, New York 10512
facsimile (845) 228-0190

For review copies, wholesale price information or account assistance, contact

Enterprise Publishing
(845) 228-0312
facsimile (845) 228-0190
e-mail martash@cloud9.net

Curriculum Directors

Enterprise Publishing also offers a companion *Student Workbook* and *Teacher's Guide* both designed to supplement this book when used as a classroom text. Information and review copies are available from the publisher.

Visit our website for updates on products, prices, and state laws nationwide:

www.CareerAtYourFingertips.com